Cardiology

FOURTH EDITION

Singh

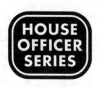

Cardiology

FOURTH EDITION

Joel W. Heger, M.D.
Foothill Cardiology
California Heart Medical
   Group, Inc.
Pasadena, California

James T. Niemann, M.D.
UCLA School of Medicine
Harbor General Hospital
Torrance, California

R. Fernando Roth, M.D.
Foothill Cardiology
California Heart Medical
   Group, Inc.
Pasadena, California

J. Michael Criley, M.D.
UCLA School of Medicine
Harbor General Hospital
Torrance, California

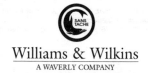

Williams & Wilkins
A WAVERLY COMPANY

BALTIMORE • PHILADELPHIA • LONDON • PARIS • BANGKOK
BUENOS AIRES • HONG KONG • MUNICH • SYDNEY • TOKYO • WROCLAW

Editor: Charles W. Mitchell
Managing Editor: Grace E. Miller
Marketing Manager: Rebecca Himmelheber
Production Coordinator: Peter J. Carley
Project Editor: Robert D. Magee
Illustration Planner: Wayne Hubbel
Cover Designer: Graphic World Publishing Services
Typesetter and Digitized Illustrations: Maryland Composition Co., Inc.
Printer Binder: World Color

Printed in the United States of America

First Edition, 1984
Second Edition, 1987
Third Edition, 1992

Library of Congress Cataloging-in-Publication Data
Cardiology / Joel W. Heger . . . [et al.]. — 4th ed.
    p. cm. — (House officer series)
  Includes bibliographical references and index.
  ISBN 0-683-30204-3
  1. Heart—Diseases. 2. Cardiology. I. Heger, Joel W.
II. Series.
RC681.H375 1998
616.1′2—dc21   97-51976
                                        CIP

The publishers have made every effort to trace the copyright holders for borrowed material. If they have inadvertently overlooked any, they will be pleased to make the necessary arrangements at the first opportunity.

To purchase additional copies of this book, call our customer service department at **(800) 638-0672** or fax orders to **(800) 447-8438.** For other book services, including chapter reprints and large quantity sales, ask for the Special Sales department.

Canadian customers should call **(800) 665-1148,** or fax **(800) 665-0103.** For all other calls originating outside ot the United States, please call **(410) 528-4223** or fax us at **(410) 528-8550.**

Visit Williams & Wilkins on the Internet: http://www.wwilkins.com or contact our customer service department at **custserv@wwilkins.com.** Williams & Wilkins Customer service representatives are available from 8:30 am to 6:00 pm, EST, Monday through Friday, for telephone access.

98 99 00
1 2 3 4 5 6 7 8 9 10

Preface

Since the first edition in 1982, *Cardiology for the House Officer* has been updated and revised. Now in this fourth edition, the authors again hope to create an easy-to-read and concise handbook for dealing with common problems in clinical cardiology.

Core material, recent research trials, and diagnostic and therapeutic advances have been summarized. A special effort has been made to give the reader visual aids, including graphs, tables, and charts, that will quickly summarize important information.

For this fourth edition, new information on cardiac imaging, interventional cardiology, and electrophysiology has been added. A completely new chapter has been added on cardiac drugs.

Joel W. Heger, M.D.

Acknowledgments

The authors wish to thank and acknowledge:

Mayer Rashtian, for his contributions to the new material on electrophysiology.

Richard Haskell, Milton Smith, Keith Bowman, and Gary Conrad for their contributions to earlier editions.

The House staff at Harbor–UCLA Medical Center and Huntington Memorial Hospital for their suggestions and criticisms.

The medical students from the University of Southern California for their fresh and stimulating ideas.

Contents

Chapter 1

Basic Electrocardiology

This chapter reviews common causes of abnormalities of atrial and ventricular depolarization and repolarization that may be recognized on the electrocardiogram (ECG). Arrhythmias may also produce changes in the morphology and/or duration of the ECG deflections and will be discussed in a separate chapter (Chapter 2).

It is beyond the scope of this text to provide a comprehensive presentation of basic electrocardiography and vectorcardiography. Discussion of electrophysiologic mechanisms underlying changes in the surface ECG are minimized in the following discussions, and it is assumed that the house officer has a basic understanding of ECG vector analysis (calculating mean axes). Emphasis has been placed on the differential diagnosis of QRS, ST, and T wave changes and on providing the house officer with readily available ECG criteria for the diagnosis of commonly encountered ECG abnormalities. Comprehensive discussions of basic electrocardiography may be found in a number of texts (1,2).

THE NORMAL ECG

The ECG is the surface representation of cardiac electrical activity. During myocardial depolarization and repolarization, deflections or waves are inscribed on the ECG. By convention, positive forces (electrical forces directed toward an ECG lead) produce upright deflections and negative forces (forces directed away from an ECG lead) are represented by downward deflections. The distances between deflections and waves are called segments and intervals, respectively.

The P Wave

- Represents atrial depolarization.
- P wave duration (width) is a measure of the time required for

depolarization to spread through the atria to the atrioventricular (AV) node. In the normal adult, maximum P wave duration is 0.10 sec.

- Mean frontal plane P wave axis (vector) is normally directed inferiorly and leftward (15–75°), and an upright deflection should be recorded in ECG leads I, II, and aVF. A negative deflection is seen in aVR. The P wave may be upright, isoelectric (flat), or inverted in III and aVL.
- Normal P wave amplitude is 0.5–2.5 mm (0.05–0.25 mV).

The PR Interval

- Represents the time required for a supraventricular impulse to depolarize the atria, traverse the AV node, and enter the ventricular conduction system.
- Measured from the beginning of the P wave to the initial deflection of the QRS complex (Q or R wave) in the frontal plane lead with the longest PR interval.
- Normal PR interval is 0.12–0.20 sec in adults in sinus rhythm. The PR interval normally shortens as the heart rate increases and lengthens at slower heart rates. First-degree AV block is said to be present if the PR interval is >0.20 sec. A PR interval of <0.12 sec may be seen as a normal variant, in hypocalcemia, with ventricular preexcitation, and in ectopic junctional or low atrial rhythms.

The QRS Complex

- Represents ventricular depolarization.
- Q wave—the first downward or negative deflection after the P wave and/or preceding the first upright deflection.
- R wave—the first positive deflection after a P wave.
- S wave—a negative deflection following an R wave.
- QS wave—a single downward deflection not preceded or followed by an upright deflection.
- R' wave—a second positive deflection after the R wave.
- Uppercase and lowercase letters are frequently used to signify approximate voltages or amplitudes of R waves.
- QRS interval (duration)—an indication of intraventricular conduction time. This measurement should be made in the frontal plane lead in which it is widest. The normal valve in the adult is <0.10 sec.

- The mean frontal plane QRS vector in the normal adult is − 30 to + 110°.

The ST Segment

- An isoelectric segment following ventricular depolarization and preceding ventricular repolarization.
- Measured from the end of the QRS complex to the beginning of the T wave.
- In contrast to the PR and QRS intervals, changes in the length of the ST segment are not as important as its deviation from baseline or the isoelectric point. The interval from the end of the T wave to the beginning of the P wave (TP interval) is usually taken as the isoelectric reference point. Elevation or depression of the ST segment by ± 1 mm (0.1 mV) from the isoelectric baseline is considered "abnormal."

The T Wave

- ECG representation of ventricular repolarization.
- T wave vector normally directed inferiorly and leftward.
- The T wave vector normally "tracks" with the QRS vector. If the QRS is predominantly negative in a frontal plane lead, an inverted T wave is usually seen and is not necessarily abnormal.
- An inverted (negative) T wave in V1 is considered normal. Inverted T waves in V2 and V3 may be normal in patients younger than 30 years of age and in patients with "funnel chest" or "straight back" body habitus.

The QT Interval

- Measured from the beginning of the QRS complex to the end of the T wave and represents duration of electrical systole. Mechanical systole usually begins during inscription of the QRS complex.
- This interval varies with heart rate. The normal QT interval, corrected for heart rate, is usually <0.425 sec and is calculated by dividing the measured QT interval (in sec) by the square root of the R-R interval (in sec). The QT interval should be measured in the lead with the most clearly defined T wave.

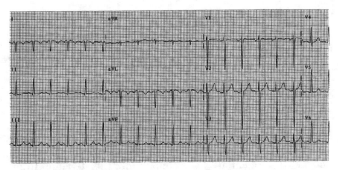

Figure 1.1. Reversed ECG Leads.

The U Wave

- A deflection following the T wave; electrophysiologic origin uncertain.
- U wave vector tracks with the T wave vector, i.e., polarity or direction similar.
- Amplitude greatest in precordial leads V2–V4.

MISPLACED ECG LEADS

Figure 1.1 is an ECG tracing obtained from the same patient as in Figure 1.2. Note the difference in the axes of the P wave, QRS complex, and T wave recorded in the standard limb leads. This

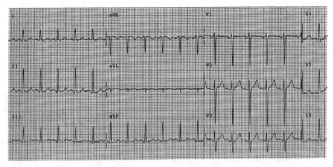

Figure 1.2. Correct Lead Placement.

is a common technician error caused by reversing the right and left arm ECG leads (Fig. 1.1). In switching the right and left arm leads, the frontal plane P, QRS, and T wave axes have been shifted rightward. Such frontal plane vector changes may also be seen in dextrocardia. However, in this example, the presence of a normal precordial (V1–V6) ECG eliminates dextrocardia as a differential possibility. With dextrocardia, horizontal-plane QRS forces should be directed anteriorly and to the right, with decreasing R wave amplitude over the left precordium.

EARLY REPOLARIZATION

Normal variant ST segment elevation may be noted in the precordial and limb leads. "Early repolarization" is the descriptive term applied to this ECG pattern (Fig. 1.3) (3). Whether accelerated subepicardial repolarization is actually responsible for the ECG variant is uncertain. ST segment elevation is most prominent in the lateral precordial leads (V4–V6). The T waves in these leads are characteristically broad-based, tall (usually >5 mm), and upright. The limb leads may also show some degree of ST elevation, but rarely more than 2 mm. The early repolarization variant has been reported in all age groups, is more common in males, and is more prevalent in the black than the white population.

This variant may be confused with the ST segment changes noted during acute pericarditis. There are no universally accepted ECG criteria that accurately or absolutely distinguish be-

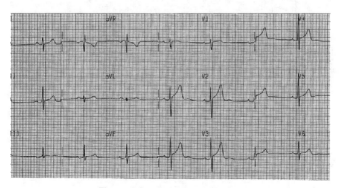

Figure 1.3. Early Repolarization.

tween the two when a single ECG is examined (4–6). However, it has been suggested that the ratio of the ST segment amplitude to the T wave amplitude in lead V6 helps to distinguish the benign variant (5). In early repolarization, the ST:T ratio in V6 is generally less than 0.25. A ratio greater than 0.25 is usually seen in acute pericarditis.

PERICARDITIS

The ECG may be of considerable value in the diagnosis of pericarditis, especially if serial tracings are obtained (6). Evolutionary changes (stages) may be noted over several days.

Stage 1 (acute phase) (Fig. 1.4)
- ST segment elevation in the precordial leads, especially V5 and V6, and in leads I and II.
- An isoelectric or depressed ST segment is commonly seen in V1.
- PR segment depression may be noted in leads II, aVF, and V4–V6.

Stage 2
- ST segment begins returning to baseline (isoelectric line).
- T wave amplitude decreases.

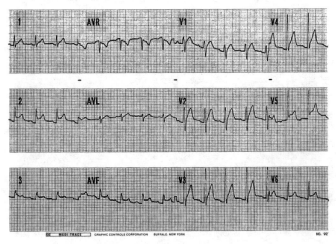

Figure 1.4.   Pericarditis (Acute Phase).

Stage 3
- ST segment isoelectric.
- T waves inverted in those leads previously showing ST segment elevation.

Stage 4
- Resolution of T wave changes.

Additional ECG abnormalities may be noted during pericarditis (see Chapter 14) and include arrhythmias, low-voltage QRS complexes (<5 mm R wave amplitude in limb leads), and electrical alternans.

THE ECG IN CHAMBER ENLARGEMENT

Atrial Enlargement

Atrial enlargement may result from:

- Valvular heart disease (e.g., mitral stenosis).
- Pulmonary hypertension.
- Congenital heart disease (e.g., tricuspid atresia).
- Ventricular hypertrophy (e.g., systemic hypertension).

The initial portion of the P wave results from right atrial depolarization and the terminal portion from left atrial depolarization. The normal mean P vector is the sum of the vectors generated by both atria and is directed leftward and inferiorly. Atrial enlargement may alter the P wave magnitude, duration, or vector orientation.

An accurate ECG diagnosis of atrial enlargement is not always possible. There is considerable normal variation in P wave amplitude, duration, and morphology. Tachycardia alone may increase P wave amplitude. Although it is not always possible to diagnose left or right atrial enlargement electrocardiographically, the following criteria may be helpful.

Right Atrial Enlargement (RAE) (Fig. 1.5)

- P wave amplitude of >2.5 mm in lead II.
- Frontal plane P wave vector shifted rightward (> + 75°).
- Rarely noted as an isolated finding, i.e., most frequently associated with ECG criteria for right ventricular hypertrophy.

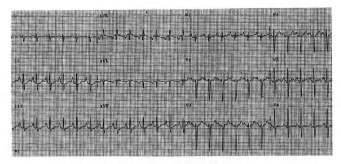

Figure 1.5. Right Atrial Enlargement.

Left Atrial Enlargement (LAE) (Fig. 1.6)

- P wave duration of >0.11 sec and P wave usually notched in lead II.
- Frontal plane P wave vector shifted leftward (0 to −30°) (terminal part of P wave may be negative in lead III and aVF).
- Biphasic P wave in lead V1 with wide, deep terminal component (>0.04 sec in duration and 1 mm in depth).

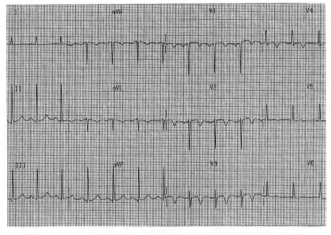

Figure 1.6. Left Atrial Enlargement.

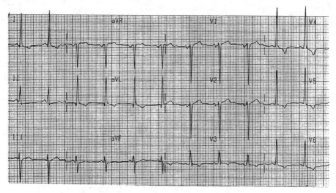

Figure 1.7. Left Ventricular Hypertrophy.

Left Ventricular Hypertrophy (LVH)

LVH manifests primarily as an increase in voltage (height of R wave) in those ECG leads that reflect left ventricular potentials (Fig. 1.7). The increase in voltage is due to an increase in muscle mass and surface area and/or the proximity of the dilated heart to the sensing ECG electrode (heart closer to chest wall). The mean QRS vector tends to be rotated leftward and posteriorly. LVH does not change the sequence of ventricular depolarization but may delay it (delayed onset of intrinsicoid deflection). Repolarization may be altered—the left precordial leads may show depressed ST segments and inverted T waves—resulting in a left ventricular strain pattern. The ECG diagnosis of LVH is based on voltage changes, ST-T wave alterations, axis deviations, and conduction delay (QRS duration of >0.08 sec but <0.12 sec). A number of ECG criteria have been advanced, all of which have varying degrees of sensitivity and specificity.

Common ECG Voltage Criteria for LVH in the Adult

• Sum of S wave in V1 or V2 and R wave in V5 or V6 is >35 mm, or
• Sum of highest R and deepest S waves in precordial leads is >45 mm, or
• R wave in V6 of >18 mm, or
• R wave in a VL of >12 mm, or

Table 1.1

Romhilt-Estes Criteria For LVH	Points
1. Amplitude of QRS	
R in V5 or V6 > 30 mm	
S in V1 or V2 > 30 mm	
Largest R or S in limb leads > 20 mm	
If any one of the above present	3
2. ST-T Strain Pattern	
In the absence of digitalis therapy	3
Digitalis therapy	1
3. LAE Present	3
4. Left Axis Duration ($\leq 30°$)	2
5. QRS Duration >0.9 sec	1
6. Intrisicoid QRS Deflection of >0.05 sec in V5 or V6	1
5 or more points = definite LVH	
4 or more points = probable LVH	

- Sum of R wave in I and S wave in III is > 16 mm, or
- R wave in I of >14 mm.

Limb lead criteria are less sensitive but highly specific.

Point Score System for Diagnosis of LVH

Because LVH may affect the amplitude, axis, and duration of the QRS complex as well as produce ST segment and T wave changes (down-sloping ST segment depression and asymmetric T wave inversion in V4–V6—strain pattern), a point score system was developed to improve diagnostic specificity (see Table 1.1) (7). This commonly referenced point score system is less sensitive than QRS voltage criteria. With the current trend toward improved or high sensitivity to prompt the physician to seek more definitive or specific confirmation (echocardiography), the contemporary value of the noted criteria is questionable. The authors do not use this point system.

Right Ventricular Hypertrophy (RVH)

The ECG diagnosis of RVH is less sensitive and less specific than that of LVH, and the ECG is frequently normal in the presence of RVH. The following ECG abnormalities are suggestive of RVH.

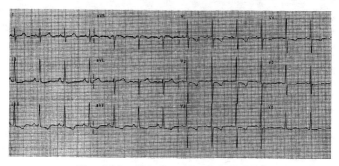

Figure 1.8. Right Ventricular Hypertrophy.

- Right axis deviation (> + 110° in an adult) in the absence of right bundle branch block (RBBB), left posterior inferior fascicular block, or anterolateral or inferior myocardial infarction.
- Dominant R wave (>7 mm) in lead V1 (may also be seen in RBBB, posterior myocardial infarction, Wolff-Parkinson-White (WPW) syndrome, and as a normal variant).
- R/S ratio in lead V1 of >1.0.
- R/S ratio in V5 or VG6 of <1.0.
- RSR pattern in lead V1 with a QRS duration of <0.12 sec.

The diagnosis of RVH is supported by the presence of RAE and/or right ventricular strain pattern (ST segment depression and T wave inversion in V1–V3) (Fig. 1.8). The ECG diagnosis of RVH may be obscured if a RBBB is also present.

Combined LVH and RVH

The value of the ECG in the diagnosis of combined ventricular hypertrophy is limited. In many instances, the ECG will demonstrate alterations suggesting hypertrophy of only one of the ventricles.

ECG Criteria Suggestive of Combined Ventricular Hypertrophy

- Voltage changes in the precordial leads "diagnostic" of both LVH and RVH.
- Voltage criteria for LVH plus:

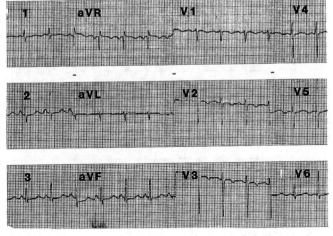

Figure 1.9. LVH and RVH (Precordial Leads ½ Standard).

right axis deviation (> + 110°), or
R/S ratio in V1 of >1.0, or
>7 mm R wave in V1, or
deep S wave in V6, or
right atrial enlargement and a vertical mean QRS axis.
• Voltage criteria for RVH plus:
R/S ratio in V2–V4 and/or in two or more limb leads of nearly
1.0 (Katz-Wachtel sign), or large R waves in V5 or V6 with strain
pattern and left atrial enlargement.

The ECG shown in Figure 1.9 demonstrates evidence of LVH
(V6 R wave >18 mm and left atrial enlargement–precordial leads
are recorded at ½ standard). However, there is also right atrial
enlargement and a right ventricular strain pattern is evident in
the anterior precordial leads. The frontal plane QRS axis is
90°—a more rightward axis would be expected with LVH alone.
The tracing is compatible with bi-atrial and biventricular hypertrophy.

RIGHT BUNDLE BRANCH BLOCK

RBBB is usually associated with organic heart disease (ischemic,
rheumatic, congenital) (Fig. 1.10) (8). In RBBB, the sequence

of ventricular activation is abnormal, resulting in a terminal QRS vector that is directed rightward and anteriorly (large R wave in V1, S wave in V6). The cardiac vector is not significantly altered during the first 0.06 sec of ventricular depolarization. The left ventricle is depolarized in a normal fashion, septal activation occurs from left to right, and the mean frontal plane QRS vector (axis) is usually normal. The site of block within the right bundle branch may be proximal or more peripheral.

The ECG Criteria for the Diagnosis of RBBB

- QRS duration of >0.12 sec in limb leads.
- Triphasic QRS complexes (RSR′ pattern) in the anterior precordial leads (V1–V3). The ST segment is often depressed and the T wave is inverted in these leads.
- Wide S wave (0.25 sec in duration) in lateral precordial leads (V5, V6) and lead I.
- Normal time of onset of the intrinsicoid deflection in lead V6.

    Associated RVH should be suspected if the secondary R wave in V1 is greater than 15 mm in amplitude or if there is right axis deviation of the mean frontal plane QRS vector.

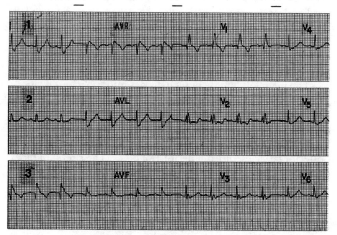

Figure 1.10.   Right Bundle Branch Block.

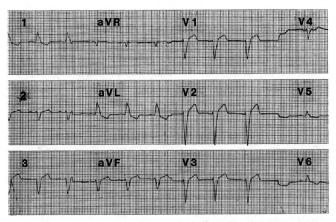

Figure 1.11. Left Bundle Branch Block (Precordial Leads ½ Standard).

LEFT BUNDLE BRANCH BLOCK

Left bundle branch block (LBBB) is almost always an indicator of organic heart disease (Fig. 1.11) (9,10). In LBBB, the entire sequence of ventricular activation is abnormal; the primary abnormality is a change in the direction of the initial QRS vector. Initial depolarization and the mean QRS vector are directed leftward and posteriorly. Septal activation occurs from right to left. There is also a change in the direction of repolarization—ST and T vectors rotate away from the mean QRS vector, resulting in ST segment depression and T wave inversion in the lateral precordial leads, lead I, and lead aVL.

The main left bundle branch divides into two major divisions (fascicles) soon after entering the interventricular septum—the left anterior superior fascicle and the left posterior inferior fascicle. Thus, LBBB may result from a lesion in the main left bundle, from simultaneous block in some portion of the anterior and posterior fascicles, or from peripheral block. The site(s) of block cannot be distinguished electrocardiographically.

Electrocardiographic Criteria for the Diagnosis of LBBB

- QRS duration of >0.12 sec.
- Large, broad, notched, or slurred R waves in the lateral precor-

dial leads, lead I, and lead aVL. Q waves and S waves are characteristically absent, the ST segment is depressed, and the T wave
is inverted in these leads.
- A small R wave precedes a deep S wave in leads II, III, and aVF.
- In most instances, left axis deviation ($< -30°$) is present. However, LBBB may be seen without left axis deviation.
- Initial R waves followed by deep S waves are present in the
  anterior precordial leads (V1–V3). The ST segment may be
  elevated in these leads.
- Onset of the intrinsicoid deflection is delayed in V6 but normal
  in V1.

From the description of the characteristic ECG findings, it
should be apparent that a diagnosis of LVH or acute infarction
is difficult in the presence of LBBB.

THE FASCICULAR BLOCKS (HEMIBLOCKS)

The main left bundle can be considered to divide into two major
divisions or fascicles soon after entering the interventricular septum—the left anterior superior fascicle and the left posterior
inferior fascicle. Conduction delay in either fascicle (hemiblock)
will alter the sequence of left ventricular depolarization and produce distinctive ECG changes (11). Left anterior superior hemiblock, either alone or in association with AV nodal or right bundle branch conduction disturbance(s), is far more common than
left posterior inferior hemiblock. This disparity may be due to:
(a) the greater length and smaller diameter of the anterior fascicle, *(b)* the location of the anterior superior fascicle within the
turbulent outflow tract of the left ventricle, and/or *(c)* the single
blood supply (left anterior descending (LAD) coronary artery)
of the anterior fascicle compared to the dual blood supply of the
posterior fascicle (LAD and right coronary artery).

Left Anterior Superior Hemiblock (LASH)

If the anterior fascicle is blocked, the wave of depolarization will
travel through the fibers of the posterior fascicle and then spread
to the portions of the left ventricular myocardium normally activated by the anterior fascicle (Fig. 1.12). The sequence of left
ventricular depolarization thus proceeds in an inferior-to-supe-
rior direction. LASH may be caused by coronary artery disease,

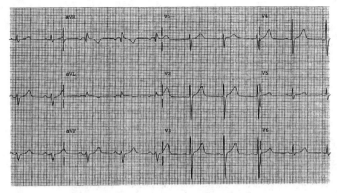

Figure 1.12. Left Anterior Superior Hemiblock.

valvular heart disease, congenital heart disease, cardiomyopathy, and myocarditis.

ECG Criteria for the Diagnosis of LASH

- Left axis deviation (mean frontal plane QRS axis of $\leq -45°$).
- QRS duration usually ≤ 0.10 sec.
- Small R waves in leads II, III, and aVF and small Q waves in leads I and aVF.
- Deep S waves in II, III, and aVF.
- Exclusion of other causes of left axis deviation: body habitus, inferior myocardial infarction, hyperkalemia, ventricular pre-excitation, etc.

Left Posterior Inferior Hemiblock (LPIH)

Ventricular activation proceeds in a superior-to-inferior direction. The mean frontal plane QRS axis will be directed inferiorly and rightward. LPIH is far less common than LASH, rarely occurs in the absence of associated AV nodal or right bundle branch conduction disturbances, and almost invariably indicates organic heart disease (Fig. 1.13).

ECG Criteria for the Diagnosis of LPIH

- Right axis deviation (mean frontal plane QRS axis of $\geq +110°$).

- QRS duration of ≤0.10 sec.
- Small R waves in leads I and aVL and small Q waves in leads II, III, and aVF.
- Tall R waves in II, III, and aVF and deep S waves in I and aVL.
- Exclusion of other causes of right axis deviation: chronic obstructive pulmonary disease (COPD), right ventricular enlargement, lateral myocardial infarction.

Bifascicular and Trifascicular Blocks

Bifascicular block refers to the combination of RBBB with either left anterior superior or left posterior inferior fascicular block. Trifascicular block refers to the combination of RBBB with either left anterior or left posterior inferior fascicular block and incomplete AV block. AV block may occur at the level of the AV node or more distally (bundle of His, main left bundle, or in the remaining fascicle) (12). The level of the AV block cannot be determined with the surface ECG—only a prolonged PR interval will be noted. Figure 1.14 demonstrates a RBBB and a left posterior, inferior fascicular block.

Bifascicular and trifascicular block may be seen with the following:

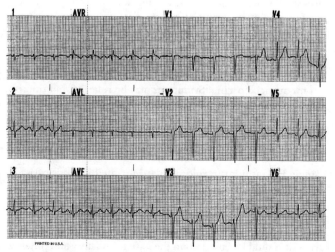

Figure 1.13. Left Posterior Inferior Hemiblock.

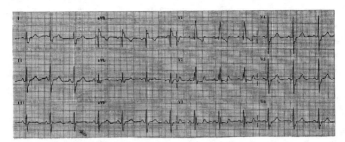

Figure 1.14. Bifascicular Block.

- Coronary artery disease.
- Cardiomyopathy.
- Valvular heart disease, especially aortic.
- Lenhgre's or Lev's disease—sclerodegenerative processes involving the cardiac conduction system.
- Cardiac surgery—repair of a ventricular septal defect or valve replacement.
- Myocarditis.

Although indicative of advanced conduction system disease, chronic bifascicular or trifascicular block alone is not an indication for permanent artificial cardiac pacing because long-term follow-up studies have not revealed a high incidence of complete heart block (12). Bifascicular or trifascicular block with clinical symptoms (syncope, dyspnea on exertion, etc.) due to documented bradyarrhythmias or complete heart block is an indication for artificial pacing. Symptoms may be relieved, but the risk of sudden death will not be significantly affected.

THE ELECTROCARDIOGRAM IN ACUTE MYOCARDIAL INFARCTION

A single ECG is not the gold standard for the diagnosis of acute myocardial infarction (AMI). The initial ECG may be nondiagnostic in 20–50% of cases of AMI. The ECG diagnosis of AMI may be obscured or mimicked by a number of conditions (13,14). The decision to admit a patient with chest pain to a coronary care unit should be based upon the patient's history and physical examination findings.

Serial ECGs during the acute phase of suspected AMI are of critical importance. Evolutionary ST segment and T wave changes during an acute transmural myocardial infarction usually persist for only 1–2 days and are followed after a variable time period by T wave inversions in those ECG leads that showed ST elevation. Persistent ST segment elevation beyond 2 weeks, especially in the anterior precordial leads, is a specific but insensitive index of a ventricular aneurysm, left ventricular dysfunction, and enhanced risk of sudden death. ST segment elevation persisting longer than 14 days after the acute event is usually permanent.

ST segment elevation (especially in anterior precordial leads) is not diagnostic of transmural AMI as it may also be seen with

- LVH with strain.
- Left bundle branch block.
- Coronary artery spasm.
- Pericarditis.
- "Early repolarization."
- Hyperkalemia.
- Use of certain drugs (digoxin, tricyclic antidepressants).
- Cerebral vascular accident.
- Ventricular aneurysm.
- Hypothermia (Osborne waves).

The presence of a LBBB may conceal changes of an acute myocardial infarction because of the repolarization changes that accompany LBBB. ECG criteria that have been found to be helpful in diagnosing acute myocardial infarction in patients with LBBB include: *(a)* ST segment elevation of ≥1 mm that is concordant with (in the same direction as) the QRS complex; *(b)* ST segment depression of ≥1 mm or more in lead V1, V2, or V3; and *(c)* ST segment elevation of ≥5 mm that was discordant with (in the opposite direction from) the QRS complex (15).

The ECG changes associated with nontransmural or subendocardial AMI are variable. The ECG changes most commonly noted include

- ST segment depression—down-sloping or "square wave" type of at least 1.0 mm (Fig. 1.15).
- T wave inversion.
- ST segment depression and T wave inversion.

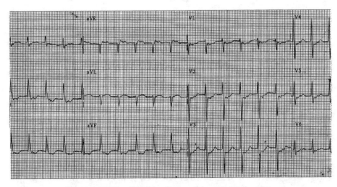

Figure 1.15. Anterior Subendocardial Infarction.

Characteristically, abnormal Q waves do not develop during the course of a nontransmural AMI. The ST-T wave changes may persist for a variable period of time but usually longer than 24 hours. The nonspecific character of these ECG changes often necessitates the use of ancillary studies (isoenzymes, radioisotopes) to confirm the diagnosis of myocardial necrosis. Patients suffering a subendocardial or nontransmural infarction may experience complications similar to those noted during transmural AMI and have a long-term prognosis not significantly different from patients with transmural necrosis (16).

ST-T wave changes that simulate those of subendocardial infarction may be noted in

- LVH with strain.
- The bundle branch blocks.
- Cardiomyopathies.
- WPW syndrome.
- Central nervous system disease.
- Late pericarditis.
- Electrolyte disturbances (especially hypokalemia).
- Association with the use of certain drugs.

The ECG is able to localize the site of infarction/injury with considerable accuracy based on which leads abnormal Q waves (>0.03 sec) or ST-T wave changes are noted.

Abnormal Q waves or ST-T wave changes in

- II, III, aVF: inferior wall infarction (Fig. 1.16).
- V1–V3: anteroseptal infarction (Fig. 1.17).
- I, aVL, V4–V6: lateral wall infarction (Fig. 1.18).
- V1 or V2–V6: anterolateral infarction.

A large R wave and ST segment depression in leads V1 and V2 are indicative of infarction of the true posterior wall of the left ventricle (Fig. 1.19). The large R wave and ST segment depressions noted in the anterior precordial leads are the surface ECG manifestations of posterior infarction/injury and may be viewed as "reciprocal" changes—if ECG leads were placed dorsally, characteristic Q waves and ST segment elevation would be noted. Isolated posterior wall infarction is infrequent. This infarction pattern is most commonly seen in association with inferior wall infarction, as these portions of myocardium share a common blood supply (right coronary artery in 90% of individuals). Infarction of the inferior and/or posterior wall of the left ventricle is often complicated by infarction of the right ventricle. In patients with an inferior infarction, a right precordial electrocardiogram should be obtained. ST elevation of ≥1 mm in lead V3R or V4R suggests right ventricular infarction (Fig. 1.20) (17).

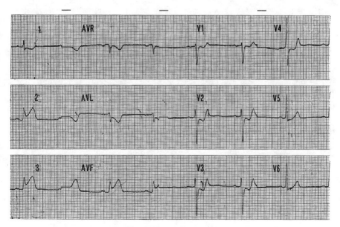

Figure 1.16. Inferior AMI.

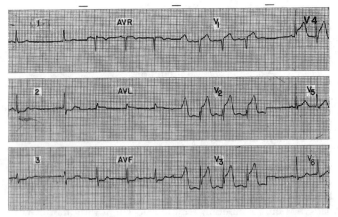

Figure 1.17. Anteroseptal AMI.

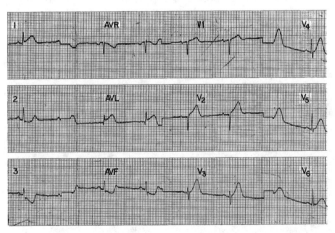

Figure 1.18. Lateral AMI.

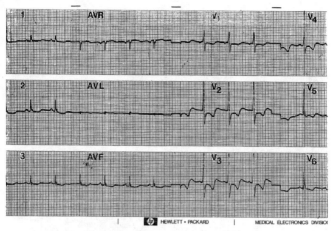

Figure 1.19.   Posterior Wall Infarction.

ELECTROLYTES AND THE ELECTROCARDIOGRAM

Cardiac electrical activity results from the movement of various ions across the sarcolemma membrane. Changes in electrolyte concentrations may, therefore, alter depolarization and/or repolarization and produce ECG abnormalities (18).

Hyperkalemia (Fig. 1.21)

1. Serum potassium, 5.5–6.6 mEq/L
   - Tall, peaked, narrow T waves in precordial leads.
   - Deep S wave in leads I and V6.
   - QRS complex usually normal.
2. Serum potassium, 7.0–8.0 mEq/L (Fig. 1.21).
   - QRS widening.
   - Slurring of both initial and terminal portions of the QRS.
   - ST segment elevation.
   - Low, wide P waves.
   - First- and second-degree atrioventricular block.
   - Sinoatrial arrest.
   - Bradycardia.
3. Serum potassium, >8.0 mEq/L
   - Marked widening of QRS complex.

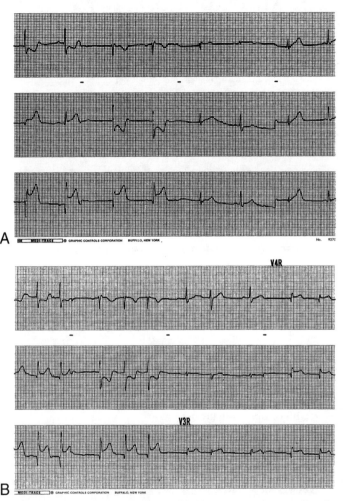

Figure 1.20. **(a)** Inferior Infarction. Standard 12-lead electrocardiogram. **(b)**Inferior Infarction. Right precordial ECG recording in the same patient.

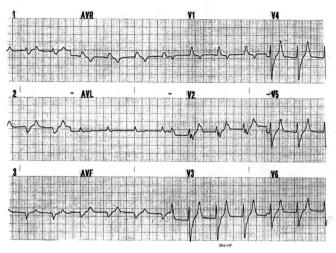

Figure 1.21. Hyperkalemia.

- Distinct ST-T wave may not be noted.
- High risk of ventricular fibrillation or a systole.

Hypokalemia

1. Serum potassium, 3.0–3.5 mEq/L
   - ECG may be normal.
   - If ECG changes are present, they are most prominent in the anterior precordial leads V2 and V3 and consist of T wave flattening and the appearance of U waves.
   - QT interval and QRS duration normal.
2. Serum potassium, 2.7–3.0 mEq/L
   - U waves become taller and T waves become smaller but do not invert.
   - The ratio of the amplitude of the U wave to the amplitude of T wave frequently exceeds 1.0 in V2 or V3.
3. Serum potassium, <2.6 mEq/L (Fig. 1.22).
   - Almost always accompanied by ECG changes.
   - ST segment depression associated with tall U waves and low-amplitude T waves.
   - QT interval normal, but accurate measurement may be dif-

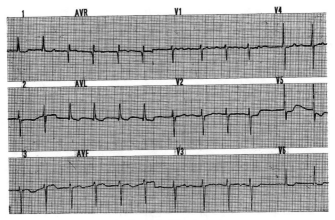

Figure 1.22. Hypokalemia.

ficult due to the proximity of the U wave. The U wave is usually smallest in lead aVL and this lead should be used to determine the QT interval.

- QRS duration rarely affected in adults.

Hypercalcemia

- Slight increase in QRS duration.
- ST segment short or absent.
- Corrected QT interval shortened.
- PR interval may be prolonged.
- T wave amplitude and duration usually normal.
- U wave amplitude may be normal or slightly increased.

Hypocalcemia (Fig. 1.23)

- Slight decrease in QRS duration.
- ST segment lengthened and corrected QT interval prolonged.
- PR interval may be shortened.
- T waves may become flat or inverted in severe hypocalcemia.

Hyponatremia or Hypernatremia

- Effects of changes in serum sodium cannot be detected electro-cardiographically.

Hypomagnesium or Hypermagnesium

- Marked magnesium deficiency is usually associated with potassium depletion, and the ECG demonstrates the characteristic changes of hypokalemia. Ventricular arrhythmias may be present.
- Hypermagnesium is uncommon clinically and is usually encountered in patients with uremia who often have other electrolyte disturbances (hypocalcemia, hyperkalemia) that produce ECG changes.
- It is uncertain whether changes in body magnesium alone affect the surface ECG.

THE ELECTROCARDIOGRAM AND NONCARDIAC DRUGS

Commonly used inotropic (digoxin) and antiarrhythmic (quinidine, procainamide) drugs produce well-defined repolarization changes that can be recognized on the surface ECG. Noncardiac drugs can also produce significant ECG changes that may be confused with organic cardiac disease (19). The phenothiazines and tricyclic antidepressants are frequently used in clinical practice and may produce a number of "benign" or significant ECG changes. These drugs share a number of electrophysiologic effects with the class 1 antiarrhythmic drugs (e.g., quinidine) and

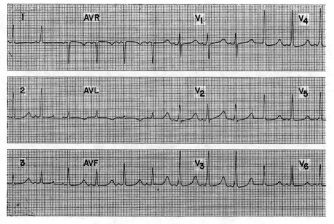

Figure 1.23. Hypocalcemia.

thus have a direct effect on the cardiac action potential. These drugs also possess variable anticholinergic properties and can affect the heart indirectly.

THE ECG IN CENTRAL NERVOUS SYSTEM DISEASE

Central nervous system (CNS) lesions, particularly subarachnoid hemorrhage, intracerebral hemorrhage, and infarction (stroke), may produce striking ECG repolarization abnormalities (20). These alterations most commonly take the form of diffuse, deep, wide, blunted T wave inversions and QT prolongation (Fig. 1.24); U waves may also be prominent. The exact incidence of ECG changes in CNS hemorrhage or infarction is undetermined but seems to be more common with frontal lobe lesions. These functional repolarization changes are believed to be caused by heightened cerebrocardiac autonomic stimuli.

ARTIFICIAL CARDIAC PACEMAKERS

The tip of a transvenous ventricular pacing catheter should lie in the apex of the right ventricle. Electrocardiographically, the mean QRS vector of paced complexes will depend on the point of electrical stimulation of the myocardium. If the catheter tip is

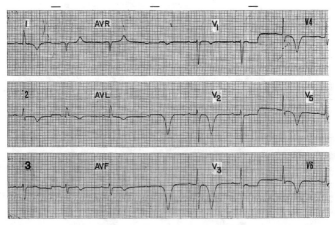

Figure 1.24. The ECG Following Massive Subarachnoid Hemorrhage.

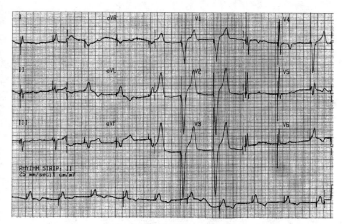

Figure 1.25. Paced Rhythm.

properly positioned, the mean QRS vector of paced complexes should be directed superiorly and posteriorly, resulting in:

- Large, wide QRS complexes with a dominant R wave in leads I, aVL, and commonly in V6.
- Large, negative deflections (QS waves) in leads II, III, aVF, and V1–V3.

The ECG pattern thus mimics that of a left bundle branch block with left axis deviation.

In Figure 1.25, each QRS complex is preceded by a pacemaker stimulus artifact ("spike"), which is seen best in leads I and II and the precordial leads. The underlying rhythm is atrial fibrillation and the patient, in this instance, is pacemaker-dependent.

WOLFF-PARKINSON-WHITE SYNDROME (PREEXCITATION)

Wolff-Parkinson-White (WPW) syndrome is a form of anomalous AV conduction or preexcitation (Fig. 1.26) (21). Ventricular preexcitation is said to exist when conduction of a supraventricular impulse to the ventricular myocardium occurs via accessory pathways that bypass the AV node. Conduction via an accessory pathway in WPW permits premature activation of ventricular myocar-

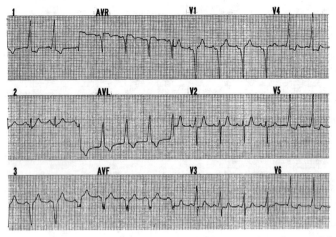

Figure 1.26. Preexcitation (short PR and delta waves-lateral precordial leads).

dium. Preexcitation can occur through a number of anatomic pathways. In classic WPW syndrome, a sinus impulse is conducted through the Kent's bundle, which bypasses the AV node, and initiates activation of the ipsilateral ventricle. A short PR interval and an initial slurring (*Δ* wave) during the inscription of the QRS complex result. The bypass tract is capable of bidirectional conduction, and reentrant tachyarrhythmias (see Chapter 2) are a feature of this syndrome.

Recent electrophysiologic studies in humans, including epicardial ECG monitoring ("mapping") during open heart surgery, have yielded a great deal of information regarding sites of bypass tracts and their electrophysiologic behavior. A new classification for the WPW syndrome has been proposed and is based on the anatomic site of the bypass tract: *(a)* right sided, *(b)* left sided, or *(c)* septal (within the membranous intraventricular septum).

ECG Criteria for the Diagnosis of WPW Syndrome

- Short PR interval (<0.12 sec).
- Normal P wave vector (to exclude junctional rhythm).

- Presence of a Δ wave—slurring or notching of first portion of the QRS complex.
- QRS duration greater than 0.10 sec.

Clinical Significance of the WPW Syndrome

- High incidence of tachyarrhythmias (usually reentrant mechanism—40–80% of patients).
- Frequently associated with organic heart disease (30–40% of cases). Disorders commonly associated with WPW syndrome include atrial septal defect, mitral valve prolapse, hypertrophic cardiomyopathy, and Ebstein's anomaly.
- ECG patterns may simulate other disease processes—myocardial infarction or ventricular hypertrophy.
- Antegrade conduction via the bypass tract and retrograde conduction through the AV node may produce regular tachyarrhythmias with wide QRS complexes, mimicking ventricular tachycardia.

References

1. Summerall CP III. Lessons in EKG interpretation. 2nd ed. New York: Churchill Livingstone, 1991.
2. Marriott HJL. Practical electrocardiography. 8th ed. Baltimore: Williams & Wilkins, 1988.
3. Eastaugh JA. The early repolarization syndrome. J Emerg Med 1989; 7:257.
4. Wanner WR, Schaal SF, Bashore TM, et al. Repolarization variant vs acute pericarditis. A prospective electrocardiographic and echocardiographic evaluation. Chest 1983;83:180.
5. Ginzton LE, Laks MM. The differential diagnosis of acute pericarditis from the normal variant: new electrocardiographic criteria. Circulation 1982;65:1004.
6. Spodick DH. Electrocardiogram in acute pericarditis. Distributions of morphologic and axial changes by stages. Am J Cardiol 1974;33: 470.
7. Romhilt DW, Estes EH. Point score system for the ECG diagnosis of left ventricular hypertrophy. Am Heart J 1968;75:752.
8. Schneider JF, Thomas E, Kreger BE, et al. Newly acquired right bundle-branch block. Ann Intern Med 1980;92:37.
9. Flowers NC. Left bundle branch block: a continuously evolving concept. J Am Coll Cardiol 1987;9:684.
10. Kreger BE, Anderson KM, Kannel WB. Prevalence of intraventricular block in the general population. Am Heart J 1989;117:903.

11. Alpert MA, Flaker GC. Chronic fascicular block. Recognition, natural history, and therapeutic implications. Arch Intern Med 1984;144:799.

12. Denes P. Atrioventricular and intraventricular block. Circulation 1987;75(Suppl III):III-19-I.

13. Goldberger AL. ECG simulators of myocardial infarction. Pathophysiology and differential diagnosis of pseudo-infarct Q wave patterns (Part I). PACE 1982;5:106.

14. Goldberger AL. Pathophysiology and differential diagnosis of pseudo-infarction ST-T patterns (Part II). PACE 1982;5:414.

15. Sgarbossa EB, Pinski SL, Barbagelata A, et al. Electrocardiographic diagnosis of evolving acute myocardial infarction in the presence of left bundle-branch block. N Engl J Med 1996;334:481.

16. Andre-Fouet X, Pillot M, Leizorovicz A, et al. "Non-Q wave," alias "nontransmural," myocardial infarction: a specific entity, Am Heart J 1989;117:892.

17. Kinch JW, Ryan TJ. Right ventricular infarction. N Engl J Med 1994;330:1211.

18. Surawicz B. Electrolytes and the electrocardiogram. Postgrad Med 1974;55:123.

19. Duke M. The effects of drugs on the electrocardiogram—a reference chart. Heart Lung 1981;10:698.

20. Strauss WE, Samuels MA. Electrocardiographic changes associated with neurologic events. Chest 1994;106:1316.

21. Prystowsky EN. Diagnosis and management of the preexcitation syndromes. Curr Probl Cardiol 1988;13:231.

Chapter 2

Arrhythmias

This chapter reviews the basic rules and principles of arrhythmia interpretation. Examples and descriptions of common arrhythmias are provided, and a basic approach to therapy is included for each arrhythmia.

BASIC RULES FOR RHYTHM INTERPRETATION

1. **Identify atrial activity—P wave.**
   - Is there evidence of atrial depolarization, i.e., are P waves present?
   - If so, do they represent normal P waves, ectopic P′ waves, the F waves of atrial flutter, or the fibrillatory waves of atrial fibrillation?
   - Do the atria depolarize in an anterograde (upright P in lead II) in a retrograde (negative P in lead II) manner?
   - Are all P waves in a single lead of similar morphology, i.e., do all P waves look the same?
   - What is the atrial rate? Is it regular or irregular?
2. **Identify ventricular activity—QRS complexes.**
   - Does ventricular depolarization arise from a supraventricular focus, i.e., is the QRS of normal duration (<0.10 sec)?
   - If the QRS is broad, is it the result of aberrant ventricular conduction or an ectopic ventricular focus?
   - What is the ventricular rate? Is it regular or irregular?
3. **Evaluate atrioventricular (AV) conduction—analyze the relationship between the P wave and the QRS.**
   - Is each P wave related to a QRS? If the PR interval is <0.10 sec or >0.40 sec, the P wave is unlikely to have "produced" the ensuing QRS complex.
   - Is each P wave conducted to the ventricles (1:1 AV conduction)?

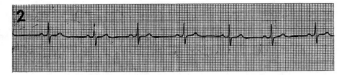

Figure 2.1. Sinus Bradycardia.

- Is the speed of AV conduction (the PR interval) normal (≤0.20 sec)?
- Is there any evidence of group beating (Wenckebach phenomenon)?

SUPRAVENTRICULAR ARRHYTHMIAS

Sinus Bradycardia

Description

Sinus bradycardia (Fig. 2.1) is the result of a decrease in the normal rate of discharge of the sinoatrial (SA) node. The atrial rate (P wave frequency) is less than 60/min, but atrial depolarization is normal (i.e., the P wave vector is directed inferiorly and leftward and upright P waves are seen in leads II, III, and aVF). The P-to-P interval is regular and each P wave is followed by a QRS complex of normal duration (1:1 AV conduction). The PR interval is fixed or constant. In the setting of an underlying interventricular conduction defect, QRS complexes may be of prolonged duration (>0.10 sec).

Causes

Normal. Increased vagal tone in the conditioned athlete.

Pathologic. Intrinsic sinus node disease—sick sinus syndrome.
Increased vagal tone—inferior myocardial infarction (MI), vasovagal response.
Drug toxicity—β-adrenergic blockade, calcium channel blockade, organophosphate poisoning.

Therapy

Therapy is dictated by the clinical circumstances in which sinus bradycardia is noted. Acute therapy is always indicated if hemodynamic compromise/hypoperfusion is present. In the setting of acute inferior myocardial infarction, acute therapy is also indicated if ventricular arrhythmias (ventricular escape beats or rhythms or premature ventricular contractions) are present.

Atropine Sulfate. Atropine is the drug of choice if sinus bradycardia is pathologic and associated with hypoperfusion. It is most effective if symptomatic bradycardia is the result of acute inferior myocardial infarction, a vasovagal response, or cholinergic drug toxicity. The drug should be administered intravenously, and 0.5-mg boluses administered at 5-min intervals (to a total dose of 2.0 mg) are recommended (1). In the setting of acute inferior myocardial infarction, a total dose of approximately 1 mg is usually successful in increasing the sinus rate. Atropine is of limited value in managing hemodynamically significant bradyarrhythmias associated with the sick sinus syndrome. It is unlikely to increase heart rate in the setting of drug toxicity caused by β-adrenergic or calcium channel blockade. Excessive use of atropine may result in sinus tachycardia and an increase in myocardial oxygen demand. This complication is of particular concern for the patient with atherosclerotic coronary artery disease (CAD).

Artificial Cardiac Pacing. If atropine fails to produce the desired response in heart rate, temporary artificial cardiac pacing should be instituted as soon as possible. Artificial pacing should initially be attempted using the transcutaneous method. Most monitor/defibrillator devices currently available have transcutaneous pacing capability. This technique is usually successful and is well tolerated by the patient at stimulus strengths of ≤ 50 milliamperes (2).

Isoproterenol Hydrochloride. Isoproterenol (Isuprel) is a pure β agonist. It will produce a decrease in peripheral arterial tone, and arterial pressure will fall if its use does not produce an increase in cardiac output (via β-1-mediated increased heart rate or improved contractility). Isoproterenol should be used with caution in the setting of acute infarction because it will increase myocardial oxygen demand that may not be met by an increase in myocardial oxygen supply. In addition, it may be arrhythmogenic and is of limited value in the setting of β-adrenergic blocker toxicity. Isoproterenol is most commonly used to treat hemodynamically significant bradyarrhythmias unresponsive to atropine. It should be administered as a continuous intravenous infusion at an infusion rate of 2–10 μg/min titrated to the hemodynamic response (1).

Dopamine (5–20 μg/min) or **epinephrine** (2–10 μg/min) may be helpful if the above interventions are ineffective (1).

Calcium Chloride. Calcium chloride may be of value in the setting of calcium channel blocker toxicity. An intravenous dose of 5–10 mL (500 mg–1 g) of a 10% calcium chloride solution may reverse peripheral dilation associated with calcium blocker toxicity but may not increase heart rate. Atropine or isoproterenol may be effective in increasing AV conduction (3).

Glucagon. Glucagon may be the drug of choice in the setting of β-blocker toxicity (3). An intravenous bolus dose of 2–4 mg is recommended.

Sinus Tachycardia

Description

Sinus tachycardia (Fig. 2.2) results from an increased rate of discharge of the sinus node and is usually a physiologic response to a demand for an increase in cardiac output. The atrial rate is 100–160/min, and the P-to-P interval is regular. P waves are upright in leads II, III, and aVF (normal atrial depolarization and P wave vector). Each P wave is usually followed by a normal QRS complex (1:1 AV conduction). However, second-degree atrioventricular block may occur, and QRS duration may be prolonged in patients with an interventricular conduction defect (fixed bundle branch block, rate-related bundle branch block, aberrant ventricular conduction). Carotid sinus massage or a properly performed Valsalva maneuver may transiently slow the SA node discharge rate and be of value in diagnosis in confusing cases (e.g., sinus discharge rate of 140–160/min with 1:1 AV conduction, which

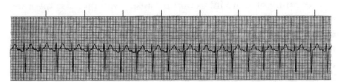

Figure 2.2. Sinus Tachycardia.

can be confused with atrial flutter with a 2:1 AV block or reentrant or automatic atrial supraventricular tachyarrhythmias). These maneuvers will not terminate this rhythm and may have no effect.

Causes

Causes include pain, anxiety, hypovolemia, left ventricular dysfunction, fever, pulmonary embolism, thyrotoxicosis, drug toxicity (e.g., cocaine, amphetamines, tricyclic antidepressants, anticholinergic drugs), drug withdrawal (e.g., narcotics, alcohol), anemia, hypoxemia, hypercarbia, and autonomic insufficiency.

If the history and physical examination fail to yield a physiologic stimulus for this rhythm disturbance, consider the following:

Pulmonary embolism: sinus tachycardia is the most frequent cardiac response to this physiologic insult, and the clinical diagnosis of pulmonary embolism is imprecise.
Hyperthyroidism: sinus tachycardia is frequently associated with this endocrine abnormality, and most other physical findings are nonspecific.
Hypovolemia: postural vital signs should be obtained during careful monitoring.

Therapy

Sinus tachycardia is a physiologic response of the sympathetic nervous system to meet a demand for an increase in cardiac output. Therapy will be effective only if the physiologic stimulus for the cardiac response can be defined. Therapy should, therefore, be directed toward correction of the physiologic stimulus. A complete history and physical examination will yield the most valuable information and will most often define the cause.

Sinus Arrhythmia

Description

This irregular supraventricular arrhythmia (Fig. 2.3) results from phasic alterations in vagal tone and is reflected by a gradual increase and decrease in the rate of sinus node discharge. The reflex arc is initiated by normal respiration. Inspiration decreases

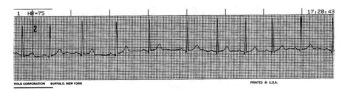

Figure 2.3. Sinus Arrhythmia.

vagal tone and produces an increase in the rate of SA discharge. Expiration results in increased vagal tone and a decrease in the rate of SA discharge. This is a normal phenomenon, especially for children and young adults. It may be accentuated by drugs (digoxin) in elderly individuals. Atrial depolarization is normal (upright P waves in leads II, III, and aVF) but irregular; there is a gradual increase and decrease in the P-P interval. The minimum difference between the longest and shortest P-P interval is usually <0.16 sec. The PR interval remains constant, and each P wave is followed by a QRS complex. The resultant rhythm is irregularly irregular and must be differentiated from other causes of an irregularly irregular rhythm (see Atrial Fibrillation).

Causes

Causes are physiologic but may be drug induced (e.g., digoxin). Marked sinus arrhythmia may be a manifestation of the sick sinus syndrome.

Therapy

The arrhythmia is physiologic and requires no therapy. Confusion may arise when it is mistaken for another rhythm disturbance.

Premature Atrial Contractions (PACs)

Description

A PAC is an electrical impulse that originates within the atrial myocardium but outside the SA node. It is premature (i.e., occurring before the next expected sinus discharge) and produces atrial depolarization and a P′ wave that differs in morphology from P waves of sinus node origin. A PAC usually depolarizes the SA node because the SA node is not "electrically isolated." The interval between the sinus P waves preceding and following a PAC is less than twice the normal P-P interval, resulting in a pause that is not fully compensatory. PACs originating from the same focus (unifocal PACs) have morphologically similar P' waves and a fixed coupling interval (the P-P' interval). When PACs are multifocal, P' waves differ in morphology and the coupling interval varies.

A PAC may be conducted normally through the AV node and ventricles. However, it may be conducted with partial AV block (PR interval >0.20 sec) or be completely blocked (nonconducted PAC) at the level of the AV node if the coupling interval is short (P' wave occurs close to T wave). Incomplete block and slow conduction at the bundle branch level may result in "aberrant" ventricular conduction (see below).

Two PACs are demonstrated in Figure 2.4. The ectopic P' waves are marked with arrowheads. The P' waves occur earlier than the next expected sinus P wave. The P'R interval is longer than the PR interval of normal sinus beats (beats 1, 2, 4, and 5) indicating conduction delay. The P' waves differ in morphology and the ectopic coupling interval also varies, suggesting that these PACs are of multifocal origin.

Causes

Causes include increased circulating catecholamines, drug toxicity (e.g., theophylline, sympathomimetics), and pericarditis (rarely).

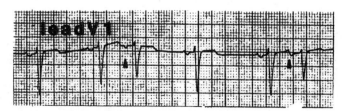

Figure 2.4. Premature Atrial Contractions.

Therapy

Treatment of isolated PACs is rarely necessary. However, if frequent PACs are associated with symptomatic episodes of sustained paroxysmal supraventricular tachyarrhythmias, quinidine, procainamide, or β blockers can be used to decrease atrial automaticity.

Multifocal Atrial Tachycardia (MFAT)

Description

MFAT is an ectopic, repetitive atrial arrhythmia that results from enhanced atrial automaticity; it frequently precedes the onset of atrial fibrillation (4,5). Ectopic atrial electrical activity from three or more foci produces an irregular atrial rate as well as an irregular ventricular rate. The atrial rate is usually 100–180/min with a varying P-P interval. The PR interval usually varies from beat to beat. The ventricular rate is also irregular (varying R-R interval). Ectopic P' waves (best seen in leads II, III, and aVF) vary in morphology. MFAT can be confidently diagnosed if three consecutive P waves of different morphology at a rate >100/min are identified in a single lead. If the atrial rate is <100/min, this rhythm is most commonly referred to as a "chaotic atrial rhythm" or "wandering atrial rhythm."

An episode of MFAT is shown in Figure 2.5. Three consecutive ectopic P' waves are indicated by arrows. The P-P, PR, and R-R intervals vary in an irregularly irregular fashion.

Causes

MFAT is most commonly encountered in patients with chronic obstructive lung disease and acute respiratory failure or patients

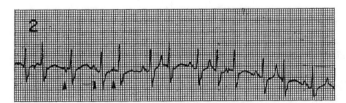

Figure 2.5. Multifocal Atrial Tachycardia.

with severe left ventricular dysfunction. Drug toxicity (sympatho-mimetics, theophylline) is a less common cause (4,5).

Therapy

Therapy should be initially directed at the underlying cause. Correction of hypoxemia and acidosis and careful use of inhaled bronchodilator therapy in the patient with chronic obstructive pulmonary disease (COPD) are essential.

Electrical cardioversion is rarely successful in producing sustained sinus rhythm. Digoxin, quinidine, and propranolol have all been reported to be of limited value in either chemical cardioversion or control of the ventricular response rate. Intravenous verapamil (5–10 mg via slow intravenous push) is a particularly effective agent in controlling the ventricular response rate. It should not be used for patients with marginal ventricular function because of its depressant effects on myocardial contractility. In patients with COPD, verapamil will not worsen airway resistance, and its effects on ventilation/perfusion mismatch (due to pulmonary vascular dilatation) are unlikely to seriously worsen hypoxemia. For patients with decreased left ventricular function, diltiazem (20 mg intravenously) should be considered. Its effect on myocardial contractility are less pronounced than that of verapamil.

Atrial Fibrillation

Description

Atrial fibrillation is the most common of the supraventricular tachyarrhythmias. It is the result of multiple atrial foci discharging nearly simultaneously, resulting in random wavelets of electrical depolarization that do not result in atrial contraction (6,7). Electrocardiographically, this chaotic electrical activity produces undulating deflections of varying sizes and shapes on the surface electrocardiogram (ECG) ("f" waves—best seen in V1, II, III, and aVF). There are no P waves. Although atrial electrical impulses are generated at frequencies of 400–700/min, the number of impulses reaching the ventricles is limited by the refractory period of the AV node. In the absence of AV node disease or drugs that alter the refractory period or conduction velocity of the AV node, 140–180 impulses/min can transverse the AV node

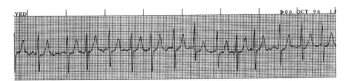

Figure 2.6.   Atrial Fibrillation.

at irregular intervals and in a random fashion. An irregularly irregular ventricular response rate (QRS complexes with varying R-R intervals) results. Atrial fibrillation with extremely low ventricular response rates (<70/min) reflecting high-grade AV block may be seen in digitalis toxicity and in patients with sick sinus syndrome.

Figure 2.6 shows an example of atrial fibrillation in a patient who was not receiving drugs that affect AV conduction. P waves are not evident, and irregular undulations ("f" waves) can be seen between R waves. The R-R interval is irregular and the ventricular response rate is 140/min.

Although atrial fibrillation is the most common cause of an irregularly irregular rhythm, it must be distinguished from other rhythm disturbances that may mimic it (see Table 2.1).

Causes

The etiology of atrial fibrillation is believed to be associated with atrial myocardial tissue injury/damage and elevated atrial pressure. The risk of developing atrial fibrillation has been related to left atrial dimension, left ventricular wall thickness, and left ventricular fractional shortenings determined by echocardiogra-

Table 2.1
Irregularly Irregular Rhythm: Differential Diagnosis

1. Atrial fibrillation
2. Atrial flutter with variable AV block
3. Multifocal atrial tachycardia or chaotic atrial rhythm
4. Sinus tachycardia with variable AV or SA block
5. Automatic atrial tachycardia with variable AV block
6. Marked sinus arrhythmia

phy (8). Similarly, successful conversion to and maintenance of sinus rhythm seems to be dependent on left atrial size and duration of atrial fibrillation (9).

Population-based data from the Framingham Study indicate that atrial fibrillation is most often associated with or caused by coronary heart disease, congestive heart failure, hypertensive cardiovascular disease, and rheumatic heart disease (10). Atrial fibrillation in the absence of clinically identifiable cardiovascular disease developed in approximately 30% of that patient population. In the absence of underlying clinical heart disease, atrial fibrillation has been termed "lone atrial fibrillation" and differs in its long-term complications and management (11).

Other causes include mitral and aortic valve disease of nonrheumatic origin, hypertrophic cardiomyopathy, hyperthyroidism, and idiopathic dilated cardiomyopathy. A paroxysmal form is commonly seen with alcohol abuse ("holiday heart syndrome").

Therapy (Atrial Fibrillation with a Rapid Ventricular Response)

For the hemodynamically unstable patient (systolic blood pressure of <90 mm Hg, cool, clammy skin, altered mentation, and/or chest pain), urgent synchronized electrical cardioversion is indicated (1). If the patient is conscious, sedation with intravenous diazepam (Valium, 5–10 mg), lorazepam (Ativan, 1–2 mg), a short-acting barbiturate (Brevital, titrated to response, with the typical dose being 1 mg/kg) should be given before cardioversion. Brevital has a 5- to 10-min half-life. If necessary, sedation with benzodiazepines can be reversed with flumazenil (0.2 mg intravenously, then 0.2 mg q 1 min to a dose of 1 mg). In the synchronized mode, **sequential countershocks** of 100, 200, 300, and 360 W/sec should be administered as necessary. If the patient is taking digoxin, atrial fibrillation with a rapid irregular ventricular response is not an arrhythmia associated with digitalis toxicity; it is a manifestation of subtherapeutic digoxin concentration. Cardioversion can be safely performed on patients with subtoxic serum digoxin concentrations (12).

If the first attempts at cardioversion are unsuccessful or atrial fibrillation recurs shortly after cardioversion to sinus rhythm, **procainamide** can be given intravenously at a rate of 30 mg/min to a maximum dose of 20 mg/kg. This regimen has been shown to be efficacious for chemical cardioversion of recent- or new-onset atrial fibrillation in patients without left atrial enlargement. Procainamide is of value in atrial fibrillation because it decreases atrial automaticity and prolongs the AV node refractory period. The patient should be closely monitored during procainamide administration because the drug may depress myocardial contractility or cause vasodilatation. The drug prolongs the QRS duration as well as the QT interval. If chemical cardioversion is successful, a procainamide infusion should be started (2–4 mg/min) (13). Alternatively, **diltiazem** (0.25 mg/kg intravenously followed by an infusion at 5–15 mg/hr) can be used. **Rapid digoxin loading** should also be performed (total dose of 0.75-1.0 mg of digoxin given over 4 hours) to control the ventricular response rate if fibrillation recurs. If atrial fibrillation with a rapid ventricular response and hemodynamic compromise persists after procainamide, electrical cardioversion can be attempted again.

Electrical cardioversion may not be necessary for the patient with clinical evidence of hypoperfusion and atrial fibrillation with a ventricular response rate of <120/min. If the ventricular response rate is irregular and between 80–120/min, other causes of hypoperfusion should be considered (e.g., myocardial infarction and ventricular dysfunction, hypovolemia, pulmonary embolism). If the response rate is <80/min and irregular or regular, digitalis toxicity should be considered if the patient is taking digoxin. Electrical cardioversion in the setting of digitalis toxicity is associated with a high complication rate.

For the hemodynamically stable patient, a number of treatment options are available (13).

Cardioversion. Attempted electrical or chemical cardioversion is most likely to be successful (i.e., conversion to and maintenance of sinus rhythm) in patients with recent-onset atrial fibrillation, those with a left atrial size of <5 cm, and those with an associated treatable illness (e.g., hyperthyroidism, infection, pulmonary embolism, acute respiratory failure). In the stable patient, initial rate control with digoxin, β-blockers, verapamil, or diltiazem and treatment of complicating illness, if present, is recommended, followed by echocardiography to assess atrial dimensions.

If left atrial size is <5 cm and the duration of atrial fibrillation is brief (less than 2 days), intravenous loading with procainamide (as described above) followed by electrical cardioversion, if needed, is often successful (13). Alternatively, quinidine (200 mg every 4–6 hours for 6–8 doses) can be added to ongoing digoxin therapy. If the addition of quinidine does not produce a chemical conversion, elective electrical cardioversion can be attempted. Digoxin levels should be monitored because quinidine decreases digoxin excretion and may precipitate digoxin toxicity (14). Transesophageal echocardiography has been proposed as a method to detect the presence of left atrial thrombi to guide anticoagulation therapy in atrial fibrillation of unknown duration (15). Left atrial thrombus formation can occur in patients with acute atrial fibrillation of <3 days in duration (16). Successful conversion to normal sinus rhythm electrocardiographically is most often not accompanied by effective atrial contraction. Spontaneous echo contrast seen after successful cardioversion is believed to be caused by "atrial stunning," which may promote new thrombus formation (17). Such data support a recommendation that all patients be considered for anticoagulation therapy in the setting of acute or new-onset atrial fibrillation (18).

If left atrial size is <5 cm and the duration of atrial fibrillation more than 3 days, anticoagulation with warfarin (Coumadin) for 3 weeks before attempted chemical or electrical cardioversion and continued for 4 weeks after cardioversion is recommended (13). Pharmacologic or electrical cardioversion of prolonged atrial fibrillation is associated with a small risk of systemic embolization (3%), which can be reduced (1%) if anticoagulants are used.

Some patients may require long-term antiarrhythmic therapy. Although β blockers are preferable due to their known safety and benefit in certain patients (e.g., post-MI), they are not always effective and contraindications to their use may exist. The class IA agents (quinidine, procainamide) have traditionally been used to maintain sinus rhythm, but several studies have identified a higher mortality in patients receiving such drugs (19,20). Amiodarone (200 mg/day) seems to be safe and effective for maintaining sinus rhythm in patients who have been cardioverted (21).

Rate Control. In the stable patient with chronic atrial fibrillation and a left atrial size of >5 cm, chemical or electrical cardioversion is unlikely to be successful. In such patients, control of the ventricular response should be the goal of therapy and many treatment options are available (13). Intravenous verapamil (5–10 mg) can be used for urgent or immediate rate control in patients with normal or slightly depressed ventricular function (22). Intravenous diltiazem (0.25 mg/kg over 2 min, followed by a 5–15 mg/hr infusion for 24 hours) causes less negative inotropy in patients with left ventricular (LV) dysfunction (23–25). Intravenous β blockers may be particularly useful for rate control of atrial fibrillation complicating hyperthyroidism, hypertrophic cardiomyopathy, and alcohol withdrawal. Digoxin has no role if urgent rate control is necessary because its onset of action is prolonged (>8 hr) and it is no more effective than placebo in the conversion of paroxysmal atrial fibrillation (26,27). However, digoxin is the drug of choice for chronic rate control, particularly in the setting of congestive heart failure secondary to myocardial dysfunction, and it can be combined with quinidine, β blockers, diltiazem, or verapamil, if necessary, for selected patients. A β blocker combined with digoxin may be efficacious for chronic therapy in patients without a contraindication to β-blocker therapy and who might benefit from other β-blocker effects, e.g., patients with essential hypertension, patients who have had a recent myocardial infarction, and patients with ventricular arrhythmias. Both verapamil and quinidine increase serum digoxin levels and drug monitoring may be necessary during early treatment with these agents. For patients unresponsive to pharmacologic therapy or who are unable to tolerate therapeutic doses of the above agents, rate control is possible with AV nodal ablation therapy and implantation of a permanent transvenous pacemaker.

Anticoagulation. Anticoagulation is recommended for most patients with chronic atrial fibrillation, especially those with increased age (>65 yr), hypertension, diabetes, and prior stroke or transient ischemic attach (TIA) (28). Chronic anticoagulation is not without risks, and its benefits and risks should be individualized for each patient. Lone atrial fibrillation in patients younger than 60 years of age is associated with a very low risk of stroke (11). Warfarin therapy to maintain an International Normalized Ratio (INR) of 2–3 should be offered to all patients with chronic atrial fibrillation without contraindications (29). For patients who are not candidates for warfarin therapy, aspirin therapy (325 mg/day) may be effective in reducing the risk of stroke or systemic embolism and may be particularly beneficial for low-risk patients (13). However, warfarin is more effective than aspirin for prevention of stroke caused by cardioembolism. Current and generally accepted recommendations include:

1. Long-term oral anticoagulation should be strongly considered for all patients older than 65 years of age with a target INR between 2 and 3. Patients younger than 65 years of age with risk factors of previous TIA or stroke, hypertension, diabetes, heart failure, clinical coronary heart disease, mitral stenosis, prosthetic heart valves, or hyperthyroidism should also be strongly considered for this therapy. Patients unwilling or unable to take warfarin should receive aspirin (325 mg/day).

2. For patients between 65 and 75 years of age without the above risk factors, the risks and benefits of warfarin versus aspirin therapy should be weighed, considering the low risk of stroke and the superior protection against stroke afforded by warfarin. Other factors, such as the inconvenience of frequent follow-up for INR monitoring, should enter into decision-making.

3. Patients older than 75 years of age should be considered for chronic anticoagulation with warfarin (INR 2–3). Age-related increased risk of bleeding should be considered.

4. Patients who have been in atrial fibrillation for more than 2 days should receive oral anticoagulation to maintain an INR of 2–3 for 3 weeks before elective cardioversion and for 4 weeks after sinus rhythm has been restored.

Atrial Flutter

Atrial flutter is a disorder of atrial impulse formation, is less commonly encountered than atrial fibrillation, and most frequently is an unstable rhythm, i.e., spontaneous conversion to sinus rhythm or atrial fibrillation often occurs. Atrial flutter may be the result of localized atrial reentry or may be of focal, ectopic origin due to enhanced automaticity (30).

Atrial depolarization occurs at a regular rate, most commonly 280–320/min, and usually is initiated by a reentry or an ectopic focus in the lower part of the right atrium. The resulting ECG deflection representing atrial depolarization is most often directed superiorly and leftward, in contrast to the normal inferior and leftward orientation. During atrial flutter, atrial depolarization produces flutter or "f" waves, which are most easily recog-

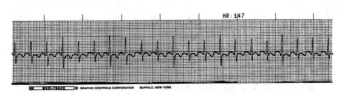

Figure 2.7. Atrial Flutter.

nized as regular negative deflections in leads II, III, and aVF. The absence of an isoelectric period between R waves may result in the typical "sawtooth" pattern in leads 2, 3, and aVF.

The ventricular rate (frequency and regularity of QRS complexes) during atrial flutter is primarily dependent on the refractory period of the AV node. Atrial flutter is almost always associated with a physiologic AV block. A physiologic 2:1 AV block occurs most often and results in QRS complexes that occur at a regular rate of 140–160/min. At this AV response rate, atrial flutter is often misdiagnosed as sinus tachycardia, as the typical sawtooth pattern in the inferior leads (II, III, aVF) is infrequently present. The sawtooth pattern is more often recognized in the inferior leads at higher degrees of AV block (Fig. 2.7). The AV conduction ratio during atrial flutter may be altered by AV node disease, autonomic nervous system variability, or drugs that affect AV node conduction velocity or refractory period (digoxin, β blockers, etc). AV block may be "fixed" (regular R-R interval) or variable (varying R-R interval, which is divisible by the inherent atrial rate, e.g., 3:1, 4:1). Atrial flutter may infrequently be conducted in 1:1, resulting in a rapid ventricular response.

The diagnosis of atrial flutter diagnostic ECG findings can be facilitated by physiologic maneuvers that increase the degree of AV block (e.g., properly performed carotid sinus massage) or the intravenous administration of adenosine, which has an extremely short half-life and effectively serves as a "pharmacologic vagal maneuver." These interventions will increase the degree of AV block and facilitate recognition of "f" waves but will not terminate atrial flutter.

Figure 2.7 shows an example of atrial flutter recorded in standard lead II. The R-R intervals are regular at a rate of 150/min (2:1 AV block).

Causes

Etiologies are similar to those of atrial fibrillation.

Therapy

The management of atrial flutter is similar to that of atrial fibrillation and is dictated by the overall hemodynamic response to the rhythm disturbance.

For the hemodynamically compromised patient (systolic blood pressure of <90 mm Hg, cool clammy skin, altered mentation, and/or chest pain) with atrial flutter and a rapid ventricular response rate, **urgent synchronized electrical cardioversion is indicated.** A conscious patient should be sedated (see atrial fibrillation management). In the synchronized mode, the first shock should be delivered at an energy dose of 50 W/sec. Conversion of atrial flutter can usually be accomplished at low energy levels. Countershock most often is followed by one of three outcomes.

1. **Sinus rhythm.** If clinical signs of hypoperfusion are absent, the patient should be closely monitored. If frequent PACs are noted, therapy with oral quinidine or procainamide can be initiated to decrease atrial automaticity as well as prolong AV conduction time if atrial flutter recurs or atrial fibrillation develops. The addition of a rate control agent such as digoxin, a β blocker, verapamil, or diltiazem can be helpful as well. If clinical signs of hypoperfusion persist after conversion to sinus rhythm, a fluid challenge with 250–500 mL of normal saline can be administered. If evidence of hypoperfusion persists, invasive hemodynamic monitoring with a flotation pulmonary artery catheter may be required. Long-term therapy with β blockers or low-dose amiodarone can be used to prevent recurrences. As discussed in the section on atrial fibrillation, concerns about the safety of long-term antiarrhythmic drugs have diminished their use. Electrophysiologic mapping and radiofrequency ablation of the atrial flutter pathway is another alternative to pharmacologic therapy .

2. **Atrial fibrillation.** Atrial flutter is an unstable cardiac rhythm and often spontaneously ''converts'' to atrial fibrillation. Countershock of atrial flutter is often followed by atrial fibrillation. It has been our experience that patients who are he-

modynamically compromised during atrial flutter at a ventricular response rate of 140–160 are unlikely to improve during atrial fibrillation at a similar ventricular response rate. Clinical signs of hypoperfusion frequently worsen, probably due to the lack of organized atrial contraction during atrial fibrillation. Electrical cardioversion of atrial fibrillation should be attempted as outlined above.

3. **Persistent atrial flutter.** Countershock energy dose should be increased at increments of 50 W/sec over the first energy dose until atrial flutter is terminated.

For the hemodynamically stable patient, several options are available.

1. **Electrical cardioversion** (see above). Similar rhythm outcomes should be expected. If pharmacologic therapy (discussed below) is not successful in producing the desired response (rhythm conversion or rate control), electrical cardioversion should be attempted, and the incidence of complications is unlikely to be increased. Electrical cardioversion is the treatment of choice for atrial flutter. Because atrial flutter is most often an unstable or transitional rhythm that does produce organized atrial contraction, the risk of systemic embolism with cardioversion is low but not zero. Because atrial flutter can recur and alternate with atrial fibrillation, anticoagulation should be considered for selected patients, especially if atrial enlargement is present.

2. **Intravenous diltiazem.** See section on rate control of atrial fibrillation.

3. **Intravenous verapamil.** This drug can be safely administered to patients without critical myocardial contractile dysfunction. The ventricular response rate usually decreases due to prolonged AV conduction of supraventricular electrical impulses. Verapamil may convert atrial flutter to sinus rhythm in some instances. A dose of 5–10 mg is usually effective. If hypotension occurs in the previously normotensive patient, a fluid challenge should be given. Alternatively, 0.5–1.0 g of calcium chloride can be administered to reverse the peripheral vascular effects of this drug. Pretreatment with intravenous calcium has also been advocated (31). Intravenous calcium administration has limited effects on the myocardial electrical response to verapamil.

4. **Intravenous esmolol.** Esmolol is an ultrashort-acting cardio-selective β blocker with a half-life of approximately 9 minutes (32). As with other β blockers, it should not be used for patients with LV dysfunction, bronchospasm, or high-grade AV block. However, because of to the short half-life of esmolol, patients in whom problems with a β blocker inadvertently develop usually recover promptly if the drug is stopped. A loading dose of 500 μg/kg/min is given over 1 minute and followed by a maintenance infusion of 500 μg/kg/min titrated to response.

5. **Intravenous digoxin.** This drug will usually decrease the ventricular response rate but is unlikely to decrease the atrial rate. Its clinical effect on the AV node is delayed in onset. The efficacy of digoxin for pharmacologic conversion of atrial flutter to sinus rhythm is variable.

REENTRANT SUPRAVENTRICULAR TACHYARRHYTHMIAS

Overview

The concept of functional or anatomic dissociation of conduction tissue into two pathways with different conduction velocities and refractory periods is postulated to explain reentry. With dissociation into two pathways, a premature impulse encounters refractoriness (unidirectional block) in one pathway and is conducted slowly in the other. During this period of delayed conduction, the blocked pathway recovers responsiveness. If the two pathways are connected, the impulse can reenter the previously blocked pathway and be conducted to the chamber of origin in a retrograde fashion. During retrograde conduction, the pathway previously used for antegrade conduction regains responsiveness. Once initiated, impulse conduction over the pathways becomes self-perpetuating. Longitudinal dissociation of conducting tissue into two pathways, one with unidirectional block and the other with prolonged conduction time, is necessary for reentry to occur. In humans, reentry has been demonstrated in the SA and AV nodes, atrium, and the His-Purkinje system (33,34).

Supraventricular Tachycardia (SVT)-AV Nodal Reentry

The pathways used for reentry lie within the AV node. An episode of SVT is initiated by a closely coupled PAC. The P′ wave produced by the premature atrial depolarization is morphologically different from the sinus P wave, and the P'R interval of the PAC is usually longer than the PR interval of sinus beats. This is due to the fact that atrial depolarization has occurred prematurely and the AV node has not completely repolarized after the preceding sinus beat. If "longitudinal dissociation" has occurred, a regular tachyarrhythmia will result. The ventricular rate is regular and usually between 160–260/min. Each impulse is conducted back to the atria, but the sequence of atrial depolarization is abnormal, proceeding superiorly and leftward. Abnormal atrial depolarization may be recognized by "inverted" P waves in the inferior ECG lead. In approximately 30% of patients with SVT and AV nodal reentry, an inverted retrograde P wave will be seen to closely follow each QRS complex. If P waves are seen, they are regular, occur at a rate equal to the ventricular rate (there is no AV block), and the R-P interval is usually less than one-half the R-R interval. However, in most cases (>60%), atrial depolarization occurs during inscription of the QRS complex and a retrograde P wave is not seen (34).

Figure 2.8 demonstrates an episode of SVT due to AV node reentry. As demonstrated in the ladder diagram, the underlying sinus rhythm is interrupted by PACs that are nonconducted. Ectopic P' waves deform the T wave and are not conducted to the ventricles because of the recovery periods of the conduction system. The third PAC induces a rapid, regular tachyarrhythmia (ventricular rate 160/min) due to AV nodal reentry. As is typical, retrograde P waves are not seen.

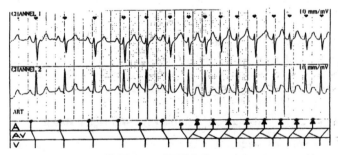

Figure 2.8.   AV Node Reentry.

SVT Reentry Using a Concealed Bypass Tract (CBT)

This mechanism is similar to that of SVT with AV node reentry; however, an extra nodal conduction pathway is used for retrograde conduction to the atria. This extra nodal pathway can conduct impulses only in a retrograde direction. Patients with Wolff-Parkinson-White (WPW) syndrome also have an extra nodal conduction pathway (bypass tract), but it can conduct impulses in both a retrograde or antegrade direction. Antegrade conduction via the extra nodal pathway during normal sinus rhythm (NSR) in WPW produces the characteristic "delta wave." Patients with an extra nodal conduction pathway capable of only retrograde conduction are said to have a CBT because a delta wave is not inscribed during sinus rhythm.

An episode of SVT is initiated in the same manner as described previously for SVT with AV node reentry. The ventricular rate is regular but slightly faster than in SVT with AV node reentry. The sequence of atrial depolarization is again abnormal or inverted P waves (leads II, III, and aVF) following each QRS complex, which will be seen in almost all patients. The R-P interval is usually less than one-half of the R-R interval. During the SVT, a negative P wave is usually seen in lead I in patients with a concealed bypass tract but not in patients with SVT and AV node reentry.

SVT with SA Node Reentry

A PAC usually depolarizes the SA node, resulting in a characteristic noncompensatory pause. However, an early PAC can encounter block in one portion of the sinus node, enter sinus nodal tissue in another portion, and traverse the nodal tissue slowly enough so that the emerging impulses are able to excite the atria. Therefore, the SA node, in a manner similar to the AV node, can provide pathways for reentry. SVT is initiated by a PAC, but subsequent P waves are normal (upright in leads II, III, and aVF) and morphologically similar to sinus beats because the SA node serves as the site of origin. The atrial rate is regular (160–260/min). AV block (fixed or variable) may occur because the AV node is not a part of the reentrant loop. A 1:1 AV conduction ratio can also occur. The R-P interval is usually greater than one-half the R-R interval. Carotid sinus massage (CSM) or a Valsalva maneuver may terminate the rhythm disturbance.

SVT with SA node reentry is uncommon and is frequently misdiagnosed because it may mimic sinus tachycardia with AV block and SVT due to an automatic atrial ectopic focus.

AUTOMATIC ATRIAL TACHYCARDIA

An episode of SVT may also result from the rapid firing of an automatic ectopic focus within the atria. This rhythm disturbance has been traditionally called "nonparoxysmal atrial tachycardia." Although it is initiated by a PAC, the coupling interval is not typically short. The ectopic P' wave electrical vector is usually normal (directed inferiorly and leftward); therefore, upright P waves will be noted in leads II, III, and aVF. P wave morphology will be slightly different from that of sinus beats. The R-P interval is usually greater than one-half the R-R interval. AV block may occur; it does not occur in SVT with AV node reentry or SVT with a CBT. The ventricular rate may be regular or irregular, depending on whether the degree of AV block is variable or fixed. 1:1 AV conduction can occur. Because this rhythm does not involve a reentry "loop," vagal maneuvers that alter AV conduction (carotid sinus massage, Valsalva maneuver) will not terminate the arrhythmias but may increase the degree of AV block.

An automatic atrial tachycardia is shown in Figure 2.9 (lead III). P' waves are shown with an "x." These P' waves deform the T wave of the preceding QRS complex, are upright in lead III (normal atrial depolarization vector), and are regular at a rate of 280/min. The ventricular rate is also regular at 140/min (2:1 AV block).

The Value of the ECG in Defining SVT Mechanism

Careful inspection of the 12-lead ECG during an episode of SVT may be of value in suggesting the underlying electrophysiologic mechanism (see Table 2.2) (35).

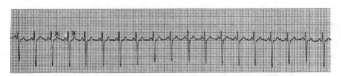

Figure 2.9. Automatic Atrial Tachycardia.

Table 2.2
Summary of ECG Findings in SVT

	SVT-AV node reentry	SVT-CBT	SVT-Automatic focus or SA node reentry
Approximate frequency as cause of SVT	70%	20%	10%
P waves in II, III, and aVF	relatively uncommon	always	always
P wave in I	upright	inverted	upright
R-P interval	<1/2 R-R	<1/2 R-R	>1/2 R-R
P wave in II, III, aVF	inverted	inverted	upright
AV block	never	never	common
Functional bundle branch block	uncommon	common	uncommon
Effect of carotid sinus massage	no change or terminates	no change or terminates	may ↑ AV block but does not terminate

Therapy

Short runs of these tachyarrhythmias are usually well tolerated and require no specific therapy other than possible PAC suppression to prevent further recurrence. Prolonged episodes may require medical therapy and/or electrical cardioversion. Because these tachyarrhythmias typically result from "reentry" within the AV node, one must interrupt the critical relation of conduction and refractoriness in the pathways of the AV node.

If the patient is hemodynamically stable, proceed with medical management as outlined below. If the patient is clinically unstable, proceed with sedation and synchronized cardioversion utilizing 100 W/sec.

Treatment of Supraventricular Tachycardia of Reentrant Origin

1. **Carotid sinus massage.** Massage either the right or left carotid independently for 10–15 sec while observing a monitor. The arrhythmia will either convert to normal sinus rhythm or will remain unchanged.

2. **Valsalva maneuver.** Frequently helpful, especially when combined with CSM. Continue CSM after Valsalva maneuver is released.

3. **Adenosine.** Adenosine is an endogenous nucleoside that inhibits AV nodal conduction (36,37). It has a very brief half-life of 10–30 sec and few side effects that are transient (most commonly flushing). It is the drug of choice for terminating an SVT, which involves the AV node as a part of the reentrant loop (1). The dose is 6 mg via rapid intravenous bolus. Two subsequent 12-mg doses can be given minutes later if the first dose is ineffective. The successful conversion rate is >90% (38). The drug must be given as a bolus (followed by a flush injection of normal saline into the intravenous tubing) due to its rapid plasma breakdown. Adenosine can also be useful in the diagnosis and treatment of wide-complex tachycardias. Adenosine can terminate SVT with aberrant conduction and yet not cause adverse effects in patients with ventricular tachycardia due to its short half-life. Adenosine, on occasion, may also convert ventricular tachycardia to sinus rhythm (39).

4. **Verapamil.** Verapamil can be given intravenously for termination of acute episodes of AV nodal reentrant tachycardia. The drug prolongs AV node conduction time via its effects on slow calcium channels. It should be given as a slow intravenous bolus at a dose of 0.1 mg/kg (5–10 mg). Conversion to sinus rhythm usually occurs within minutes of administration. Verapamil terminates AV nodal reentrant tachycardia in >90% of patients (38). The drug is contraindicated in patients with moderate to severe LV dysfunction, those taking β blockers, and patients with a systolic BP of <90 mm Hg during the tachyarrhythmia. Intravenous administration is not uncommonly complicated by hypotension due to the effects of verapamil on peripheral vascular resistance. This side effect can be minimized by pretreatment with intravenous calcium chloride (500–1000 mg). The AV nodal effects of verapamil are not substantially affected by CaCl2.

5. **Diltiazem.** The recommended dose is 0.25 mg/kg or 20 mg intravenously for the typical adult patient. Conversion usually occurs within 3–7 minutes.

6. **β blockers.** Currently, propranolol, metoprolol, esmolol, and atenolol are available for intravenous injection in the United States. As with other drugs, these should be titrated carefully

to effect with close monitoring and blood pressure determinations. Contraindications include LV dysfunction, asthma, high-degree AV block, and sick sinus syndrome.

7. **Digoxin.** Intravenous doses are generally of little value in acute therapy because of the slow onset of action.

8. **Atrial pacemaker.** This method frequently will capture the atria and lead to normal sinus rhythm. Set the atrial pacer to a rate faster than the SVT and then abruptly terminate pacing, looking for resumption of normal sinus rhythm. This method is especially helpful after open-heart surgery for patients who may have atrial epicardial wires in place postoperatively.

9. **AV node ablation.** Catheter-based techniques in the electrophysiology laboratory allow for the precise analysis and localization of the mechanism of tachycardia. AV nodal reentry mechanisms can be treated by ablating one of the pathways and thereby interrupting the reentry circuit. Some supraventricular rhythms that are difficult to define on the 12-lead ECG can be definitively diagnosed and treated, such as atrial flutter and concealed bypass tracts.

ATRIOVENTRICULAR CONDUCTION DEFECTS

A disturbance in impulse conduction from atria to ventricles may occur at the level of the SA node, internodal pathways, AV node, His bundle, bundle branches, or Purkinje network. Although the terms "AV block" and "AV dissociation" are often used interchangeably, they are separate entities with markedly differing mechanisms.

AV block may be due to an organic lesion along the conduction pathway, an increase in inherent refractoriness of the conduction pathway, or marked shortening of the supraventricular cycle with encroachment on the normal refractory period. The first two causes are pathologic; the last is physiologic (as exemplified by atrial flutter). AV block may be classified as partial or complete, permanent or temporary, or according to the site of the block (AV nodal or infranodal) (40,41).

First-Degree AV Block (1° AVB)

Description

Each supraventricular impulse is conducted to the ventricles but more slowly than normal. Electrocardiographically, 1° AVB is re-

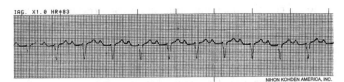

IAG. X1.0 HR+83

NIHON KOHDEN AMERICA, INC.

Figure 2.10.   1° AV Block.

flected by a prolonged PR interval (>0.20 sec) that is constant from beat to beat. In Figure 2.10, the PR interval is 0.32 sec. The AV node is usually the site of block, but delay may occur at the level of the internodal pathways, His bundle, or bundle branches (one bundle branch may be completely blocked, with delay occurring in the opposite bundle branch). The intensity of the first heart sound tends to decrease as the PR interval becomes longer.

Causes

Causes include increased parasympathetic tone, drugs that prolong AV conduction (e.g., digoxin, propranolol, verapamil), and conduction system disease (e.g., fibrosis, inflammation associated with myocarditis).

Therapy

First-degree AVB alone does not produce symptoms and requires no therapy. Digoxin may cause 1° AVB, but this ECG finding is usually not considered a sign of digoxin toxicity unless the PR interval exceeds 0.24 sec.

Second-Degree AV Block (2° AVB)

Some supraventricular impulses are conducted to the ventricles, whereas others are blocked. There are two types of 2° AVB, and this distinction is prognostically and therapeutically important.

Second-Degree AVB, Mobitz Type I (Wenckebach)

Description   Type I 2° AVB is characterized by progressive prolongation of the PR interval, indicating a progressive decrease in conduction velocity ("decremental conduction") before a P wave is completely blocked. This form of block almost always occurs at the level of the AV node, but the phenomenon of decremental conduction and "Wenckebach periodicity" has been reported in other conducting tissue. Usually, only a single impulse is blocked and the cycle is repeated. Longer pauses may be interrupted by escape beats (junctional, ventricular). Repetition of such cycles results in "group beating," e.g., three sinus beats are conducted with progressively increasing PR intervals and the fourth sinus beat is completely blocked and a QRS complex is not inscribed. Such a "group" would be referred to as 4:3 conduction. The conduction ratio is usually constant but may vary, e.g., 4:3 to 3:2.

In addition to gradual prolongation of the PR interval, typical Wenckebach periodicity is characterized by a decreasing R-R interval before the blocked sinus impulse. This is because the increment of PR prolongation becomes progressively less with each conducted beat, i.e., whereas the absolute length of the PR interval increases with each beat, the amount of increase is less with each beat after the second beat of the cycle. The P-P interval is usually constant.

In Figure 2.11, 4:3 Wenckebach periodicity is demonstrated. Relevant intervals are shown in seconds. The atrial rate is regular (constant P-P interval). The PR interval increases from beat to beat. The fourth sinus impulse of the cycle is not conducted to the ventricles. During the Wenckebach cycle, the R-R interval can be seen to decrease before the dropped beat, because the increment in the PR interval is decreasing. The increment from 0.28 to 0.40 sec is 0.12 sec, whereas the next increment is only 0.06 sec; the R-R thus decreases by 0.06 sec.

Atypical Wenckebach

Description Rhythms that manifest all the features outlined above represent the typical Wenckebach phenomenon. If many but not all of these features are found, then atypical Wenckebach is said

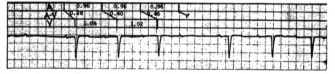

Figure 2.11.   Typical Wenckebach (Mobitz I AVB).

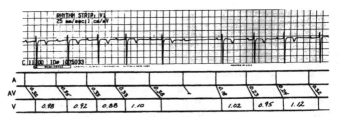

Figure 2.12.   Atypical Wenckebach.

to be present and is due to inconsistent change in the degree of conduction delay from beat to beat. In typical Wenckebach conduction, each impulse is progressively delayed, but with a progressive decrease in the increment of that delay. In atypical Wenckebach, the increment may fail to decrease (PR interval does not change between two consecutive beats), the increment may increase, or a PR interval may be less than the one preceding it. In atypical Wenckebach, conduction delay will tend to increase through the cycle as a whole but will not demonstrate progression from beat to beat. The frequency of atypical Wenckebach conduction increases as the conduction ratio increases—at a conduction ratio greater than 6:5, Wenckebach conduction is almost always atypical.

Figure 2.12 demonstrates a Mobitz I AVB with a 9:8 conduction ratio. PR and R-R intervals are included in the ladder diagram. The first four QRS complexes from the right represent the start of the sequence. QRS complexes 2, 3, 4, and 5 from the left represent the end of the cycle. The PR interval does not progressively increase from beat to beat, but over the sequence, increases from 0.18 sec to 0.38 sec.

Causes

Causes for 2° AVB, Mobitz type I are the same as for 1° AVB. In addition, this arrhythmia frequently occurs during acute inferior MI due to AV nodal ischemia, resulting in increased vagal tone at this level of conduction (in approximately 90% of hearts, the right coronary artery supplies the inferior wall as well as the AV node). This rhythm is a sign of digoxin toxicity in patients taking the medication.

Therapy

Acute therapy is not indicated for the hemodynamically stable patient. Intensive care unit (ICU) observation with ECG monitoring is suggested for patients with acute infarction, suspected drug toxicity, or suspected acute myocarditis. In the setting of acute inferior infarction, this arrhythmia is usually transient and well tolerated.

Acute intervention is required for the hemodynamically unstable patient. Signs and symptoms of hypoperfusion caused by this rhythm disturbance are usually not encountered until the ventricular rate falls below 60/min.

Intravenous atropine should be given in 0.5-mg increments at 5-min intervals until the ventricular response rate increases or a total dose of 2 mg is administered.

Temporary pacing should be instituted as soon as possible for patients who do not respond to atropine. Atrial pacing is not likely to be effective because the block is at the level of the AV node. However, it may be of value in selected cases in which Wenckebach AV conduction is accompanied by profound sinus bradycardia.

If temporary artificial pacing is not immediately available, an **isoproterenol infusion** (2–20 μ/min) titrated to hemodynamic response can be used with caution. In the setting of acute infarction, the drug may increase myocardial oxygen demand and extend the zone of infarction if demand is not accompanied by an increase in coronary blood flow. In the setting of digoxin toxicity, isoproterenol may worsen ventricular irritability due to its β-1 effects.

If hypoperfusion persists after an effective ventricular rate increase (>70/min) with atropine or pacing in the setting of acute inferior MI, associated right ventricular infarction should be suspected and diagnosed and appropriate interventions should be started (see Chapter 9).

Second-Degree AVB, Mobitz Type II

Description Block usually occurs below the level of the AV node (infranodal and within the His-Purkinje system). The PR interval is usually normal but may be slightly prolonged. PR intervals do not change measurably from beat to beat, although the PR interval after a blocked impulse may be somewhat shorter. The QRS

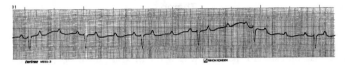

Figure 2.13. 2° AVB, Mobitz Type II.

complexes may be wide (QRS duration, >0.10 sec) because fascicular or bundle branch block (or both) is often present, because the infranodal block commonly occurs within the bundle branches. On occasion, QRS complexes of normal duration may be encountered (Fig. 2.13). The conduction ratio may be fixed or variable.

Figure 2.13 demonstrates Mobitz type II second-degree block (lead II). The sinus rate is 90/min and the ventricular rate is 30/min (3:1 AV block).

When AV block occurs with a conduction ratio of 2:1, the distinction between type I or type II 2° AVB may be difficult because there is no progressive prolongation of the PR interval in 2:1 type I block. Type I should be suspected if the QRS duration of conducted beats is normal and the presence of more typical Wenckebach periodicity is noted at other times; 2:1 AVB and wide QRS complexes are most often caused by infranodal type II 2° AVB if the PR interval is normal.

Causes

This arrhythmia is most commonly encountered in chronic degenerative diseases (e.g., Lev's disease). It may be seen in acute myocarditis, following cardiac surgery, and in acute anterior MI due to distal conduction system ischemia/necrosis.

Therapy

This arrhythmia is usually not a transient phenomenon; it tends to be persistent or recurrent and may progress to complete heart block. It has a more serious prognosis because it is associated with extensive structural damage to the ventricular conduction system. Artificial demand ventricular pacing will be required in most instances. Atropine administration in the acute management is unlikely to be successful but can be attempted as described in Mobitz type 1 AVB.

Third-Degree AV Block (3° AVB), Complete Heart Block

Description

Third-degree AVB indicates complete absence of atrioventricular conduction. There are two types, which represent a progression in severity from type I and type II 2° AVB.

Third-Degree AVB at AV Nodal Level

When conduction of supraventricular impulses is blocked completely at the AV node, a "junctional" or AV nodal escape pacemaker initiates ventricular depolarization. This is a stable pacemaker with an inherent firing rate of 40–60 min. Because the escape pacemaker is located above the His bundle, the sequence of ventricular depolarization is normal, resulting in a normal QRS (QRS duration of <0.10 sec). This type of 3° AVB is not uncommon after acute inferior MI caused by an increase in vagal tone at the level of the AV node. It is usually transient but may last up to 1 week.

Infranodal 3° AVB

The ventricles are depolarized by an intrinsic pacemaker located in the bundle branch-Purkinje system. Because the pacemaker lies below the site of the block and the bifurcation of the His bundle, ventricular depolarization does not occur via the normal conducting system and QRS complexes will have a wide configuration (Fig. 2.14). A ventricular escape pacemaker has an inherent firing rate of 30–40/min and is relatively unstable, i.e., episodes of ventricular asystole may occur (Fig. 2.4).

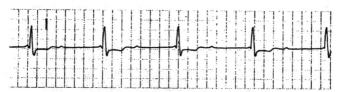

Figure 2.14. Infranodal 3° AVB.

Infranodal 3° AVB is indicative of extensive conduction system disease and is often a complication of acute anterior MI.

In both types of 3° AVB, atrial and ventricular depolarization are independent, the PR intervals vary in a random fashion, and the atrial rate is faster than the ventricular rate. The ventricular rate is regular. The atrial rate is usually regular but may show sinus arrhythmia (ventriculophasic sinus arrhythmia: P-P intervals that bracket a QRS are shorter than those that do not). Critical differentiating features are QRS morphology and escape pacemaker rate.

Therapy

1. 3° AVB at AV node level
   Same as for 2° AVB, Mobitz type I.
2. Infranodal 3° AVB
   An artificial demand pacemaker will almost always be required.
   Acutely, intravenous atropine or isoproterenol can be given, but neither is likely to be of value for the hemodynamically compromised patient.

Atrioventricular Dissociation

Description

Atrioventricular dissociation (AVD) is never a primary diagnosis; it is always secondary to some other rhythm disturbance. In AVD, the atria and ventricles are depolarized by separate pacemakers. The atria are activated by the sinus node. The ventricles are depolarized by a lower-level pacemaker at the level of the AV node or within the ventricular conduction system. The ventricular rate is either equal to the atrial rate (isorhythmic AVD) or greater than the atrial rate. In AV block, the atrial rate is faster than the ventricular rate. The lower pacemaker depolarizes the ventricles because it encounters a nonrefractory myocardium. Atrioventricular dissociation may be passive or active.

Passive AVD

When the sinus node fails to depolarize within approximately 1 sec, a junctional or ventricular escape beat or rhythm may emerge. If a sinus impulse should reach the AV junction between

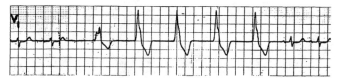

Figure 2.15. Passive AVD.

escape beats when the AV node is not refractory, the sinus beat will be conducted to the ventricles. Therefore, AV block is not present.

Figure 2.15 demonstrates the passive type of AV dissociation. The first two sinus beats are conducted normally to the ventricles. A long pause follows the second QRS due to sinus arrest. The pause is interrupted by a fusion beat and then an accelerated idioventricular rhythm. Sinus rhythm resumes at the end of the strip.

Active AVD

The discharge rate of the lower pacemaker exceeds or usurps that of the sinus node in the absence of bradycardia. Therefore, it is caused by an accelerated junctional or idioventricular rhythm or ventricular tachycardia.

Therapy

For the asymptomatic patient, therapy is often unnecessary. Therapy should be directed at the underlying cause—the primary rhythm. Atropine may be effective in increasing the sinus rate in passive AVD. Suppressing an accelerated idioventricular rhythm in the presence of a slow sinus rhythm may be deleterious.

VENTRICULAR ARRHYTHMIAS

① Ventricular Extrasystole (Premature Ventricular Contraction)

Description

A premature ventricular contraction (PVC) is a premature impulse of ventricular origin occurring before the next expected sinus beat. It may arise from a ventricular focus with enhanced automaticity or may represent a form of reentry within the His-

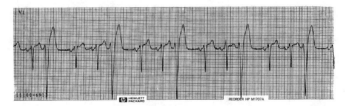

Figure 2.16. Unifocal PVCs.

Purkinje system. Both mechanisms may be operative under different circumstances. PVCs may be unifocal (identical or nearly identical QRS morphology with a fixed coupling interval) (Fig. 2.16) or multifocal (varying QRS morphology and coupling intervals).

Because a PVC originates in the ventricle, ventricular depolarization and repolarization are abnormal, resulting in a wide QRS complex (>0.12 sec) and an ST segment and T wave directed opposite the QRS complex. The SA node is anatomically and "electrically" separated from the ventricles, and a PVC usually does not depolarize the SA node because of refractoriness to retrograde conduction in the AV node. Therefore, the rhythm of the SA node is not disturbed and there is usually a fully compensatory pause. On occasion, the SA node may be depolarized, and a noncompensatory pause will result. In the presence of a slow sinus rhythm, a PVC may occur between two sinus beats, resulting in an "interpolated" PVC (the P-P interval remains unchanged because there is no pause). The sinus impulse after an interpolated PVC usually has a prolonged PR interval, because the AV node is still refractory from incomplete penetration (concealed conduction) by the PVC.

The second, fifth, eighth, eleventh, and fourteenth QRS complexes in Figure 2.16 are PVCs of unifocal origin (same morphology and coupling interval) followed by a fully compensatory pause (R-R interval of sinus beats bracketing a PVC is twice that of the basic sinus rate). This is an example of ventricular trigeminy.

Causes

Causes include acute and chronic myocardial ischemia, cardiomyopathy, electrolyte disturbances (hypokalemia, hypomagnesium), and drug toxicity (sympathomimetics, digoxin).

Therapy

For the acutely ill patient with an acute infarction, suspected infarction, acute respiratory failure or after cardiac surgery, etc., lidocaine, given as an intravenous bolus followed by continuous intravenous infusion, should be administered (see Chapter 9). Indications for therapeutic intervention in the management of ''chronic'' PVCs are discussed in Chapter 15.

 Ventricular Escape Beats (Idioventricular Rhythm)

Description

A ventricular escape beat is an impulse originating from a pacemaker within the His-Purkinje network. It occurs after the next expected supraventricular impulse has failed to occur or be conducted to the ventricles. Such a pacemaker has an intrinsic rate of 30–40/min, and the interval preceding the escape beat is usually greater than 1.5 sec. If more than one escape beat occurs in succession, a ventricular escape (or idioventricular) rhythm and atrioventricular dissociation are present. If the rate is greater than 40/min but less than 100/min, an accelerated idioventricular rhythm (AIVR) is said to be present (Fig. 2.17). Escape beats and rhythms have wide QRS complexes, abnormal ST segments, and secondary T waves changes as seen in PVCs.

Figure 2.17 demonstrates AIVR on the top strip, which is interrupted by a PVC. The last beat on the top strip is the beginning of a 3-beat interlude of sinus bradycardia, which is, in turn, interrupted by the resumption of AIVR when the sinus rate be-

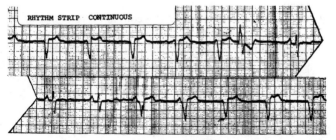

Figure 2.17. Accelerated Idioventricular Rhythm.

comes slower than the AIVR rate. The rhythm disturbance is similar to that shown in Figure 2.15.

Therapy

Ventricular escape beats and accelerated idioventricular rhythms are not uncommon after acute MI. Suppressant drugs such as lidocaine should not be used because they may represent the only reliable pacemaker. Intravenous atropine sulfate given in 0.5-mg increments every 5 min (total dose, 2 mg) may accelerate the SA node or allow the atria to "capture" the ventricles. Artificial pacing may be required if the dominant rhythm is too slow for adequate perfusion.

Ventricular Parasystole

Description

Ventricular parasystole refers to the presence of concurrent impulse formation by two pacemakers, one in the SA node and the other in the ventricle (42). Independent pacemakers may also be noted during AVD, but differences exist between AVD and parasystole. The ventricular parasystolic pacemaker has three important properties not shared by a lower pacemaker in AVD.

1. **Entrance block.** An electrical impulse cannot enter the parasystolic focus and depolarize it; therefore, the parasystolic pacemaker fires at a fixed rate and is not reset by ventricular depolarization.
2. **Intermittent exit block.** Despite the fact that impulses are repetitively generated by the parasystolic pacemaker, impulse conduction to the surrounding myocardium does not always occur.
3. **Constant rate of discharge.** The constant rate of discharge is evidenced by the fact that the interval between parasystolic beats (interectopic interval) remains constant or is a multiple of a basic interval. Each impulse may not produce a QRS complex due to existing block or refractoriness of the myocardium from a preceding depolarization.

Parasystolic beats are ventricular ectopic beats with constant QRS morphology, but the coupling interval is usually variable. "Fusion beats" may be seen if the sinus beat reaches the ventricle

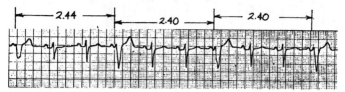

Figure 2.18.   Ventricular Parasystole.

at approximately the same time that the parasystolic focus discharges.

In the following example of ventricular parasystole (Fig. 2.18), the interectopic interval is nearly constant (varies by less than 2%). The first ectopic beat immediately follows the P wave and there is no fusion. The subsequent three ectopic beats demonstrate fusion with progressively more influence from the conducted beat—the QRS complex narrows and the T wave amplitude declines—because the ectopic beat is occurring progressively later after the P wave.

Therapy

Ventricular parasystole frequently occurs in the presence of severe underlying heart disease. Suppressive drugs (lidocaine) are less effective than in fixed-coupled PVCs. Parasystole can lead to ventricular tachycardia or fibrillation, particularly in the setting of myocardial ischemia or infarction. In the absence of ischemia, the rhythm can be stable for many years.

Ventricular Tachycardia (VT)

Description

VT is a ventricular arrhythmia that may be caused by either an abnormality of impulse generation (automatic arrhythmia focus or triggered activity) or impulse propagation (reentry within the His-Purkinje system) (43,44). PVCs usually presage its occurrence (see Chapter 15). An episode of VT is constituted by at least three successive ventricular ectopic beats at a rate in excess of 100/min (usual rate, 140–220/min). Because the sequence of ventricular depolarization and repolarization is abnormal, QRS complexes

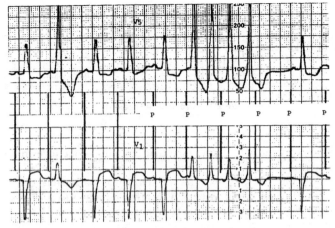

Figure 2.19. Ventricular Tachycardia.

during VT are wide, and distinct ST segments and T waves may not be evident. The basic sinus rhythm may remain intact, leading to antegrade atrial depolarization with AV dissociation. On occasion, the sinus node may "capture" the ventricle (capture beat) or cause fusion beats if the AV node and ventricular myocardium are not refractory. VT is usually a regular rhythm, except when a capture beat occurs. Conduction from the ventricle to the atria may occur, resulting in retrograde atrial depolarization. Therefore, AV dissociation is not necessary for the diagnosis of VT. Capture and fusion beats will not occur during ventriculoatrial conduction.

In Figure 2.19, simultaneous V5 and V1 equivalent leads from a Holter monitor recording reveal a single PVC followed by a four-beat burst of VT. The P waves are marked by vertical lines. There is AV dissociation with a constant atrial rate of 94 during the VT, which occurs at a rate of 165. The P waves are too close to the ectopic ventricular beats to cause fusion beats.

Causes

Causes are similar to those of PVCs.

Therapy

If the patient is hemodynamically stable, a lidocaine bolus may be given and a constant infusion of lidocaine may be initiated.

If the patient has clinical signs of hypoperfusion or is in cardiopulmonary arrest, countershock should be administered immediately and CPR would be initiated (1).

Ventricular Ectopy Versus Aberrant Ventricular Conduction

Premature, morphologically bizarre QRS complexes may result from discharge of a ventricular ectopic focus (PVC) or from abnormal or "aberrant" ventricular conduction of a supraventricular impulse. Aberrant ventricular conduction (AVC) occurs when a premature impulse encounters partially refractory ventricular conduction tissue, usually the right bundle branch. The right bundle branch has a longer refractory period than the left bundle branch. The more premature the supraventricular impulse, the more likely that AVC will occur. Because of the disparity in refractory periods of the bundle branches, AVC usually takes the form of a right bundle branch block (RBBB) pattern. Left bundle branch aberration may also occur but is infrequent (45).

The length of the refractory period of the bundle branches is determined by the preceding R-R interval—the refractory period is longer with slow heart rates (long R-R interval) and shorter with fast rates (short R-R interval). A long R-R interval preceding a PAC will facilitate AVC.

Close inspection of the ECG may allow differentiation of a PVC from AVC of a supraventricular impulse, usually a PAC (45).

The following ECG features are suggestive of a PAC with AVC (Fig. 2.20):

- An rSR' pattern in lead V1.
- A premature P' wave preceding the bizarre QRS complex. The P wave morphology may be different from that of sinus P waves, and the PR interval of the PAC is usually longer than that of the normally conducted sinus beats. The premature P wave may be "hidden" in the preceding T wave.

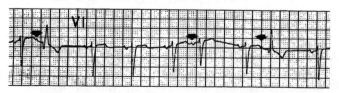

Figure 2.20. PACs with Aberrant Ventricular Conduction.

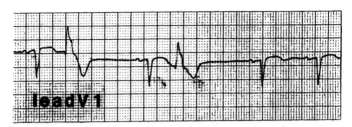

Figure 2.21. Ventricular Ectopy.

- A noncompensatory pause follows the bizarre QRS complex.
- A QRS duration of <0.12 sec.
- In atrial fibrillation or in MFAT, aberrantly conducted beats resembling PVCs may be seen when short R-R intervals follow long R-R intervals ("long-short cycle sequence"). These beats are often called Ashman beats in recognition of their characterization by Gouaux and Ashman in 1947.

In Figure 2.20 (lead V1), wide QRS complexes are shown to interrupt sinus rhythm. These complexes are triphasic (rSR' or RBBB morphology), and the QRS duration is <0.12 sec. Premature P waves (arrows) can be recognized on the downslope of the preceding T wave, and the PR intervals of the PACs are greater than those of normally conducted sinus beats. The wide QRS complexes are, therefore, the result of aberrant conduction of PACs. Note that the second PAC is less premature than the first and third, and there is no aberrancy.

The following ECG features are suggestive of a PVC (Fig. 2.21):

- A monophasic or biphasic QRS complex in lead V1.
- If the QRS complex is notched ("rabbit ear" pattern), the amplitude of the R wave is greater than that of the R' wave in V1. If R' wave amplitude is greater than that of the R wave, a PVC may not be confidently distinguished from a PAC with AVC.
- A QRS wave in V6.
- A P wave does not precede the bizarre QRS complex.
- QRS duration of >0.16 sec.
- Bizarre QRS complex followed by a fully compensatory pause.

Table 2.3
SVT with Aberration Versus Ventricular Tachycardia

	SVT-AVC	V TACH
QRS morphology in V1	triphasic (rSR′)	mono- or biphasic
R/S ratio in V6	>1.0	<1.0
Frontal plane QRS axis	normal or rightward	<-30°
QRS duration	≤0.14 sec	>0.14 sec
Ventricular rate	>170/min	<170/min
Fusion beats	no	yes
AV dissociation/VA dissociation	no	yes

An algorithmic approach has also been proposed to differentiate regular, wide QRS complex tachyarrhythmias. This algorithm has been demonstrated to have a sensitivity and specificity of >95% in delineating the origin of the rhythm disturbance (48).

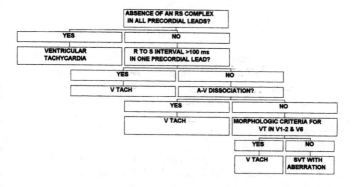

Two PVCs are shown in Figure 2.21 (the second and fourth QRS complexes). These complexes have a QRS duration of 0.14 sec, are biphasic, and have a rabbit ear pattern (notch on QRS down stroke). Each is followed by a fully compensatory pause.

Similar criteria have been reported to aid in the differentiation of sustained ventricular tachycardia (VT) from a sustained supraventricular tachyarrhythmia with aberrant ventricular conduction (SVT-AVC). These are summarized in Table 2.3 (46,47).

This useful algorithm requires only the identification and measurement of an RS complex in the precordial leads, recognition of AV dissociation (or fusion beats), and using morphologic criteria in the precordial leads. Morphologic criteria for VT in V1 or V2 include a monophasic R wave, a QR or RS complex, or

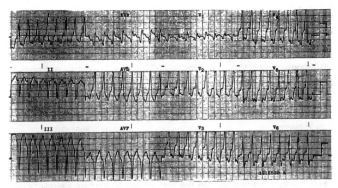

Figure 2.22. Ventricular Tachycardia (12-lead ECG).

R wave >0.30 sec. Criteria in V6 include an R to S wave ratio of <1, a QS or QR complex, or a monophasic R wave.

Careful inspection of the 12-lead ECG with the above differences in mind will most often lead to a correct diagnosis. In more difficult cases, the physical examination may be of help. The presence of AV dissociation during VT may produce "cannon a" waves in the jugular venous pulse pattern and a first heart sound of varying intensity. The presence or absence of hypotension is of no differential diagnostic value (49).

Figure 2.22 is an example of ventricular tachycardia. The 12-lead recording meets the criteria for VT as noted in the algorithm.

Therapy

In the hemodynamically unstable patient, cardioversion is the treatment of choice, regardless of the origin of the rhythm. In the stable patient, without classic ECG findings for VT or SVT with aberrant conduction, intravenous procainamide (10–12 mg/kg over 30 min) should be administered. Procainamide will not only slow or terminate VT but can also interrupt a supraventricular tachycardia due to reentry (47).

Torsade de Pointes

Description

The term torsade de pointes ("twisting of the points") was chosen by Dessertenne in 1966 to describe a new ventricular arrhythmia with unusual characteristics. As initially described, the limb leads show cycles of alternating QRS polarity such that the peaks of the QRS complexes appear to be twisting around the isoelectric line of the recording. In each cycle, the amplitude of consecutive ventricular complexes increases and decreases in a sinusoidal fashion. However, these sinusoidal cycles make up only a portion of the arrhythmia. At other times, the rhythm is that of typical ventricular tachycardia (uniform morphology and polarity of wide ventricular complexes in the monitor lead) (Fig. 2.23). This rhythm is also characterized by frequent spontaneous conversion and recurrence. If spontaneous conversion occurs, it usually does so within 30 sec of onset of the arrhythmia. Electrical cardioversion may be required to terminate the arrhythmia. **Current opinion is that torsade de pointes should be diagnosed only if the above morphologically distinct ECG pattern is associated with a prolonged correct QT interval between occurrences.** In most instances, the corrected QT interval will be >0.60 sec. In the absence of QT prolongation, a diagnosis of polymorphous or atypical ventricular tachycardia is suggested. This distinction is extremely important for acute and chronic management of this unusual ventricular arrhythmia (50).

Most data indicate that torsade de pointes is a reentrant ventricular tachyarrhythmia due to increased temporal dispersion of myocardial recovery times (repolarization rates). The arrhythmia is usually precipitated by a ventricular premature beat occurring in late diastole and usually falling on the summit of a prolonged T-U wave.

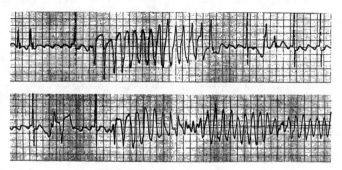

Figure 2.23.   Torsade de Pointes.

Causes

Causes include *(a)* congenital QT prolongation syndromes; *(b)* drug-induced acquired QT prolongation (class IA antiarrhythmics (quinidine, procainamide), phenothiazines, tricyclic antidepressants); *(c)* complete heart block; *(d)* hypokalemia; *(e)* hypomagnesemia; *(f)* intrinsic heart disease (ischemic heart disease, myocarditis); and *(g)* CNS disease (51).

Therapy

A correct diagnosis is critical in acute and chronic management. Use of class IA antiarrhythmics for this rhythm disturbance may adversely affect outcome. Treatment aims are to remove or correct the predisposing cause when possible (e.g., stop drugs, correct electrolyte disturbances) and to suppress the arrhythmia until either the QT interval decreases or a diagnosis of congenital QT prolongation is confirmed.

Cardioversion should be used for prolonged episodes. However, because this arrhythmia tends to recur, the therapeutic objective should be to prevent recurrence (51).

Intravenous magnesium sulfate (effective dose approximately 2 g) has been shown to be of value in preventing recurrence, even in patients with normal serum magnesium levels. Its mechanism of effect has not been conclusively established. Because this drug has not produced adverse effects and can be rapidly administered in the acute setting, magnesium may be the drug of first choice for management of this arrhythmia.

An **isoproterenol infusion** $(2-10 \,\mu/\text{min})$ can be used for acute control. Isoproterenol reduces the dispersion of myocardial recovery by a direct effect and indirectly by increasing the sinus node discharge rate. The QT interval decreases with increasing heart rate. However, this drug increases myocardial oxygen demand and decreases peripheral vascular resistance. It should be used with caution, especially for patients with intrinsic heart disease.

Temporary overdrive pacing has been particularly successful in preventing recurrence. If AV conduction is intact, atrial pacing is the preferred technique. Most agree that overdrive pacing is the definitive method for preventing recurrence.

Temporary blockade of the left stellate ganglion by injection of lidocaine may also be effective. However, this intervention requires skill and is only a temporary measure.

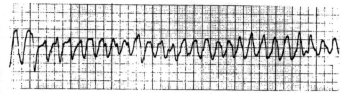

Figure 2.24. Ventricular Fibrillation.

Bretylium (5 mg/kg) has also been successfully used in a limited study population.

The class IA antiarrhythmics should not be used because they will further increase the QT interval. Lidocaine produces inconsistent results.

For patients with acquired QT prolongation, overdrive pacing can be discontinued when the predisposing cause has been corrected and the QT interval has returned to normal. Prophylactic drug therapy is not needed.

For patients subsequently diagnosed as having congenital QT prolongation, long-term treatment with oral propranolol has been shown to be effective for symptomatic patients. Complete electrophysiologic studies with possible implantation of an automatic defibrillator should be considered.

Ventricular Fibrillation

Description

This is a chaotic ventricular rhythm (Fig. 2.24) that is believed to be caused by multiple reentrant foci within the ventricle. Organized electrical activity is not present and because the ventricle does not depolarize as a unit, no ventricular contraction occurs.

References

1. Guidelines for Cardiopulmonary Resuscitation and Emergency Cardiac Care. Adult advanced cardiac life support. JAMA 1992;268: 2199–2241.
2. Zoll PM, Zoll RH, Falk RH, et al. External noninvasive temporary cardiac pacing: clinical trials. Circulation 1985:937–944.
3. Cox J, Wang RY. Critical consequences of common drugs: manifestations and management of calcium-channel blocker and β-adrenergic antagonist overdose. Emerg Med Rep 1994;15:83–90.

4. Scher DL, Arsura EL. Multifocal atrial tachycardia: mechanisms, clinical correlates, and treatment. Am Heart J 1989;118:574–580.
5. Kastor JA. Multifocal atrial tachycardia. N Engl J Med 1990;322: 1713—1717.
6. Waldo AL. Mechanisms of atrial fibrillation, atrial flutter, and ectopic atrial tachycardia—a brief review. Circulation 1987;75(Suppl III):III-37–III-40.
7. Flegel KM. From delirium cordis to atrial fibrillation: historical development of a disease concept. Ann Intern Med 1995;122:867–873.
8. Vaziri SM, Larson MG, Benjamin EJ, et al. Echocardiographic predictors of nonrheumatic atrial fibrillation. The Framingham Heart Study. Circulation 1994;89:724–730.
9. Golzari H, Cebul RD, Bahler RC. Atrial fibrillation: restoration and maintenance of sinus rhythm and indications for anticoagulation therapy. Ann Intern Med 1996;125:311–323.
10. Kannel WB, Abbott RD, Savage DD, et al. Epidemiologic features of chronic atrial fibrillation: the Framingham Study. N Engl J Med 1982; 306:1018–1022.
11. Kopecky SL, Gersh BJ, McGoon MD, et al: The natural history of lone atrial fibrillation. A population-based study over three decades. N Engl J Med 1987;317:669–674.
12. Mann DL, Maisel AS, Atwood JE, et al. Absence of cardioversion induced ventricular arrhythmias in patients with therapeutic digoxin levels. J Am Coll Cardiol 1985;5:883.
13. Prystowsky EN, Benson DW, Fuster V, et al. Management of patients with atrial fibrillation. A statement for healthcare professionals from the Subcommittee on Electrocardiography and Electrophysiology, American Heart Association. Circulation 1996;93:1262–1277.
14. Mungall DR, Robichaux RP, Perry W, et al. Effects of quinidine on serum digoxin concentration. Ann Intern Med 1980;93:689–696.
15. Manning WJ, Silverman DI, Gordon SPF, et al. Cardioversion from atrial fibrillation without prolonged anticoagulation with use of transesophageal echocardiography to exclude the presence of atrial thrombi. N Engl J Med 1993;328:750–755.
16. Stoddard MF, Dawkins PR, Prince CR, et al. Left atrial appendage thrombus is not uncommon in patients with acute atrial fibrillation and recent embolic event: a transesophageal echocardiographic study. J Am Coll Cardiol 1995;25:452–459.
17. Fatkin D, Kuchar DL, Thornburn CW, et al. Transesophageal echocardiography before and during direct current cardioversion of atrial fibrillation: evidence for atrial stunning as a mechanism of thromboembolic complications. J Am Coll Cardiol 1994;23:307–316.
18. Blackshear JL, Kopecky SL, Litin SC, et al. Management of atrial fibrillation in adults: prevention of thromboembolism and symptomatic treatment. Mayo Clin Proc 1996;71:150.

19. Flaker GC, Blackshear JL, McBride R, et al. (for the Stroke Prevention in Atrial Fibrillation Investigators). Antiarrhythmic drug therapy and cardiac mortality in atrial fibrillation. J Am Coll Cardiol 1992;20: 527–532.

20. Falk RH. Proarrhythmia in patients treated for atrial fibrillation or flutter. Ann Intern Med 1992;117:141–150.

21. Gosselink AT, Crijns HJ, Van Gelder IC, et al. Low-dose amiodarone for maintenance of sinus rhythm after cardioversion of atrial fibrillation or flutter. JAMA 1992;267:3289–3293.

22. Tammaso C, McDonough T, Parker M, et al. Atrial fibrillation and flutter. Immediate control and conversion with intravenously administered verapamil. Arch Intern Med 1983;143:877.

23. Ellenbogen KA, Dias VC, Plumb VJ, et al. A placebo-controlled trial of intravenous diltiazem infusion for 24 hour heart rate control during atrial fibrillation and atrial flutter: a multicenter study. J Am Coll Cardiol 1991;18:891–897.

24. Goldenberg IF, Lewis WR, Dias VC, et al. Intravenous diltiazem for the treatment of patients with atrial fibrillation or flutter and moderate to severe congestive heart failure. Am J Cardiol 1994;74:884–889.

25. Ellenbogen KA, Dias VC, Cardello FP, et al. Safety and efficacy of intravenous diltiazem in atrial fibrillation or atrial flutter. Am J Cardiol 1995;75:45–49.

26. Falk RH, Leavitt JI. Digoxin for atrial fibrillation: a drug whose time has gone? Ann Intern Med 1991;114:573–575.

27. Roberts SA, Diaz C, Nolan PE, et al. Effectiveness and costs of digoxin treatment for atrial fibrillation and flutter. Am J Cardiol 1993;72: 567–573.

28. Atrial Fibrillation Investigators. Risk factors for stroke and efficacy of antithrombotic therapy in atrial fibrillation. Arch Intern Med 1994; 154:1449–1457.

29. Laupacis A, Albers GW, Dalen JE, et al. Antithrombotic therapy in atrial fibrillation. Chest 1995;108(Suppl):352S–395S.

30. Waldo AL. Atrial flutter. New directions in management and mechanism. Circulation 1990;81:1142–1143.

31. Haft JI, Habbab MA. Treatment of atrial arrhythmias. Effectiveness of verapamil when preceded by calcium infusion. Arch Intern Med 1986;146:1085–1089.

32. Platia EV, Michelson EL, Porterfield JK, et al. Esmolol versus verapamil in the acute treatment of atrial fibrillation or atrial flutter. Am J Cardiol 1989;63:925–929.

33. Ganz LI, Friedman PL. Supraventricular tachycardia. N Engl J Med 1995;332:162–173.

34. Pieper SJ, Stanton MS. Narrow QRS complex tachycardias. Mayo Clin Proc 1995;70:371–375.

35. Akhtar M, Jazayeri MR, Sra J, et al. Atrioventricular nodal reentry.

Clinical, electrophysiological, and therapeutic consideration. Circulation 1993;88:282–295.

36. Shen W, Kurachi Y. Mechanisms of adenosine-mediated actions on cellular and clinical cardiac electrophysiology. Mayo Clin Proc 1995; 70:274–291.

37. Gamm AJ, Garratt CJ. Adenosine and supraventricular tachycardia. N Engl J Med 1991;325:1621–1629.

38. DiMarco JP, Miles W, Akhtar M, et al. Adenosine for paroxysmal supraventricular tachycardia: dose ranging and comparison with verapamil. Assessment in placebo-controlled, multicenter trials. Ann Intern Med 1990;113:104–110.

39. Wilber DJ, Baerman J, Olshansky B, et al. Adenosine-sensitive ventricular tachycardia. Clinical characteristics and response to catheter ablation. Circulation 1993;87:126–134.

40. Gomes JAC, El-Sherif N. Atrioventricular block. Mechanism, clinical presentation, and therapy. Med Clin North Am 1984;68:955–967.

41. Denes P. Atrioventricular and intraventricular block. Circulation 1987;75(Suppl III):III-19–III-25.

42. Castellanos A, Moleiro F, Saoudi NC, et al. Parasystole. In: Zipes DP, Jalife J, eds. Cardiac electrophysiology. from cell to bedside. Philadelphia: WB Saunders, 1990:619–626.

43. Akhtar M. Clinical spectrum of ventricular tachycardia. Circulation 1990;82:1561–1573.

44. Binah O, Rosen MR. Mechanisms of ventricular arrhythmias. Circulation 1992;85(Suppl I):I-25–I-31.

45. Marriott HJL, Conover MHB. Differential diagnosis in the broad QRS tachycardia. In: Marriott & Conover. Advanced concepts in arrhythmias. St. Louis: Mosby, 1983:218–246.

46. Wellens HJJ, Bar FWHM, Lie KI. The value of the electrocardiogram in the differential diagnosis of a tachycardia with a widened QRS complex. Am J Med 1978;64:27.

47. Wellens HJJ. The wide QRS tachycardia. Ann Intern Med 1986;104: 879.

48. Brugata P, Brugata J, Mont L, et al: A new approach to the differential diagnosis of a regular tachycardia with a wide QRS complex. Circulation 1991;83:1649–1659.

49. Garratt CJ, Griffith MJ, Young G, et al. Value of physical signs in the diagnosis of ventricular tachycardia. Circulation 1994;90:3103–3107.

50. Tan HL, Hou CJY, Lauer MR, et al. Electrophysiologic mechanisms of the long QT interval syndromes and torsade de pointes. Ann Intern Med 1995;122:701–714.

51. Stratmann HG, Kennedy HL. Torsades de pointes associated with drugs and toxins: recognition and management. Am Heart J 1987; 113:1470–1482.

Exercise Stress Testing

Exercise stress testing (EST) is a sensitive and informative examination of the cardiovascular response to exercise. EST is particularly useful in the detection and quantitation of ischemic heart disease (IHD) in patients who are at increased risk for its occurrence. For the purposes of this discussion, IHD is used to represent impairment of coronary perfusion usually caused by, but not limited to, atherosclerotic coronary artery disease (CAD).

The electrocardiogram is the most common parameter used to evaluate the ischemic response during exercise. This may be combined with cardiac imaging (echocardiography, nuclear perfusion scintigraphy, etc.) to increase the sensitivity and specificity of the test (see Chapters 4 and 5) (1–4). Additionally, exercise testing combined with cardiac imaging can be used to evaluate physiological responses in certain valvular abnormalities (e.g., mitral stenosis).

Exercise Physiology—Basic Principles (5)

1. The heart extracts 70% of the oxygen carried by each unit of blood perfusing the myocardium, and myocardial metabolism is nearly entirely aerobic. Therefore, an increase in myocardial oxygen demand during exercise must be matched by an increase in coronary blood flow (supply) or ischemia will result.
2. Major factors affecting myocardial oxygen demand:
   - Heart rate (HR)
   - Contractility (inotropic state)
   - Wall tension (directly proportional to ventricular pressure × radius)
3. There is a good correlation between the "double product" (blood pressure × HR) and measured myocardial oxygen consumption during dynamic exercise. Angina occurs as a

Table 3.1
Expected HR Response to Graded Exercise

Age	Mild	Moderate	Moderately severe	Near maximal	Maximal
20–29	115	135	155	175	195
30–39	110	130	150	170	190
40–49	106	126	146	166	186
50–59	102	122	142	162	182
>60	98	118	138	158	178

remarkably constant double product in a given patient with IHD and is often independent of duration, intensity, or type of exercise performed. In practice, EST is designed to produce an increase in HR of known magnitude, defined as a percentage of the maximal predicted HR of a normal population of matched age and sex (Table 3.1).

4. In the presence of IHD, coronary blood flow cannot increase adequately to meet the demands of the myocardium for oxygen, resulting in ischemia and manifested by *(a)* pain (angina), *(b)* electrocardiogram (ECG) ST segment changes, *(c)* ventricular dysfunction, *(d)* arrhythmias, or *(e)* a combination of the above.

5. Types of exercise
   • Static: isometric sustained muscular contraction against a fixed resistance, for example, hand grip.
   • Dynamic: rhythmic contractions of extensor and flexor muscle groups, for example, a bicycle or treadmill exercise.
   • Combination of static and dynamic exercise.

6. There are several reasons why dynamic exercise is preferred in EST:
   a. Isometric exercise can produce exaggerated blood pressure (BP) response, which may be detrimental to patients with high blood pressure or CAD.
   b. HR response is variable in isometric exercise, although it will reliably increase during dynamic exercise.
   c. Angina pectoris is less reliably provoked during isometric exercise.
   d. Isometric exercise frequently provokes ventricular arrhythmias.

e. ECG changes during isometric exercise may be subtle and obscured by muscle tremor artifact.

7. Alternatives to conventional EST for patients who cannot exercise include the following (1,2,6). Pharmacologic agents (dobutamine, adenosine, or dipyridamole) can be administered in conjunction with cardiac imaging (echo, nuclear scanning) to determine the physiological consequences of ischemia (wall motion abnormalities, areas of reversible hypoperfusion) (see Chapters 4 and 5).

Indications for EST(5)

- Differential diagnosis of chest pain, i.e., evaluation of patients with symptoms suggestive of IHD.
- Assessment of the level of exercise at which ischemic manifestations occur in a patient with known IHD.
- Evaluation of therapy for arrhythmias and angina.
- Evaluation of functional disability secondary to organic heart disease, e.g., valvular heart disease.
- Evaluation of the asymptomatic patient older than 40 years of age who has multiple risk factors for IHD.

Contraindications to EST

- Recent acute myocardial infarction (MI) (4–6 weeks), except for submaximal (65% of predicted maximum HR) or symptom-limited EST before hospital discharge.
- Angina at rest.
- Rapid ventricular or atrial arrhythmias.
- Advanced atrioventricular (AV) block (unless chronic).
- Uncompensated congestive heart failure.
- Acute noncardiac illnesses.
- Severe aortic stenosis.
- BP greater than 170/100 before the onset of exercise.

Safety of EST

Serious complications (acute MI, cardiac arrest, arrhythmias requiring treatment, stroke, or death) of EST are extremely uncommon (0.8 complications per 10,000 maximal tests) (7). Therefore, EST is a safe procedure when performed under proper supervision and with the necessary safeguards and equipment (8). These include the following:

1. Physician's knowledge of the patient's history and physical findings before the EST.
2. Physician, qualified physician's assistant, or a nurse present for the entire test.
3. Continuous monitoring of HR and rhythm and frequent BP determinations during the procedure and for 6–10 min thereafter.
4. Emergency equipment readily available, including a defibrillator, airway management equipment, and emergency drugs.
5. Termination of the EST at the appropriate time (see below).

Terminating the EST

1. Achievement of predicted HR (see Table 3.1).
2. Patient unable to continue due to symptoms of excessive fatigue, claudication, and/or dyspnea.
3. Premature ventricular contractions (PVCs) increasing in frequency and/or ventricular tachycardia.
4. Onset of advanced AV block.
5. Severe angina occurs.
6. Diagnostic ST segment changes clearly obtained on ECG.
7. BP criteria: systolic greater than 220, diastolic greater than 120 during exercise, or during exercise BP drops to a level below baseline (may indicate left ventricular (LV) dysfunction).
8. Failure of the ECG monitoring system.

After termination of the EST, the patient should be observed for 6–10 min with continuous ECG monitoring. Obtain BP frequently and look for ECG ST segment changes and arrhythmias, which commonly occur postexercise. The ECG should return to baseline before releasing the patient.

The EST Procedure

1. Protocols are used that use dynamic exercise on a treadmill up to a predicted maximal heart rate for age. There are many multistage protocols that use increments in treadmill elevation and speed; each protocol has its advantages, depending on the patient being tested (5). Small increments in work-

Table 3.2
Exercise Stress Test Protocols

Bruce Protocol:

3 min	1.75 mph	10% grade
3 min	2.5 mph	12% grade
3 min	3.4 mph	14% grade
3 min	4.2 mph	16% grade
3 min	5.0 mph	18% grade

Ellestad Protocol:

3 min	1.6 mph	10% grade
3 min	2.2 mph	10% grade
2 min	2.6 mph	10% grade
2 min	3.0 mph	10% grade
2 min	3.6 mph	10% grade

loads of short duration (Ellestad protocol) may be better tolerated than larger workloads of longer duration (Bruce protocol), especially for older patients in poor physical condition. To obtain the maximal amount of information from the EST, a protocol can be altered somewhat to meet the clinical situation. The Bruce and the Ellestad protocols are shown in Table 3.2.

2. ECG monitoring in EST: if a single lead is to be used for ECG monitoring in EST, lead V5 usually provides the largest R wave and, therefore, the greatest likelihood for detecting ECG changes. Sensitivity is enhanced by 15% by using a 12-lead ECG system, which also detects ST segment changes from the anterior and inferior walls (Fig. 3.1).

ECGs are routinely performed supine and standing before the EST, at each step in the EST protocol, immediately postexercise, and at 2-min intervals thereafter for 6–10 min.

Interpretation

1. ST segment changes are the most reliable electrocardiographic indicators of myocardial ischemia (5). Six major types of ST segments may occur in response to exercise (Fig. 3.2).

2. A horizontal or down-sloping ST segment that is depressed at least 1 mm below the isoelectric at the J point and persists for 80 msec thereafter is interpreted as a positive test (see

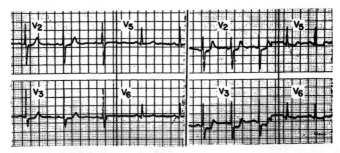

Figure 3.1. Control and Immediate Postexercise ECGs in a Patient with IHD. Note the 2-mm horizontal ST segment depression in lead V3. This diagnostic change would not have been detected if only lead V5 had been monitored.

Fig. 3.2, patterns C and D). The incidence of false positives is significantly reduced when a 2-mm ST segment depression requirement is used for a positive test. Three consecutive beats without baseline variation are required for reliable measurement of ST segments. Two examples of a positive EST are shown in Figures 3.1 and 3.3. Most modern treadmill equipment has filtering software to assist in correcting for artifact.

3. The depth of the ST segment depression correlates roughly with the extent of coronary artery disease, i.e., patients with

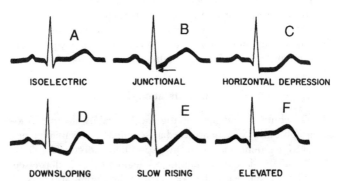

Figure 3.2. ST Segment Response to Exercise.

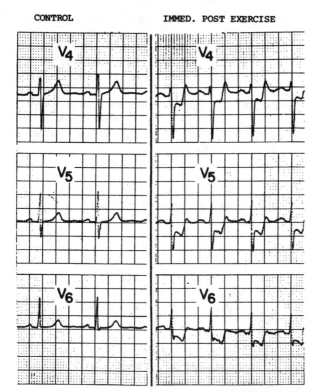

Figure 3.3. Control and Immediate Postexercise ECGs in a Patient with IHD. Note the 3-mm down-sloping ST segment depression in leads V5 and V6.

a 3-mm or greater ST segment depression 80 msec after the J point have a high incidence of triple-vessel disease. In addition, ST segment changes that occur during the first 3 min of exercise and/or persist past 8 min during recovery correlate with an 85% prevalence of two- and three-vessel disease (7).

4. Other patterns of ST segment depression (see Fig. 3.2).
   Pattern B. Depression of the J point with a rapid rise in the ST segment is a normal occurrence with exercise and correlates poorly with IHD.

Pattern E. Depression of the J point with a slow-rising ST segment and 2.0-mm ST depression at 80 msec from the J point has been shown to correlate well with IHD, but there is a high incidence of false positives (32%). Therefore, this pattern is not widely used for the diagnosis of IHD.

Pattern F. ST segment elevation occurs rarely in EST and probably represents a severe degree of myocardial ischemia or an LV aneurysm. No quantitative criteria are established for EST interpretation.

5. Interpretation of the EST must also include the following:
   - An evaluation of the workload performed.
   - The heart rate and BP response.
   - The presence or absence of arrhythmias.
   - The presence or absence of symptoms.
6. ST segments changes can be difficult to interpret for the following reasons:
   a. The resting ECG demonstrates a left bundle branch block (LBBB), left ventricular hypertrophy (LVH) with repolarization abnormalities, Wolff-Parkinson-White (WPW) syndrome, changes of digitalis, or significant ST segment depression.
   b. The patient does not achieve his or her 85% maximum heart rate and the ST segments do not change. However, if a patient develops ST segment depression or angina at a submaximal pulse rate, this may indicate significant ischemia.

Physiology of ST Segment Depression

The electrophysiologic basis for ST changes during EST is an intracellular potassium loss resulting from an imbalance between myocardial oxygen supply and demand. The subendocardial layer of the left ventricle is most vulnerable because it is subjected to a high wall tension, which adversely affects tissue perfusion. Subendocardial loss of potassium ion results in an ST segment shift toward the affected subendocardial area, which is manifest on the surface ECG as ST depression.

Other Causes of ST Segment Depression

1. Supply/demand imbalance due to anemia, aortic stenosis, coronary spasm, severe hypertension, left ventricular hypertrophy, and/or hypertrophic cardiomyopathy.

2. LBBB induces secondary repolarization changes unrelated to supply/demand imbalance.
3. Drugs—digitalis (this drug is usually discontinued 10 days before the EST if atrial fibrillation is not present), and antihypertensives.
4. Miscellaneous—cardiomyopathies, mitral valve prolapse, syndrome X (chest pain with angiographically normal coronary arteries), and autonomic dysfunction.
5. Hypokalemia, recent glucose or food ingestion, and vasoregulatory asthenia.

Diagnostic Accuracy of EST in Detection of IHD

The predictive value of any test will vary with the prevalence of the disease in the population being tested. Therefore, the greater number of patients with IHD in the population being tested, the greater the predictive value. Therefore, populations tested with few risk factors for IHD will have a larger number of false-positive responses and a decreased predictive value. Females of any age have a high incidence of false-positive tests as compared with males of the same age group (5).

Using the criterion of 1 mm of ST segment depression (patterns C and D) as an indicator of IHD, conventional EST has a sensitivity of approximately 68% (the proportion of people who truly have coronary artery disease who are identified by EST), a specificity of approximately 77% (the proportion of people who are truly free of coronary artery disease who are so identified by EST), and a predictive value of 70–80% (the likelihood of IHD if EST is positive) (9).

Results are also influenced by the severity of CAD present; for example, only 9% of patients with triple-vessel disease had false-negative tests, whereas 63% of patients with single-vessel disease had a false-negative EST.

Common Misconceptions About EST

1. *EST is the definitive tool to verify the existence of IHD.* Overall sensitivity is 64%; therefore, 36% of patients with CAD will have a false-negative test.
2. *There is little benefit from the EST in subjects with known IHD, especially those considered stable post-MI.* The treadmill may be used to determine those patients at high risk for

future coronary events, i.e., a patient with a positive EST 2 months post-MI is twice as likely to have a future coronary event as a patient with a negative EST post-MI. In addition, EST is useful to establish efficacy of drugs (antianginal agents/antiarrhythmics) and to establish an exercise prescription in cardiac rehabilitation programs.

3. *ST segment depression is the only manifestation of IHD.* Many other aspects of EST may correlate with the presence and severity of IHD. Look for the following:
   a. Submaximal pulse response (chronotropic incompetence correlates with LV dysfunction)
   b. Decrease in blood pressure.
   c. Exercise-induced chest pain.
   d. Ventricular ectopy.
   e. Magnitude and configuration of ST segment depression.
   f. Time of onset of ST segment depression, i.e., earlier onset correlates with more severe disease.
   g. Length of time ST segment abnormalities persist in recovery phase; longer-lasting abnormalities correlate with more severe disease.

References

1. Chou TM, Amidon TM. Evaluating coronary artery disease noninvasively—which test for whom? West J Med 1994;161:173.
2. Mayo Clinic Cardiovascular Working Group on Stress Testing. Cardiovascular stress testing: a description of the various types of stress tests and indications for their use. Mayo Clin Proc 1996;71:43.
3. Jain A, Murray DR. Detection of myocardial ischemia. Curr Probl Cardiol 1995;20:773.
4. Botvinick EH. Stress imaging. Current clinical options for the diagnosis, localization, and evaluation of coronary artery disease. Med Clin North Am 1995;79:1025.
5. Fletcher GF, Balady G, Froelicher VF, et al. Exercise standards. A statement for healthcare professionals from the American Heart Association. Circulation 1995;91:580.
6. Stratmann HG, Kennedy HL. Evaluation of coronary artery disease in the patient unable to exercise: alternatives to exercise stress testing. Am Heart J 1989;117:1344.
7. Gibbons L, Blair SN, Kohl HW, et al. The safety of maximal exercise testing. Circulation 1989;80:846.
8. Pina IL, Balady GJ, Hanson P, et al. Guidelines for clinical exercise

testing laboratories. A statement for healthcare professionals from the Committee on Exercise and Cardiac Rehabilitation, American Heart Association. Circulation 1995;91:912.

9. Gianrossi R, Detrano R, Mulvihill D, et al. Exercise-induced ST depression in the diagnosis of coronary artery disease. A meta-analysis. Circulation 1989;80:87.

Chapter 4

Echocardiography

BASIC PRINCIPLES

Echocardiography encompasses an array of related procedures that use ultrasound to provide moving two-dimensional images of the cardiac chambers and valves, accurate dimensions of these structures, and flow-velocity profiles. All of these modalities are integrated in time and space, so that it is possible to depict diseased valves, abnormal chamber dimensions, altered wall motion, and abnormal flow-velocity patterns simultaneously. These noninvasive procedures do not use harmful ionizing radiation and are therefore invaluable in the initial assessment of patients with suspected cardiac valve disease as well as in serial examinations in long-term follow-up (1,2).

Ultrasound waves are propagated in a liquid medium (e.g., blood) or through tissues with high water content (e.g., muscle and liver,) and reflect off interfaces between dissimilar structures (blood versus valves, blood versus myocardium, etc.). To create an image, a wave must be reflected back to the receiver so that its distance from the receiver can be computed from the time delay between emitted and received ultrasound. Objects with reflecting surfaces are at approximately right angles relative to the ultrasound produce clear images and Doppler waves, whereas those that are nearly parallel will not return the signals to the receiver and will drop out.

Ultrasound waves cannot penetrate dense media such as bone, heavily calcified valves, or metallic devices, e.g., prosthetic valves. Gas-filled organs, e.g., the lung and gut, scatter the waves. In addition, structures within 1–2 cm of the transducer are poorly defined ("near field effect"). Objects at a distance greater than 15 cm from the transducer are also poorly seen. Another limitation of echo is the paucity of suitable "windows" through which the cardiac structures can be imaged. Diagnostic images can usu-

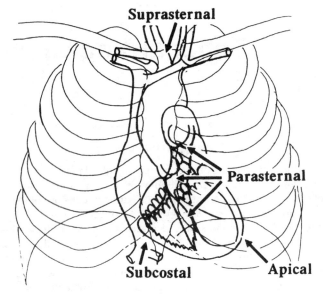

Figure 4.1. Echocardiographic Windows. The location of echocardiographic access points on the chest wall. The heart and vascular structures are accessible to imaging because they underlie the chest wall without intervening lung tissue or bone at the locations indicated by arrows. The right ventricle (shaded) is the first structure traversed by the echo beam and is therefore poorly visualized because of the near field effect described in the text.

ally be obtained through one or more of the transthoracic windows illustrated in Figure 4.1.

M-Mode Echocardiography

M-mode echo plots depth against time through an "ice pick" path. It is primarily used to measure chamber dimensions and to establish the timing of events such as valve or cardiac wall motion. M-mode echocardiography provides high-resolution one-dimensional images of cardiac structures, usually from a left parasternal window. The images display vertical dimension (depth) on the y axis and time on the x axis. The rate of depth sampling is greater than 1000/sec, compared to 30/sec imaging frequency of two-dimensional echocardiograms, ideally suited to tracking rapidly moving structures such as the opening and closing motions of cardiac valves. The relationship between M-mode and two-dimensional echocardiograms is depicted in Figure 4.2.

The two-dimensional depictions in Figure 4.2 represent four phases of the cardiac cycle. The M-mode cursor is calibrated in centimeters. At the *e* point, the anterior mitral leaflet is less than 1 cm from the interventricular septum and 2 cm from the posterior mitral leaflet, and the mitral valve is widely open. The ventricular walls move progressively away from each other during diastolic filling. The anterior mitral leaflet motion describes the letter "M," and the posterior mitral leaflet a mirror-image "W." During ventricular systole, the mitral leaflets are pressed together and the walls of the ventricle move closer together. The right ventricle is not well seen because of the near field effect of the echocardiogram described previously.

The M-mode echocardiographic landmarks have correlates in other recording techniques representing intracardiac events

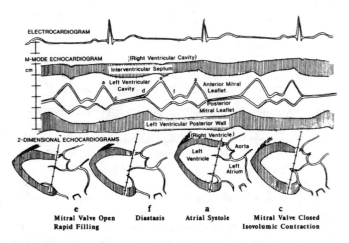

Figure 4.2. Normal M-Mode and Two-Dimensional Echo. The heart is imaged through a left parasternal window. The two-dimensional images demonstrate the position of the mitral valve leaflets during four phases of the cardiac cycle. The letters on the M-mode echocardiogram represent landmark positions of the mitral valve: **a–c**, mitral closure; **d–e**, the opening of the mitral valve; and **e–f**, the drift toward partial closure during diastasis.

(see Chapter 11). The *a* wave correlates with the atrial and ventricular *a* waves, and the *c* point with the *c* wave of the atrial pressure and first heart sound. The *e-f* slope mirrors the rate of left atrial emptying, with *f* representing the end of rapid filling. In the illustrations of valvar pathology in Chapter 11, the M-mode mitral valve echocardiograms depict the abnormal motion of the valves that are characteristic of specific disease conditions.

M-mode echocardiograms can be diagnostic of certain valve conditions, myocardiopathies, and pericardial diseases. Because of the high-frequency response of the M-mode images, phono-echocardiograms are useful in defining correlates of abnormal heart sounds and murmurs. Figures 4.3 and 4.4 depict diagnostic phonoechocardiograms in distinct forms of valve disease.

TWO-DIMENSIONAL ECHOCARDIOGRAPHY

Two-dimensional images of the cardiovascular structures can be generated by mechanically or electronically sweeping the echo beam in a manner similar to a windshield wiper, building a sector image of up to 90° at the end of each sweep and updating the image 30 times per second. The windows illustrated in Figure 4.1 can be used to visualize each of the cardiac chambers and valves, as well as a limited portion of the aortic root (from the parasternal window) and the aortic arch (suprasternal window).

TRANSESOPHAGEAL ECHOCARDIOGRAPHY

In approximately 5% of examinations, transthoracic images may be very difficult to acquire. This may be due to emphysema, severe obesity, or chest wall deformities that prevent the ultrasound waves from reaching the structures of interest. Additionally, acoustic shadowing may occur when the ultrasound beam is directed toward an echoreflective object such as a prosthetic heart valve. To obtain better views of the heart, transesophageal echocardiography (TEE) has been developed, whereby a small transducer is attached to an endoscopy device. This apparatus can then be inserted through the patient's mouth and down the esophagus. Because the esophagus lies just behind and contiguous with the left atrium, superb images of the heart can be obtained without interference from the lungs, bones, or prosthetic valves. Additionally, the esophagus is closely positioned near the aorta, allowing superb views of the thoracic aorta. Var-

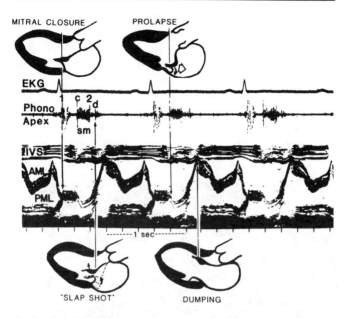

Figure 4.3. Phonoechocardiogram in Mitral Prolapse. A mitral valve echo-cardiogram reveals thickened leaflets with midsystolic dorsal excursion (prolapse) of the mitral leaflets (AML = anterior mitral leaflet, PML = posterior mitral leaflet) in midsystole. This dorsal coincides with a click (c) on the apical phonocardiogram, followed by a late systolic murmur (sm). Two-dimensional drawings above the ECG depict the position of the valve during systole at the time of mitral valve closure and prolapse and regurgitation (white arrow) through the prolapsed valve. The figures below depict two diastolic events: 1) the early diastolic contact of the separated leaflets as the posterior leaflet moves ventrally and forcibly impacts the anterior leaflet ("slap shot") to produce a diastolic sound (d); and 2) the maximal opening of the valve with septal apposition of the anterior leaflet.

ious views of the heart and aorta can then be acquired. Transducers can image in single plane, biplane (transverse and horizontal), and multiplane dimensions. Multiplane transducers can be steered or directed from 0° to 180° by the operator and allow a greater degree of flexibility and image-specific orientation. Imaging of the transverse aorta is also facilitated with multiplane transducers, because single and biplane probes have a "blind

spot" where the air-filled trachea interferes with ultrasound waves
(3). The standard scan planes for single plane imaging are illustrated in Figure 4.6.

Common indications for using transesophageal echocardiography include the following:

- Dysfunction of prosthesis, especially mitral.
- Suspected cardiac source of an embolus, such as the left atrial appendage thrombus or tumor, a patent foramen ovale with right to left shunting and resultant "paradoxical" embolus

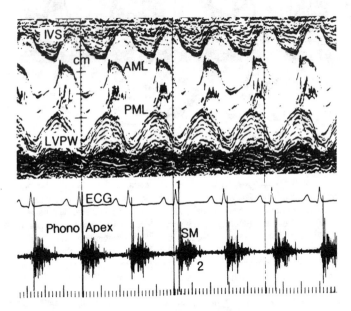

Figure 4.4. Phonoecho in Acute Mitral Regurgitation. The M-mode echo reveals exaggerated excursions of the interventricular septum (IVS) and left ventricular posterior wall (LVPW), with normal ventricular chamber size and a flail posterior mitral leaflet (PML) typical of acute mitral regurgitation. The systolic murmur (SM) does not extend to the second sound (2) because of the greatly elevated left atrial systolic pressures (see Chapter 11). The M-mode cursor can be moved leftward (apically) to better record the wall thickness, dimensions of the cavity, and movement of the ventricular walls at midventricle or rightward to depict the aortic valve and left atrium as shown in Figure 4.5.

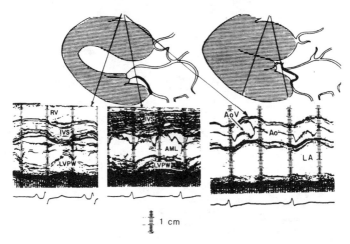

Figure 4.5. M-Mode Echo in Hypertrophic Cardiomyopathy. The echo beam is swept to the left to record the dimensions at midventricle (left), through the mitral valve (center), and through the aortic valve and left atrium (right) to reveal a thick-walled, small chamber left ventricle with complete emptying (cavitary obliteration). There is asymmetrical septal thickness (IVS = 2.4 cm versus LVPW = 1.4 cm), systolic anterior motion of the mitral valve, premature closure of the aortic valve (AoV), and left atrial enlargement (0.5 cm), characteristic of hypertrophic cardiomyopathy.

from a venous source, or an ulcerated aortic plaque. Atherosclerotic plaques >4 mm in thickness located in the aortic arch are associated with a significant risk of stroke and other vascular events (4).

- Endocarditis and its complications, such as aortic and mitral annular abscesses, fistulas, and vegetations.
- Diagnosis and evaluation of atrial septal defect. TEE can define the location and size of the defect, aiding with management and treatment decisions.
- Attachment site and qualitative features of cardiac tumors. Some tumors have characteristic appearances, such as myxomas.
- Extent and degree of mitral regurgitation with color flow imaging. Eccentric or "wall-hugging" jets on transthoracic imaging can be underestimated, leading to an inaccurate quantitative assessment.

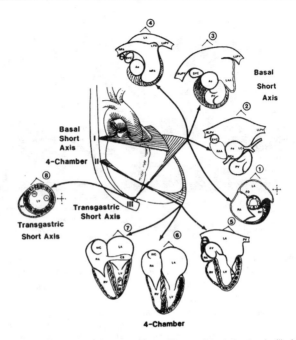

Figure 4.6. Diagram of Common Scan Planes. Basal short axis (I), four-chamber (frontal long axis) (II), and transgastric short axis (III) and resultant tomographic planes of section (1 through 8). Basal short axis sections: aortic root (1), coronary arteries (2), left atrial appendage (3), and pulmonary artery bifurcation (4). Four-chamber sections: left ventricular outflow view (5), four-chamber view (6), and coronary sinus view (7). Transgastric short axis section: ventricular short axis view (8). AL = anterolateral papillary muscle, Ao = aorta, AV = aortic valve, CS = coronary sinus, FO = fossa ovalis, IVC = inferior vena cava, L = left coronary cusp, LA = left atrium, LAA = left atrial appendage, LCA = left coronary artery, LLPV = left lower pulmonary vein, LPA = left pulmonary artery, LUPV = left upper pulmonary vein, LV = left ventricle, MPA = main pulmonary artery, N = noncoronary cusp, PM = posteromedial papillary muscles, PV = pulmonary valve or pulmonary vein, R = right coronary artery, RLPV = right lower pulmonary vein, RPA = right pulmonary artery, RUPV = right upper pulmonary vein, RV = right ventricle, SVC = superior vena cava. Directional axes: A = anterior, L = left; P = posterior, R = right. (With permission from Seward JB, Khandheria BK, Freeman WK, et al. Multiplane transesophageal echocardiography: image orientation, examination technique, anatomic correlations, and clinical applications. Mayo Clin Proc 1993;68:523.)

- Morphology of mitral valve in mitral stenosis and mitral valve prolapse in patients anticipating surgery. The extent of calcification, mobility, and subvalvular involvement can be evaluated.
- Postoperative evaluation of mitral and aortic valve prosthesis.
- Intraoperative evaluation of left ventricular function in patients undergoing noncardiac surgery with suspected cardiac disease.
- Intraoperative evaluation of aortic and mitral valve repair or replacement.
- Diagnosis of acute aortic dissection.
- Management of critically ill patients who have inadequate transthoracic (or surface) echocardiograms (5).
- Assessment of complex congenital heart disease.

DOPPLER ULTRASONOGRAPHY

The Doppler shift—the change in pitch that affects sound emanating from a structure approaching or receding from the point where sound is received—can be used to denote direction and velocity of flowing blood elements. The modified Bernoulli equation permits estimation of the pressure change that occurs when blood flows between high- and low-pressure chambers or sites (for example, across a stenotic or regurgitant valve or a septal defect). The pressure gradient, or P_1 P_2, can be calculated by:

$$P_1 - P_2 = 4 \times velocity^2$$

The ultrasound waves are emitted and the reflected waves are received by the transceiver; the location of the reflected signal scan be determined by simultaneous two-dimensional imaging of the heart. There are three Doppler techniques currently in use:

1. **Pulsed wave (PW).**
2. **Continuous wave (CW).**
3. **Color flow (CF) Doppler.**

Each depicts flow and velocity relative to the transducer but is progressively less able to detect flow as the angle (between the path of the target element and the emitted/received sound waves) approaches 90° because the reflecting targets (the blood cells) are neither moving toward nor away from the transducer.

Figures 4.7 through 4.9 demonstrate the use of each of the techniques in assessing a patient with aortic regurgitation.

Pulsed wave or PW Doppler samples from a specific point in a cardiovascular chamber (the sample volume) as though the

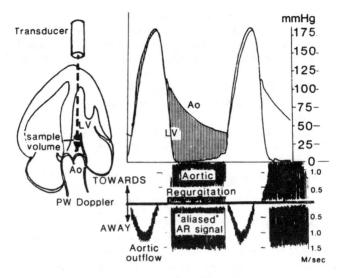

Figure 4.7. PW Doppler in Aortic Regurgitation. The transducer is placed at the cardiac apex, with the sample volume below the aortic valve in the regurgitant stream. The direction of flow is indicated on the PW Doppler signal relative to the thick center line. The aortic regurgitation (AR) jet (toward the apex) exceeds the Nyquist limit of 1.5 M/sec because the aortic diastolic pressure exceeds the left ventricular pressure by >80 mm Hg (velocity >4.5 M/sec) in early diastole and 25 mm Hg (2.5 M/sec) in late diastole, as indicated by the shaded area on the pressure tracings. The aortic regurgitant signal wraps around the zero line to indicate "aliasing." There is a small (5 mm Hg) systolic gradient between the rising LV and Ao pressures; the Doppler velocity (1.4 M/sec) is below the zero line because outflow is away from the transducer.

sensors were positioned in a selected spot to detect the direction and velocity of flow relative to that site. The transducer alternately sends and receives ultrasound pulses, so that by appropriate positioning of the sample volume within the two-dimensional image, regurgitant flow from a valve or shunts can be detected. PW Doppler is limited by its inherent sampling rate (the Nyquist limit) in its ability to quantitate high-velocity flow; when high-velocity flow is encountered, "aliasing" of the signal occurs and the Doppler signal wraps around the zero line.

Continuous wave or CW Doppler transducers continuously

emit and receive ultrasound so CW is not limited in high-velocity tracking, but it cannot localize the depth from which the signals emanate. All velocity signals along the path of the beam are super-imposed, with the highest velocity dominating the signal. With sequential use of PW and CW Doppler techniques, the site of high-velocity signals can be localized by PW and the magnitude by CW (Fig. 4.8).

Color flow or CF Doppler is based on PW Doppler. Hundreds of sampling sites, similar to pixels, are assigned a color code that

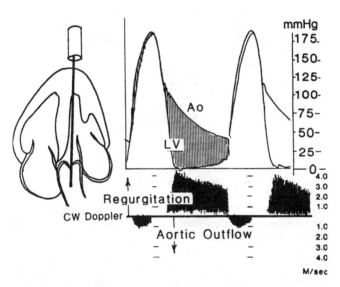

Figure 4.8.   CW Doppler in Aortic Regurgitation. The transducer is on the chest wall at the left ventricular apex. CW Doppler signals along the path of the regurgitant stream (above the zero line) reveal velocities of 4.5 M/sec in early diastole, which decline to 2.5 M/sec in late diastole. The initial diastolic pressure gradient between the aorta (Ao) and the left ventricle (LV) can be approximated by the Bernoulli equation (4×4.5^2) to be 81 mm Hg, and the late diastolic gradient to be (4×2.5^2) 25 mm Hg, closely approximating the pressure difference directly recorded in the left ventricle and aorta, shown immediately above the Doppler signal. When the flow vectors are within 20° of the Doppler beam, accurate estimates of pressure gradients can be made by this noninvasive technique.

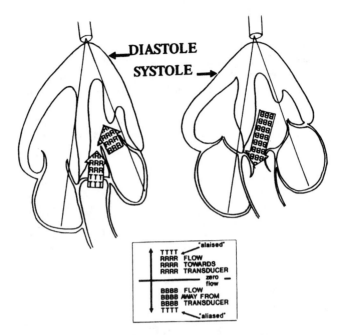

Figure 4.9. Color Flow (CF) Doppler in Aortic Regurgitation. Flow toward the left ventricular apical transducer is red (R) and flow away is blue (B). "Aliasing" is shown by a turquoise (T) hue emanating from the high-velocity diastolic transvalvar jet. The turquoise and red regurgitant flow as well as red mitral inflow are seen during diastole. Only blue aortic outflow is seen during systole.

permits detection of the direction of blood flow at each specific site (Fig. 4.9).

USE OF DOPPLER METHODS TO ASSESS HEMODYNAMIC PARAMETERS

Noninvasive estimation of intracardiac pressures is made possible by combining Doppler recordings of velocity and measurements of blood pressure and/or estimates of jugular venous pressure. These estimates of intracardiac pressure are dependent upon the ability to measure accurately high-velocity anterograde or regurgitant flow across valves, which is not always possible. Almost all hearts, normal or abnormal, will manifest regurgitant flow across the tricuspid valve. These estimates can be extremely useful in the management of patients.

The following examples will illustrate the estimation of pressures (Fig. 4.10).

The jugular venous pressure in Figure 4.10 is estimated by inspection to be 5 mm Hg (normal) and there is a tricuspid regurgitant jet velocity (V) of 2 M/sec. The systolic pressure difference (RV − RA) is, therefore:

$$4 \times V^2, \quad \text{or} \quad 4 \times 2^2 = 16 \text{ mm Hg}$$

Therefore the right ventricular systolic pressure is

$$16 + 5 = 21 \text{ mm Hg}$$
$$(\text{JVP})$$

The pulmonary artery systolic pressure is equivalent to right ventricular systolic pressure. These estimates obviously require the presence of a tricuspid regurgitant jet. Tricuspid regurgitation, usually of trivial degree, can be detected in many normal

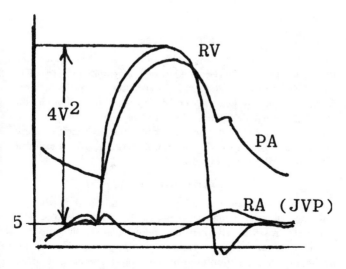

Figure 4.10. Estimation of Right Ventricular (and Pulmonary Artery) Systolic Pressure.

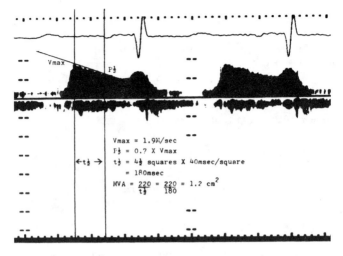

Figure 4.11. Mitral Stenosis Half-Time.

hearts and in most hearts with elevated systolic pressures in the right ventricle.

Mitral Stenosis

The concept of the pressure half-time, or the time required for the peak velocity to be reduced by one-half, can be used to calculate the severity of mitral stenosis with relative ease and reliability. By multiplying the peak velocity of mitral inflow at the e point by 0.7 and then calculating the time required to drop to that point, one can derive the **pressure half-time.** Dividing this number into an empirically derived number (220) gives the mitral valve area (MVA) (see Fig. 4.11) (6).

Aortic Stenosis

Peak systolic aortic valve velocities can be acquired using continuous wave Doppler signals in patients with aortic stenosis. The gradient across the valve can then be calculated using the Bernoulli equation (pressure gradient = $4 \times [\text{velocity}]^2$). Several problems can be encountered in assessing the severity of aortic stenosis. First, a patient with a very low cardiac output (such as a severely depressed left ventricular ejection fraction [LVEF]) may not be able to generate much of a gradient and the value would be very low, giving the false impression that the stenosis may be mild when in fact it is very severe. Additionally, the aortic stenosis jet may be difficult or impossible to record due to body habitus or other technical difficulties. Last, the angle of the Doppler signal may not be parallel to the flow of the jet, again giving a value that may be lower than the actual gradient. For situations in which the cardiac output may be low, the continuity equation has been reported to be more accurate in reflecting the severity of aortic stenosis. The principle behind this equation states that flow on one side of an orifice must equal flow on the other side of the orifice. This can be expressed as $A_1 \times V_1 = A_2 \times V_2$, where V_1 and V_2 are the flow velocities proximal and distal to the orifice and A_1 and A_2 are the areas at the sites in which the velocities where measured.

This can be rearranged to the following:

$$A_2 = \frac{A_1 \times V_1}{V_2}$$

A_1 can be calculated using $\pi \times R^2$ and measuring the diameter of the LV outflow tract. V_1 is obtained by sampling with the pulsed wave Doppler just proximal to the aortic valve. The V_2 is obtained by using continuous wave Doppler interrogation to measure the peak velocity at or beyond the valve. Limitations of this method include the technical difficulty in obtaining accurate measurements (7–9).

An example using the continuity equation is as follows. Since the area (A) is equal to $\pi \times R^2$, this is equivalent to $3.14 \times$ (diameter/2)^2, which simplifies to $d^2 \times 0.785$. If the diameter of the left ventricular outflow tract is 2.3 cm, $V_1 = 0.7$ m/sec, and $V_2 = 3.5$ m/sec, then the area of the aortic valve area (AVA) can be calculated as follows (see Figs. 4.12 and 4.13):

$$AVA = d^2 \times 7.85 \times V_1/V_2$$

$$AVA = (2.1)^2 \times 0.785 \times (0.7/3.5)$$

$$AVA = 3.46 \times (0.2) = 0.7 \text{ cm}^2$$

DOPPLER EVALUATION OF DIASTOLIC DYSFUNCTION

Mitral inflow and pulmonary vein Doppler velocity patterns can be helpful in assessment of abnormalities of left ventricular filling. The four phases of diastole are the isovolumic relaxation

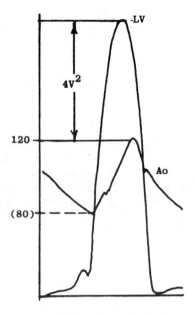

Figure 4.12. Estimation of Left Ventricular Systolic Pressure in Aortic Stenosis. If the systolic Doppler velocity across the aortic valve is converted into mm Hg and added to the systolic blood pressure (cuff), the left ventricular systolic pressure can be estimated. If the blood pressure is 120/80, and the Doppler velocity across the aortic valve 5 M/sec, the left ventricular systolic pressure would be: systolic BP + 4 × (52) = 120 + 100 = 220 mm Hg.

period (after aortic closure but before mitral opening), early rapid filling (dependent on the pressure difference between the left atrium and the left ventricle), diastasis (minimal filling occurs), and atrial contraction (dependent on active contraction of the atrium). Mitral inflow Doppler sampling is performed at the mitral leaflet tips with pulsed wave Doppler in the apical four chamber view. The pulmonary veins can usually be interrogated in this view as well. Parameters that are measured include the **E wave,** which corresponds to the peak early filling velocity, the **A wave,** which corresponds with the peak atrial filling velocity, the **deceleration time (DT),** which is a measure of the time it takes to go from the peak of the E wave to the point at which early filling diminishes to baseline, and the **isovolumic relaxation** period **(IVRT)**. The pulmonary vein flow normally has a **systolic flow phase (S)**, a **diastolic flow phase (D)**, and an **atrial reversal wave (AR)** (10).

Three abnormalities can be seen with abnormal diastolic function. First, **abnormal relaxation** results in an initial decrease in the E:A ratio due to a decrease in the early transmitral pressure gradient and an increase in the atrial contribution to filling. Then, as myocardial disease progresses, filling pressures increase, increasing the transmitral pressure gradient and creating a **pseudonormal pattern.** This can be distinguished from the normal pattern by the presence of an increased atrial reversal velocity and duration on the pulmonary venous flow pattern. Also, the venous systolic/diastolic ratio is <1. Finally, with advanced disease, the left ventricular compliance is severely decreased; most filling occurs early and little filling occurs during atrial contraction, creating a **restrictive pattern.** This can also be seen in peri-

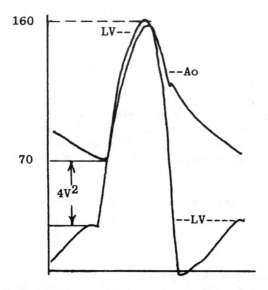

Figure 4.13. Estimation of Left Ventricular Diastolic Pressure in Aortic Regurgitation. If the cuff blood pressure is 160/70 mm Hg and the diastolic Doppler velocity across the aortic valve (aorta—left ventricle) is 3 M/sec, the left ventricular diastolic pressure can be derived in the following manner: diastolic BP − 4(32) = 70 − 36 = 34 mm Hg.

cardial and restrictive diseases in which left atrial pressure is elevated (11).

Myocardial ischemia, left ventricular hypertrophy, and normal aging can result in abnormal left ventricular relaxation. This is characterized by a reduced early filling wave (E velocity) due to a lower pressure gradient between the left atrium and left ventricle, a prolonged deceleration time, a stronger atrial contraction velocity (increased A velocity), and E:A ratio of <1, and a prolonged IVRT due to the longer time it takes for the mitral valve to open after aortic valve closure. The pulmonary venous velocities reflect an increased S:D ratio and an increased atrial reversal velocity and duration.

Elevated left atrial pressures result in earlier mitral valve opening with an increased E wave velocity, a lower A wave velocity, an increased E:A ratio (>2), a shortened IVRT, and a shorter DT. This characterizes the **restrictive pattern.** The pulmonary venous flow pattern shows a decreased systolic wave, an increased diastolic wave, a decreased systolic:diastolic ratio, and an increased atrial reversal wave. For patients with dilated cardiomyopathy, this implies a worse prognosis. Another disease with this pattern is the late stage of cardiac amyloidosis. Restrictive myocardial and constrictive pericardial disease can demonstrate restrictive patterns of flow. However, there are marked respiratory changes in flow with constrictive disease that are not present with restrictive disease (12,13).

Certain factors must be considered when interpreting these data. Increased heart rates, atrial arrhythmias, prosthetic mitral valves, mitral stenosis, aortic and mitral regurgitation, and sample volume position may significantly affect the value, making them difficult to interpret.

CLASSIC ECHOCARDIOGRAPHIC FINDINGS

Certain cardiac diseases have classic echocardiographic findings. Some of the more common disease states are presented in the flowing examples.

A. **Infective Endocarditis** (Fig. 4.14)
B. **Dilated Cardiomyopathy** (Fig. 4.15)
C. **Hypertrophic Cardiomyopathy** (Fig. 4.16)
D. **Pericardial Effusion** (Fig. 4.17)
E. **Atrial Septal Defect** (Fig. 4.18)

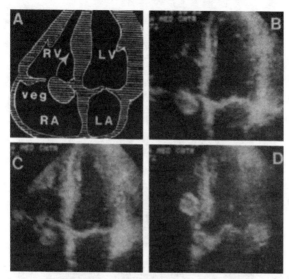

Figure 4.14.   Infective Endocarditis. Two-dimensional echocardiography in the apical four-chamber view demonstrates a large mobile vegetation attached to the septal leaflet of the tricuspid valve. **(A)** A diagram depicting the vegetation (veg) in systole; its diastolic motion is indicated by the arrow. **(B)** A systolic frame corresponding to the diagram demonstrates the vegetation in the right atrium. **(C)** An early diastolic frame shows the slinglike attachment to the tip of the septal leaflet as the vegetation is being flung toward the right ventricular cavity. **(D)** The vegetation is in the right ventricle, adjacent to the interventricular septum in mid-diastole.

F. Transesophageal Echovegetation (Fig. 4.19)

ECHOCARDIOGRAPHY IN ISCHEMIC HEART DISEASE

Echocardiography may be useful in the evaluation of acute myocardial infarction and its complications. Ischemic manifestations of acute coronary thrombosis may include wall motion abnormalities (hypokinesis, akinesis, or dyskinesis), acquired ventricular septal defect, mitral regurgitation due to papillary muscle dysfunction or rupture, and left ventricular thrombi. In chronic ischemic cardiomyopathies, myocardial thinning or scarring may commonly be seen in the area of a previous infarction. Left ven-

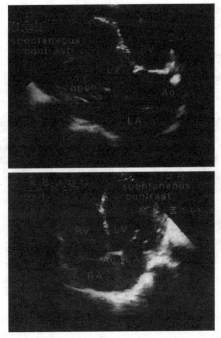

Figure 4.15. Dilated Cardiomyopathy with Spontaneous Contrast. **(A)** Parasternal long axis, diastole. The left ventricle (LV) is massively dilated (8 cm) and a swirling cloud of "spontaneous contrast" is seen in the body of the ventricle. This phenomenon represents the settling of blood elements resulting from sluggish flow. The right ventricle is also dilated (>4 cm). **(B)** Apical five-chamber diastole. Spontaneous contrast is seen in the body of the left ventricle. Both ventricular chambers are dilated (calibration marks = 1 cm).

tricular ejection fraction can be accurately determined and can be very useful in determining the future prognosis of the patient. The presence of segmental wall motion abnormalities in a patient with a dilated cardiomyopathy favors ischemia as an etiology in the differential diagnosis.

EXERCISE STRESS ECHOCARDIOGRAPHY

Combining an imaging modality such as echocardiography with an exercise stress test has many advantages. A wall motion defect is the final common pathway for the physiological response to a significantly ischemic region of myocardium. The echocardiographic equipment is a portable system that can be used easily in the office or in the hospital. It provides immediate information without using ionizing radiation. Intravenous lines are not necessary, as they are with other nuclear scanning techniques (see Chapter 5). Additionally, stress echo compares favorably in cost-effectiveness when compared with nuclear imaging. Many of the indications of stress echo are similar to those of stress thallium,

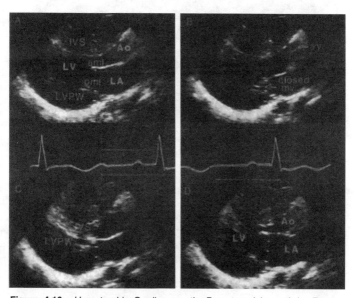

Figure 4.16.   Hypertrophic Cardiomyopathy-Parasternal Long Axis. Four phases of the cardiac cycle are depicted in a patient with hypertrophic cardiomyopathy; the timing of each frame is related to the electrocardiogram. **(A)** Late diastole: the interventricular septum (IVS) and left ventricular posterior wall (LVPW) are 2.8 and 2.0 cm thick, the mitral valve is open with the anterior mitral leaflet (aml) and posterior mitral leaflet (pml) widely separated. The left ventricular (LV) cavity is small. **(B)** Isovolumic systole: the mitral valve (mv) and aortic valve (av) are closed. **(C)** Midsystole: the cavity of the left ventricle is obliterated, and the mitral valve is pressed against the interventricular septum. **(D)** Early diastole: the mitral valve is open and ventricular filling has begun (calibration marks = 1 cm).

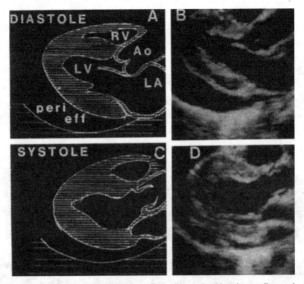

Figure 4.17. Pericardial Effusion. Two-dimensional echocardiography in the parasternal long axis view (corresponding to Fig. 4.16) in a patient with a large pericardial effusion with tamponade demonstrates an echo-free space behind the left ventricle which represents the pericardial effusion (peri eff). **(A)** A diagram depicting the diastolic appearance of the heart with the anterior leaflet approaching the interventricular septum and the aortic valve closed. **(B)** This diastolic frame corresponds to **(A)**. **(C)** A diagram depicting the heart in systole, with the mitral valve closed and the aortic valve open. Systolic collapse of the left atrium is seen as an indentation of the posterior atrial wall. **(D)** This systolic frame corresponds to **(C)**. A rocking motion of the heart can be appreciated by noting the ventral position of the heart in diastole and the dorsal position in systole.

isonitrile (technetium-99m sestamibi), and radionuclide angiography. These include the following:

- Patients with abnormal resting electrocardiograms (left ventricular hypertrophy [LVH], left branch bundle block [LBBB] digitalis effect, ST segment depression).
- Patients with a high likelihood of false-positive electrocardiogram (ECG) results (middle-aged women).
- Patients for whom a therapeutic procedure is planned (such

as angioplasty or bypass surgery) so that the physiologic significance of the lesion can be assessed and followed.

The disadvantages of stress echo include difficulty in obtaining a good image (due to body habitus or technician inexperience), the need to image during or as close to peak exercise as possible, and difficulty in interpreting new wall motion defects in the presence of resting hypokinesis or akinesis. However, the use of digitized, on-line cine loop technology has greatly facilitated the interpretation of stress echo images. Whereas the specificity of stress echo is high, the sensitivity may not be as high as

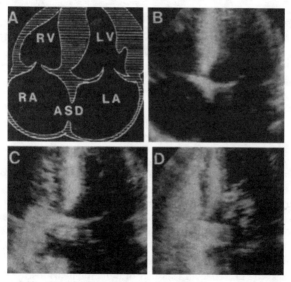

Figure 4.18. Atrial Septal Defect. Two-dimensional echocardiography in the apical four-chamber view demonstrates a large ASD. **(A)** A diagram demonstrates the location of the cardiac chambers and the echo dropout in the midatrial septum, suggesting an ASD. **(B)** This echo frame corresponds to **A. (C)** Immediately after an antecubital vein injection of indocyanine green dye, a cloud of echo-dense microbubbles fills the right heart chambers and a negative washout (encroachment of echo-lucent blood into the microbubbles) is seen in the region of the ASD, demonstrating a left-to-right shunt. **(D)** A later frame after the injection of microbubbles demonstrates right-to-left shunting into the left atrium and left ventricle.

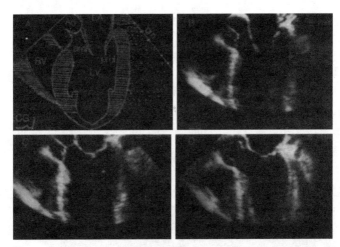

Figure 4.19. Transesophageal Echocardiogram. The patient had a small vegetation on the anterior aortic cusp (arrow) but had normal size cardiac chambers and valve motion. **(A, B)** Late diastole: the mitral valve is open and the aortic valve is closed. The two leaflets of the mitral valve are well seen (aml = anterior mitral leaflet, pml = posterior mitral leaflet). **(C)** Isovolumic systole: the mitral valve has closed. **(D)** Midsystole: the aortic valve is open, and the ventricular cavity size has decreased.

thallium or isonitrile techniques. Certain groups of investigators, however, have achieved excellent results when compared to nuclear imaging (14,15). Intravenous injection of sonicated albumin can enhance the visualization of the endocardium in patients who are difficult to image with standard ultrasound (16). For patients unable to perform exercise, pharmacological stress with dobutamine can be used in conjunction with echocardiography to assess the presence and severity of ischemic heart disease (see Chapter 3). Dipyridamole and adenosine have also been used, but less so than dobutamine. Exercise echo remains the best modality for predicting the extent of coronary artery disease, followed by dobutamine stress ultrasound imaging, and lastly, dipyridamole (17).

DOBUTAMINE ECHO FOR ASSESSMENT OF MYOCARDIAL VIABILITY

Dobutamine echocardiography can also be used in the assessment of myocardial viability before anticipated coronary revascularization. Both acute and chronic ischemia can impair contractility of viable myocardium. Revascularization of viable but ischemic myocardium can significantly improve the morbidity and mortality of patients with coronary disease and left ventricular dysfunction. A biphasic response to dobutamine stimulation with improvement in wall motion and increased systolic thickening at low doses (5–7.5 μg/kg/min) with worsening at higher doses (>7.5 μg/kg/min) suggests dysfunctional but viable myocardium. Continued improvement in wall motion can be seen in myopathic ventricles of nonischemic etiology and has poor predictive value. Nonviable, scarred myocardium would not show improvement in wall motion with either low- or high-dose dobutamine (18). Myocardial contrast echocardiography involves injecting sonicated albumin into a coronary artery during cardiac catheterization and observing by transthoracic echo the distribution of the agent into the myocardium. Collateral flow to ischemic myocardium indicates viability (19).

References

1. Feigenbaum H. Echocardiography. 4th ed. Philadelphia: Lea & Febiger, 1994.
2. Popp RL. Echocardiography (Part 1). N Engl J Med 1990;323:101; (Part 2) N Engl J Med 1990;323:165.
3. Seward JB, Khandheria BK, Freeman WK, et al. Multiplane transesophageal echocardiography: image orientation, examination technique, anatomic correlations, and clinical applications. Mayo Clin Proc 1993;68:523.
4. Amarenco P, Cohen A, Tzourio C, et al. Atherosclerotic disease of the aortic arch and the risk of ischemic stroke. N Engl J Med 1994; 331:1474.
5. Seward JB, Khandheria BK, Oh JK, et al. Transesophageal echocardiography: technique, anatomic correlations, implementation, and clinical applications. Mayo Clin Proc 1988;63:649.
6. Hatle L, Angelsen B. Doppler ultrasound in cardiology: physical principles and clinical applications. 2nd ed. Philadelphia: Lea & Febiger, 1985.
7. Richards KL, Cannon SR, Miller JF, et al. Calculation of aortic valve area by Doppler echocardiography: a direct application of the continuity equation. Circulation 1986;73:964.
8. Harrison MR, Gurley JC, Smith MD, et al. A practical application of Doppler echocardiography for the assessment of severity of aortic stenosis. Am Heart J 1988;115:622.
9. Nishimura RA, Miller FA, Callahan MJ, et al. Doppler echocardiogra-

phy: theory, instrumentation, technique, and application. Mayo Clin Proc 1985;60:321.

10. Nishimura RA, Housmans PR, Hatle LK, et al. Assessment of diastolic function of the heart: background and current applications of Doppler echocardiography. Part I. Physiologic and pathophysiologic features. Mayo Clin Proc 1989;64:71.

11. Appleton CP, Hatle LK, Popp RL. Relation of transmitral flow velocity patterns to left ventricular diastolic function: new insights from a combined hemodynamic and Doppler echocardiographic study. J Am Coll Cardiol 1988;12:426, 1988.

12. Cohen GI, Pietrolungo JF. A practical guide to assessment of ventricular diastolic function using Doppler echocardiography. J Am Coll Cardiol 1996;27:1753.

13. Nishimura RA, Abel MD, Hatle LK, et al. Assessment of diastolic function of the heart: background and current applications of Doppler echocardiography. Part II. Clinical studies. Mayo Clin Proc 1989; 64:181.

14. Armstrong WF, O'Donnell J, Dillon JC, et al. Complementary value of two-dimensional exercise echocardiography to routine treadmill exercise testing. Ann Intern Med 1986;105:829.

15. Armstrong WF. Stress echocardiography for detection of coronary artery disease. Circulation 1991;84(Suppl 1):I-43.

16. Yvorchuk KJ, Sochowski RA. Sonicated albumin in exercise echocardiography: technique and feasibility to enhance endocardial visualization. J Am Soc Echocardiogr 1996;9:462.

17. Dagianti A, Penco M, Agati L, et al. Stress echocardiography: comparison of exercise, dipyridamole, and dobutamine in detecting and predicting the extent of coronary artery disease. J Am Coll Cardiol 1995; 26:18.

18. Hansen TH, Segar DA. The use of dobutamine stress echocardiography for the determination of myocardial viability. Clin Cardiol 1996; 19:607.

19. Sabia PJ, Powers ER, Rogosta M, et al. An association between collateral blood flow and myocardial viability in patients with recent myocardial infarction. N Engl J Med 1992;327:1825.

Chapter 5

Nuclear Cardiology

During the last 25 years, nuclear cardiology has developed rapid, accurate, noninvasive means for evaluating regional myocardial perfusion and quantitating cardiovascular performance. The technical advances that have made this possible include the availability of appropriate radiopharmaceutical agents, high-performance γ-scintillation cameras, and low-cost computer equipment that allows rapid data acquisition and analysis. The noninvasive nature of these techniques has resulted in widespread applicability and acceptance.

Nuclear cardiology procedures can be separated into four broad categories:

- Myocardial perfusion imaging.
- Infarct avid imaging.
- Radionuclide angiography.
- Positron emission tomography

MYOCARDIAL PERFUSION IMAGING

Myocardial perfusion imaging assesses myocardial blood flow by using radiopharmaceutical agents that are injected into the bloodstream and accumulate in the myocardium (1). **Thallium-201** and **technetium-99 sestamibi** are radioisotopes that are delivered to all organs of the body in relative proportion to the blood flow each organ receives. The heart accumulates thallium-201 in areas of viable myocardium in proportion to blood flow to those regions. The greater the perfusion of blood to a region of the myocardium, the greater the uptake of thallium-201 to that region. Regions with decreased blood flow are represented by decreased or absent thallium uptake and are seen as "cold spots." Imaging can be performed either in planar or tomographic format; the latter procedure is referred to as **single photon emission computed tomography (SPECT).**

The most widely used clinical applications for myocardial perfusion imaging is stress testing with either thallium-201 or technetium-99 sestamibi (discussed later) (2). During this procedure, the patient undergoes stress testing with an intravenous line in place. Approximately 1 min before stopping exercise, thallium-201 is injected intravenously, and soon thereafter, the patient is taken to the nuclear medicine department where the γ-scintillation camera is used to image the myocardium (stress phase). In areas of decreased myocardial blood flow, diminished uptake of thallium-201 can be seen (2). If repeat images are obtained 3 or 4 hours later at rest (redistribution phase), changes from the stress images will reflect changes in regional myocardial blood flow occurring with exercise. Thus, "cold spots" that are seen with maximal exercise and disappear with rest indicate regions of the myocardium that have decreased blood flow with exercise but adequate blood flow at rest. Areas of reversible hypoperfusion, corresponding to reversible ischemia, indicate areas of significant obstructions to coronary artery blood flow. A "fixed defect" is an area of hypoperfusion that is seen on both rest and stress imaging and implies that there is myocardial scarring. Homogeneous uptake of the radioisotope on both rest and stress imaging suggests normal myocardial perfusion.

The standard treadmill stress test has specificity of 70–80%, depending on the population under study. A thallium-201 stress test has a specificity higher than 90% (depending on the experience and quality control of the laboratory). Soft tissue attenuation can be seen in patients with large breasts, elevated diaphragms, or obesity. This can lead to a significant incidence of false-positive results. A normal thallium-201 stress test makes the diagnosis of significant coronary artery disease very unlikely. However, balanced coronary stenosis (such as significant left main as well as right coronary stenosis) can appear as homogeneous hypoperfusion and may be missed by thallium scintigraphy. The sensitivity of the thallium-201 stress testing is higher than 85%. In contrast, the sensitivity of standard electrocardiogram (ECG) treadmill testing is approximately 60–70% (3–6).

Thallium "cold spot" imaging is useful in a number of conditions, including the following:

1. Diagnosis of coronary artery disease, particularly in patients with a conflicting database (e.g., suspected false-positive stress ECG, false-negative stress ECG with a convincing history for angina, patients with preexisting ST-segment and T-wave ECG abnormalities such as left bundle branch block [(LBBB), digitalis therapy, left ventricular hypertrophy (LVH), etc.].

2. Evaluation of patency of coronary artery bypass grafts, particularly in patients with chest pain after bypass surgery.

3. Determination of the physiologic significance of coronary artery stenosis discovered by coronary angiography.

4. Detection of additionally jeopardized myocardium after a myocardial infarction suggesting multivessel coronary artery disease.

5. Acute myocardial infarction can be diagnosed, sized, and localized with an accuracy approaching 100% if a resting thallium study is performed within 6 hours of the onset of symptoms. "Cold spot" defect resolution strongly suggests coronary artery spasm. Small infarcts, subendocardial infarcts, and scans performed later than 24 hours after the onset of symptoms can all result in negative scans.

6. Patients with dilated cardiomyopathy may have characteristic thallium-201 scans. Patients with ischemic disease as an etiology for their dilated cardiomyopathy typically demonstrate multiple large perfusion defects. In contrast, patients with idiopathic dilated cardiomyopathy generally have homogeneous uptake of thallium-201 in the myocardium.

7. Patients with sarcoidosis and myocardial involvement may have thallium-201 scans with multiple patchy left ventricular perfusion defects.

8. Assessment of viable myocardium is helpful for ischemic cardiomyopathy with depressed left ventricular function as well as for fixed perfusion defects. In the former, determination of viable myocardium is helpful when deciding whether a patient would be a suitable candidate for myocardial revascularization versus cardiac transplantation. In the latter, imaging can assist in deciding if revascularization is indicated for infarcted myocardium, which may be viable or have significant peri-infarction ischemia. Although positron emission tomography (PET) scanning (discussed later) is more accurate, thallium can be used when PET scanning is unavailable (7).

Several protocols can be used. In one method, the patient is injected at peak exercise and scanned at 4–6 hours. If a fixed scar is seen, then rescanning at 24 hours may show redistribution suggesting viability and potential benefit from revascularization. Another method of assessing viability is by injecting thallium at peak exercise with scanning 3–4 hours later followed by reinjection of thallium the following day and rescanning at 24 hours. Early and delayed rest thallium imaging (performed at 3 and 24 hours) without exercise is yet another way to assess myocardial viability and may be the most accurate of the techniques using thallium.

Technetium-99m (Tc-99m) sestamibi (Tc-99m complexed with 2-methoxy isobutyl isonitrile), is a substance that accumulates in the myocardium in proportion to blood flow (1). It is also known as Cardiolyte (produced by Du Pont), RP-30, Tc99m-MIBI, Tc-99m-isonitrile and Tc-99m-hexamibi. Tc-99m sestamibi is rapidly accumulated in proportion to regional blood flow by passive diffusion and binds to mitochondrial membranes. It remains in myocardium for several hours but is cleared from the blood rapidly, allowing for excellent contrast. Logistically, the patient is exercised and the agent is administered intravenously 1 min before exertion. The patient is then taken to the nuclear medicine department (or the nuclear camera) for image acquisition. If a defect is seen in the myocardium (indicative of regional hypoperfusion due to coronary narrowing), then the patient must return the following day for a reinjection and repeat image acquisition. If the defect remains on repeat scan, then this would indicate myocardial scar or old infarction. However, if on repeat injection, the defect is no longer present, then this would indicate that the patient has ischemia and probably a high-grade stenosis in the coronary artery supplying that segment of the myocardium.

Dual isotope imaging using thallium-201 at rest and sestamibi with exercise allows same day imaging and obviates the need for the patient to return on the second day (8).

The advantages that Tc-99m sestamibi has over thallium include the following:

1. Because Tc-99m sestamibi has no redistribution and slow washout, image acquisition can be performed up to 4 hours after the injection. In contrast, thallium imaging must be

performed within minutes of injection so that redistribution does not begin and potential perfusion defects do not fill in.

2. The photon energy of Tc-99m sestamibi is higher (140 keV) than that of thallium (80 keV), allowing better contrast and potentially fewer false-positive results due to artifact or soft tissue attenuation.

3. If administered while the patient is under the nuclear camera, Tc-99m sestamibi can be used for first-pass ventriculography of the right and left ventricle (see below). This allows for the determination of wall motion and biventricular function as well as regional perfusion with the same agent. Thallium does not provide adequate counts for radionuclide angiography.

4. Tc-99m sestamibi can be prepared easily, whereas thallium must be generated in a linear accelerator and then delivered to the institution.

5. Tc-99m sestamibi can be used to assess the efficacy of thrombolysis in the setting of acute myocardial infarction (9).

Technetium-99m teboroxime (Tc-99m teboroxime) is another isonitrile perfusion agent that has high myocardial extraction and washout. Two injections must be made, as in the Tc-99m sestamibi examination. However, because of the rapid washout, the patient must be imaged within 2 min of exercise and image acquisition must be completed within 10 min. Although Tc-99m teboroxime may have an advantage in pharmacological vasodilator imaging studies, in which the patient is usually near the scintillation camera, it may be impractical when patients cannot be transported or imaged quickly. Because it is a technetium compound, first-pass wall motion and ejection fraction can be performed. Due to the rapid washout, reinjection and imaging can be performed within 2 hours of the initial injection, allowing for a more expeditious examination (10,11).

Some patients are unable to perform adequate exercise due to severe claudication, orthopedic disability, poor exercise tolerance, or chronotropic incompetence. The use of intravenous vasodilator substances in conjunction with nuclear perfusion imaging (thallium or Tc-99m sestamibi) can assist in the evaluation of patients who cannot exercise (12–14). Dipyridamole is a phosphodiesterase inhibitor that dilates the resistance coronary vessels and produces a relative hypoperfusion in the myocardium served by stenotic coronary arteries. Dipyridamole is contraindicated for patients with asthma or bronchospastic lung disease. Adenosine is a purine molecule that is naturally produced intracellularly in the body and is used in various metabolic pathways. When administered intravenously, it is a potent coronary vasodilator and can be used with perfusion agents to detect relative areas of hypoperfusion. Adenosine is contraindicated in patients with significant conduction system disease. Vasodilator perfusion imaging has been demonstrated to be useful in the evaluation of cardiac patients anticipating noncardiac surgery as well as predicting postmyocardial infarction complications (15,16).

Dobutamine administered intravenously with or without atropine can also be used to increase the heart rate and simulate exercise, especially for patients who cannot tolerate dipyridamole or adenosine. Generally, an infusion is started at a rate of 10 μg/kg/min for 3 min and then increased by 10-μg/kg/min increments every 3 min to a maximum of 40 μg/kg/min. If the heart rate is not 85% predicted maximum for age, then atropine (0.2 mg) is given incrementally to a maximum of 1 mg (17).

INFARCT AVID IMAGING

The second type of myocardial imaging is the infarct avid imaging or **technetium pyrophosphate** scan. Pyrophosphate forms complexes with deposits of calcium. Infarction results in the influx of calcium and phosphate ions. In infarcted areas, interaction of the pyrophosphate and calcium occurs in the damaged myocardial tissue and is subsequently detected as a "hot spot" when viewed with a γ camera (1,2). The central area of an infarct typically has very reduced blood flow, and therefore, deposition of the radiopharmaceutical pyrophosphate is less than that in the peripheral areas. This results in a so called doughnut pattern of pyrophosphate deposition, with a central area with almost no pyrophosphate uptake as a result of very low flow at the center of the infarct and a circular surrounding zone of high uptake corresponding to the peripheral areas of the infarct with lesser reductions in coronary blood flow.

Pyrophosphate is normally used as a bone imaging agent, and a normal pyrophosphate scan image demonstrates no activity in the region of the heart, with activity seen in the ribs, sternum, and vertebral column. A positive pyrophosphate scan results in one of two types of uptake:

1. Focal uptake in one anatomic region of the heart.
2. Diffuse uptake in the entire heart not limited to any specific anatomic region.

Patients can be imaged at the bedside using a portable scintillation camera. Maximal uptake of pyrophosphate occurs between 48 and 72 hours and most scans revert to normal in 7–17 days.

Occasionally, scans can remain persistently positive for weeks or months, possibly related to ongoing cellular necrosis or aneurysm formation. Transmural infarcts result in a positive scan in more than 90% of cases if imaging is performed 2–3 days after infarction. Nontransmural, subendocardial infarctions are detected less frequently (perhaps 50% of the time).

Acute myocardial infarction is the most common cause for a positive technetium pyrophosphate scan, but there are a number of other conditions that infrequently can result in a positive scan, including the following:

1. Left ventricular aneurysms.
2. Myocardial contusions.
3. Valvular calcifications (believed to be caused by pyrophosphate binding to calcium).
4. Cardiomyopathy (diffuse uptake).
5. Unstable angina pectoris (diffuse uptake).
6. Myocarditis.
7. Cardiac amyloidosis.

Technetium pyrophosphate scanning is often useful in conditions that suggest myocardial infarction but in which the usual noninvasive tools are not helpful. Examples include the following:

1. After cardiac or other forms of surgery in which high levels of creatine kinase will be present. The pyrophosphate scan can determine whether infarction has occurred.
2. Atypical chest pain in patients with equivocal ECG or enzyme changes.
3. Patients with chest pain and ECGs that do not allow assessment of transmural injury (e.g., LBBB).
4. Patients with preexisting infarcts and evidence for infarct extension.
5. Myocardial contusion.

RADIONUCLIDE ANGIOGRAPHY

The third class of nuclear cardiology procedures is radionuclide angiography, sometimes called radionuclide ventriculography. This technique allows visualization of the atria and ventricles using radioactive intravascular indicators to create pictures of the great vessels and chambers of the heart (18–21).

There are two types of radionuclide ventriculography: the first-pass method and the gated-equilibrium method. In the first-pass method, a bolus of a technetium compound, e.g., technetium sodium pertechnetate, is injected intravenously and sequential cardiac images are obtained at a rapid rate during the initial passage of the radiotracer through the great vessels and chambers of the heart. The tracer first passes through the superior vena cava and the right-sided chambers of the heart. Because the tracer moves through the lungs rapidly, good separation of the right and left heart chambers can be achieved. Background activity is minimized because most of the radiopharmaceutical is in the heart itself during imaging. The first-pass study can be performed rapidly.

Using the gated-equilibrium method of blood pool imaging, red blood cells are labeled with technetium, which allows continuous imaging of the heart chambers. Gating means obtaining a repetitive image of the heart at a predetermined time after the QRS complex. Each cardiac cycle is divided into a series of segments by the computer, and tracer counts from corresponding segments of the cardiac cycle from multiple heartbeats are added together to create one summed picture of the cardiac chambers at one set time in the cardiac cycle. This allows for an averaged picture of the cardiac chambers from systole to diastole.

Both methods allow the calculation of end-systolic and end-diastolic counts. Therefore, calculation of ventricular ejection fractions can be performed using the end-diastolic counts minus end-systolic counts (stroke count) divided by end-diastolic counts. The ejection fractions so calculated are highly correlated with values obtained by standard contrast ventriculography at cardiac catheterizations.

Regional wall motion abnormalities can be detected by displaying the end-diastolic and end-systolic images in a static format. In addition, sequential frames of the cardiac cycle can be displayed on a video monitor to create a "movie" of ventricular function over an entire cardiac cycle. This helps in the precise localization of regional wall motion abnormalities.

Ventricular volumes can be determined using data from gated radionuclide ventriculograms. Geometric formulas usually used with routine contrast ventriculograms have been used to approximate ventricular volumes. Another technique for volume determination compares the isotope activity in a known volume of the patient's blood drawn at the time of the radionuclide ventriculogram. This allows conversion of isotope counts in the ventricle to volume in the ventricle.

A priori, the right ventricular (RV) stroke volume and left ventricular stroke volume should be equal. In the presence of aortic regurgitation (AR) or mitral regurgitation (MR), however, left ventricular stroke volume will be greater than right ventricular stroke volume and the difference will represent the regurgitation fraction.

Left ventricular aneurysms can be detected using radionuclide ventriculography. Left ventricular aneurysms result in systolic images protruding beyond diastolic images and the regional difference representing aneurysmal dilatation.

Right ventricular ejection fractions can be calculated from both first-pass and gated studies. Radionuclide ventriculograms revealing dilation of the right ventricle and a reduced RV ejection fraction are seen in RV infarcts.

In normal hearts, exercise results in an increase in the left ventricular ejection fraction. On the other hand, coronary artery disease results in a decline or no change in ejection fraction with exercise. Radionuclide ventriculography detects this decrease in ejection fraction as well as regional wall motion abnormalities with exercise. The sensitivity of exercise radionuclide ventriculography for detecting coronary disease is better than that using exercise electrocardiography alone and is similar to exercise thallium-201 scans. The specificity of the technique is similar to that of the stress ECG. Advantages of radionuclide ventriculography include a lower cost for Tc-99m than for thallium-201 and the ability of radionuclide ventriculography to assess ventricular function, information thallium scans cannot provide. Disadvantages include the requirement for computer acquisition and processing of the study information. Tc-99m sestamibi, however, can provide both perfusion and wall motion information and has essentially replaced radionuclide ventriculography in the assessment of patients with suspected coronary artery disease in many centers.

Radionuclide ventriculography provides useful information about chronic valvular heart disease, particularly regarding aortic and mitral regurgitation. These data may be useful in the timing of valve replacement surgery. Compensated regurgitant lesions (AR, MR) result in an increased stroke volume. There is an increased end-diastolic volume with a normal end-systolic volume. With time, chronic valvular regurgitant lesions result in progressive dysfunction of the left ventricle marked by a decrease in resting ejection fraction and failure to increase ejection fraction with exercise. In addition, an increase in end-systolic volume is seen. These very sensitive indicators of worsening left ventricular function may be of value in assessing a patient's need for valve replacement.

The first-pass method of radionuclide ventriculography can accurately predict the presence and extent of left-to-right cardiac shunts. A technetium compound is injected intravenously and followed as it passes through the right heart, the lungs, and then through the left heart. A computer-derived region of interest is placed over the lung and the computer plots the counts that occur in that region over time. In normal patients, the pulmonary time-activity curve shows an initial peak as the tracer moves through the lungs, followed by a later smaller secondary peak due to "recirculation" as part of the tracer bolus reappears in the lungs after having traveled through the systemic circulation. A left-to-right intracardiac shunt results in the early and prominent reappearance of the secondary peak curve because of the early reappearance of the tracer that took a "short cut" through the shunt back to the right heart rather than the longer route through the systemic circulation. A normal shunt study effectively excludes an intracardiac left-to-right shunt of any clinical significance. Right-to-left shunts may be detected by early appearance of tracer in the left-sided chambers or in the aorta.

Echocardiography (with transesophageal imaging if necessary) has been more useful in the qualitative detection of intracardiac shunts. However, in larger shunts, nuclear-derived shunt ratios can be complementary in the evaluation of patients who have undergone echocardiographic examinations.

POSITRON EMISSION TOMOGRAPHY

Positron emission tomography (PET scan) imaging is useful in the detection of coronary artery disease and in the assessment of myocardial viability in patients with coronary disease and left ventricular dysfunction. Rubidium-82 and ammonia labeled with nitrogen-13 are tracers used for the evaluation of regional myocardial blood flow. Fluorodeoxyglucose (FDG) and carbon-11 acetate are used for evaluation of glucose and fatty acid metabolism, respectively. If perfusion testing with rubidium-82 and nitrogen-13 ammonia demonstrate decreased flow and metabolic testing with FDG and carbon-1 acetate demonstrate absent metabolic activity, then that region of myocardium would be considered nonviable or necrotic (matched depression of perfusion and metabolism). On the other hand, if flow appeared reduced by the perfusion tracers but metabolic activity was preserved, then that region of myocardium would be considered ischemic and viable (mismatched depression of perfusion with preserved metabolism) (7). Limited widespread availability and cost have prevented general use of PET scanning (22,23).

Although PET is considered the gold standard for assessment of viability, thallium techniques are a cost-effective alternative (see section above). **Fluorine-18** (F-18) injection combined with **SPECT** imaging allows the use of a metabolic agent with a standard SPECT camera, which is more widely available than PET. Perfusion assessed by thallium-201 imaging combined with F-18 metabolic imaging compares favorably when compared to thallium-201 stress-reinjection and dobutamine echo in assessing myocardial recovery after revascularization (24).

Dobutamine echocardiography is another technique that can be used in the assessment of myocardial viability (see Chapter 4).

ELECTRON BEAM COMPUTED TOMOGRAPHY

Although not a nuclear cardiology technique, electron beam computed tomography (EBCT) has been used to quantify and localize coronary calcium. Because atherosclerotic plaque is commonly associated with calcium, detection of coronary artery calcium may be helpful in screening patients at risk for coronary artery disease. This is a rapid test that can be performed quickly, noninvasively, and with no need for contrast injection. The absence of calcium in the coronary arteries has a high negative predictive value (95%) for significant lesions of greater than 50% luminal diameter stenosis. However, the specificity of an abnormal scan is not good, ranging from 45 to 66% for significant disease. Many atherosclerotic plaques have calcium but are not flow limiting. EBCT may be useful for screening high-risk individuals to help guide risk factor modification as well as for the evaluation of patients at low risk for coronary disease who have atypical features for angina. Because this test does not exclude the presence of obstructive or unstable plaques, it should not be used as an alternative for angiography in the definition of coronary anatomy (25,26).

References

1. Zaret BL, Wackers FJ. Nuclear cardiology. Part 1. N Engl J Med 1993; 329:775.

2. Mayo Clinic Cardiovascular Working Group on Stress Testing. Cardiovascular stress testing: a description of the various stress tests and indications for their use. Mayo Clin Proc 1996;71:43.

3. Kotler TS, Diamond GA. Exercise thallium-201 scintigraphy in the diagnosis and prognosis of coronary artery disease. Ann Intern Med 1990;113:684.

4. American College of Physicians. Position paper. Efficacy of exercise thallium-201 scintigraphy in the diagnosis and prognosis of coronary artery disease. Ann Intern Med 1990;113:703.

5. Beller GA. Diagnostic accuracy of thallium-201 myocardial perfusion imaging. Circulation 1991;84(Suppl I):I-1.

6. Ritchie JL, Bateman TM, Bonow RO, et al. Guidelines for clinical use of cardiac radionuclide imaging. A report of the American Heart Association/American College of Cardiology Task Force on Assessment of Diagnostic and Therapeutic Cardiovascular Procedures, Committee on Radionuclide Imaging, developed in collaboration with the American Society of Nuclear Cardiology. Circulation 1995; 91:1278.

7. Hendel RC, Chaudhry FA, Bonow RO. Myocardial viability. Curr Probl Cardiol 1996;21:145.

8. Berman DS, Kiat H, Friedman JD, et al. Separate acquisition rest thallium-201/stress technetium-99m sestamibi dual-isotope myocardial perfusion single-photon emission computed tomography: a clinical validation study. J Am Coll Cardiol 1993;22:1455.

9. Gibbons RJ. Perfusion imaging with 99mTc-sestamibi for the assess-

ment of myocardial area at risk and the efficacy of acute treatment in myocardial infarction. Circulation 1991;84(Suppl I):I-37.

10. Berman DS, Kiat H, Maddahi J. The new 99m-Tc myocardial perfusion imaging agents: 99mTc-sestamibi and 99mTc-teboroxime. Circulation 1991;84(Suppl I):I-7.

11. Johnson LL. Clinical experience with technetium 99m teboroxime. Semin Nucl Med 1991;21(3):182.

12. Chou TM, Amidon TM. Evaluating coronary artery disease noninvasively—which test for whom? West J Med 1994;161:173.

13. Coyne EP, Belvedere DA, Vande Streek PR, et al. Thallium-201 scintigraphy after intravenous infusion of adenosine compared with exercise thallium testing in the diagnosis of coronary artery disease. J Am Coll Cardiol 1991;17:1289.

14. Taillefer R, Amyot R, Turpin S, et al. Comparison between dipyridamole and adenosine as pharmacologic coronary vasodilators in detection of coronary artery disease with thallium-201 imaging. J Nucl Cardiol 1996;3:204.

15. Eagle KA, Brundage BH, Chaitman BR, et al. Guidelines for perioperative cardiovascular evaluation for noncardiac surgery. Report of the American College of Cardiology/American Heart Association Task Force on Practice Guidelines (Committee on Perioperative Cardiovascular Evaluation for Noncardiac Surgery). Circulation 1996;93:1278.

16. Heller GV, Herman SD, Travin MI, et al. Independent prognostic value of intravenous dipyridamole with technetium-99m sestamibi tomographic imaging in predicting cardiac events and cardiac-related hospital admissions. J Am Coll Cardiol 1995;26:1202.

17. Geleijnse ML, Elhendy A, VanDomburg RT, et al. Prognostic value of dobutamine-atropine stress technetium-99m sestamibi perfusion scintigraphy in patients with chest pain. J Am Coll Cardiol 1996;28:447.

18. Zaret BL, Wackers FJ. Nuclear cardiology. Part 2. N Engl J Med 1993;329:855.

19. Gibbons RJ. Rest and exercise radionuclide angiography for diagnosis in chronic ischemic heart disease. Circulation 1991;84(Suppl I):I-93.

20. Aurigemma GP, Gaasch WH, Villegas B, et al. Noninvasive assessment of left ventricular mass, chamber volume, and contractile function. Curr Probl Cardiol 1995;20:361.

21. Johnson LL. Radionuclide assessment of ventricular function. Curr Probl Cardiol 1994;19:589.

22. Council on Scientific Affairs. Report of the Positron Emission Tomography Panel: application of positron emission tomography in the heart. In: Topics in Radiology/Council Report. JAMA 1988;259:2438.

23. Bonow RO, Berman DS, Gibbons RJ, et al. Cardiac positron emission tomography. A report for health professionals from the Committee

on Advanced Cardiac Imaging and Technology of the Council on Clinical Cardiology, American Heart Association. Circulation 1991; 84(1):447.

24. Bax JJ, Cornel JH, Visser FC, et al. Prediction of myocardial dysfunction after revascularization. Comparison of fluorine-18 fluorodeoxy-glucose/thallium-201 SPECT, thallium-201 stress-reinjection SPECT, and dobutamine echocardiography, J Am Coll Cardiol 1996;28:558.

25. Rumberg JA, Sheedy PF, Breen JF, et al. Electron beam computed tomography and coronary artery disease: scanning for coronary artery calcification. Mayo Clin Proc 1996;71:369.

26. Wexler L, Brundage BB, Crouse JC, et al. Coronary artery calcification: pathophysiology, epidemiology, imaging methods, and clinical applications. A statement for health professions from the American Heart Association. Circulation 1996;94:1175.

Chapter 6

Cardiac Catheterization

Many cardiac problems can be properly diagnosed and treated without the need for invasive procedures. In some clinical situations, cardiac catheterization may be required to manage the cardiac patient. The decision to study a patient invasively is one that should be carefully considered. The clinician must take into consideration the clinical setting, the patient's age, and past medical and/or surgical history of the suspected cardiac problem. The individual performing the procedure is, in fact, performing a high-level consultation and not merely a laboratory test. He or she should have a thorough knowledge of the patient and, most importantly, of what questions must be answered by the procedure in the specific patient undergoing the study.

Before the patient consents to an invasive study, he or she must be informed of the risks of the procedure. Although the risks vary depending on the type of case, cardiac catheterization in a stable patient is very safe with competent personnel and carries a less than 1% probability of morbidity. The risks are amplified for more elderly or more infirmed patients and for patients who are not physiologically or psychologically stable at the time of the procedure. Coronary angiography is a safe procedure with the risks of a major adverse event (e.g., stroke, myocardial infarction (MI), major bleeding) being <0.5%. Overall mortality is <0.2% (1). Other complications include local thrombosis, embolism, cardiac perforation, significant arrhythmias, and allergy to contrast media.

The referring physician should be satisfied that the procedure can be performed safely and adequately and that the laboratory has the ability to answer the clinical questions. Not all catheterization laboratories are properly equipped with a wide range of laboratory equipment, and not all catheterization personnel have adequate training and experience.

Patients with ischemic heart disease constitute most cases in the average cardiac catheterization laboratory. The principal information needed in these cases is an angiographic demonstration of the nature and extent of disease in the coronary arteries, the left ventricular filling pressure, ejection fraction, size, wall motion, and valvular competence. Patients with congenital or valvular heart disease require more elaborate physiologic studies to identify the anatomical relationships, pressures, and regional flood flow in the central circulation (2,3).

During the 1980s, the cardiac catheterization laboratory was the site of significant changes as it evolved from strictly a diagnostic arena to the place of therapeutic interventions. Balloon angioplasty was the backbone of the interventional procedures in the 1980s. Percutaneous transluminal coronary angioplasty (PTCA) changed extensively since the first procedure by Gruentzig in 1977. Initially, PTCA was limited to single-vessel lesions in patients with coronary artery disease (CAD) who were symptomatic on medical therapy. Later, this evolved to a much broader spectrum of patients undergoing this nonsurgical technique, including those with multivessel CAD, patients who have undergone previous coronary artery bypass grafting (CABG) surgery and stenosis in the native or graft vessels, patients with acute MI who present early in their course to a properly equipped facility, patients with total occlusions, and certain high-risk surgical cases (elderly patients with renal failure, systemic disease, and some with severe left ventricular dysfunction).

In experienced hands, PTCA is a low-risk procedure with 1% or less mortality and approximately 5% morbidity including MI, arrhythmia, infection, bleeding, and the need for emergency CABG because of dissection or acute closure (4). The success rate for experienced operators is 90% per vessel dilated. Certain advantages of PTCA make it an attractive alternative to surgery, e.g., it is less expensive and does not necessitate general anesthesia and thoracotomy, and duration of hospitalization is shorter. The major pitfall of PTCA is restenosis, which is a complex problem that occurs in some 30–50% of cases. Restenosis occurs to a variable degree in virtually all lesions (5). The terms *acute gain, late loss,* and *net gain* have been used to describe the relationship between lumen diameter at baseline, immediately after intervention and during follow-up. *Acute gain* is the difference in lumen diameter before and immediately after intervention and is due to arterial expansion or plaque removal. *Late loss* is the difference in lumen diameter after intervention and at follow-up; late loss is due to intimal hyperplasia, elastic recoil, and vascular remodeling.

In most cases of restenosis, the clinical presentation of restenosis is recurrent angina and not MI or sudden death. This may be explained by the fact that restenotic lesions, which consist of intimal hyperplasia and fibrous tissue, are less prone to rupture and acutely thrombose. Angiographic analysis suggests that early recoil is associated with a high incidence of restenosis. It seems that restenosis involves not only intimal proliferative hyperplasia but also remodeling (both positive and negative remodeling). Whatever the mechanisms involved, the most powerful indicator of restenosis is a high degree of residual plaque.

DEVICES FOR CORONARY INTERVENTION

From 1979 to 1990, balloon angioplasty was the only modality for coronary intervention. Despite an explosive growth in the use of the procedure (>300,000 cases annually), PTCA is still plagued by a number of limitations.

- Difficulty in crossing certain lesions such as total occlusions.
- Difficulty dilating rigid lesions such as densely calcified lesions or dilating osteal or elastic lesions such as vein grafts.
- Difficulty in preventing dissection-induced abrupt closure of the dilated vessel.
- 30–50% incidence of restenosis in 6 months of follow-up.

Interest in alternative modes of luminal enlargement grew with increasing recognition of the limitations of standard balloon angioplasty. Devices entered clinical testing in the late 1980s and then gained Food & Drug Administration (FDA) approval between 1990 and 1994.

STENTS

Stents serve as endoluminal scaffolds that resist elastic recoil and "tack up" dissections. Introduction of the intracoronary stent has revolutionized transcatheter intervention.

Kuntz and Baim postulated that a larger postprocedural lumen will favorably affect restenosis rates, i.e., "bigger is better" (5). The Palmaz-Schatz stent achieves the greatest acute gain and is the only device that has been proven to reduce the incidence of restenosis compared to PTCA. Randomized trials such as the STRESS trial (6,7) and the BENESTENT trial (8) have shown a decrease in restenosis for de novo lesions in native coronary arteries. The SAVED trial (*S*tenting of *A*ngioplasty in *VE*in graft *D*isease) has demonstrated lower restenosis in saphenous vein grafts (9). Along with treating de novo lesions and saphenous vein (SV) graft lesions, stents have shown to be highly effective in the treatment of actual or threatened closure. Stenting success rates of >90% and reduced stent thrombosis rates of 1–3% with optimal higher pressure deployment techniques has catapulted the stent to the most valuable available tool for the interventional cardiologist (10).

Approved Stents

Palmaz-Schatz Stent—slotted tube
Gianturco-Roubin Stent—flexible coil
ACS Multilink Stent—slotted tube
Wiktor Stent—coil

Investigational Stents

AVE Micro Stent
Strecker Stent
Cordis Stent
Wallstent
Sci-Med Stent

Stenting has also been observed to be valuable in certain aorto-ostial lesions, restenotic lesions, long lesions, chronic occlusions, and some cases of acute MI.

ATHERECTOMY

Atherectomy refers to removal rather than displacement of the plaque that comprises the lesion under treatment. Various atherectomy approaches have been developed.

Directional atherectomy (DVI Simpson AtheroCath) involves extracting plaque that has been excised by advancing a blade that is pushed down into a collecting nose cone. Early suboptimal directional atherectomy resulted in the disappointing results of the CAVEAT trial (*C*oronary *A*ngioplasty *V*ersus *E*xcision *A*therectomy *T*rial) (11). Optimal directional atherectomy (aggressive tissue removal plus postdilatation) has been shown by the BOAT trial (12) (*B*alloon versus *O*ptimal *A*therectomy *T*rial) and the OARS Trial (*O*ptimal *A*therectomy *R*estenosis *S*tudy) (13) to provide significantly larger luminal diameters than seen in CAVEAT without sacrificing procedural safety. The major niche for this seems to be in the osteal lesions, which are not calcified, and in bifurcation lesions. Although the alternative stenting technique is the preferred technique in most laboratories, directional atherectomy is still used in a small number of interventions nationwide (<5%).

Rotational atherectomy involves a diamond-chip-coated burr that rotates at speeds of 160,000–180,000 rpm that is advanced over a guidewire. This device preferentially ablates hard or calcified tissue with resulting particles <5–10 μ being liberated into the distal coronary circulation. Because of its unique niches in the calcified, osteal, and longer lesions, the rotablator accounts for up to 20% of interventions in the most modern interventional laboratories (14,15).

Rotational coronary atherectomy combined with stenting (rotastenting) is an extremely effective approach in some cases by combining the benefits of debulking a lesion and then providing a maximal lumen scaffold to prevent recoil. Improvements in the technique and equipment have significantly decreased problems of spasm, bradycardia, slow flow, and the "no flow" problems.

Extraction atherectomy is performed with the transluminal extraction catheter (*TEC*) and uses suction to remove thrombi. The device is believed to have some niche in removing thrombi in degenerated vein grafts (16); however, its cumbersome technology and complication rates have diminished its appeal. It is used in less than 5% of current interventions.

Laser atherectomy photochemically ablates plaque by using high-energy laser pulses transmitted through a catheter containing multiple optical fibers. Persistent problems of dissection, perforation, and high restenosis rates of greater than 50% have markedly diminished the enthusiasm for this device and it accounts for less than 3% of interventions nationwide (17).

VALVULOPLASTY

Balloon valvulotomy is another example of a therapeutic tool used in the cardiac catheterization laboratory. Pulmonary valvulotomy is now a well-established technique for the treatment of severe pulmonary stenosis in all age groups (18). A successful procedure results in a dramatic relief of the pressure gradient with excellent long-term clinical results. Balloon dilatation of the mitral valve is an acceptable alternative to surgical valvotomy, and data indicate that the results of this procedure are similar to closed surgical valvotomy (19). The largest group of patients with severe rheumatic mitral stenosis likely to benefit from this procedure live in the developing countries. The use of aortic valvu-

Table 6.1
Normal Values and Pressures

	Normal
O_2 consumption (VO_2)	110–150/mL/min/M^2
Pulmonary arteriovenous (AV) O_2 difference	3.5–4.7 vol. %
Systemic AV O_2 difference	3.5–4.7 vol. %
Systemic O_2 saturation	≥94%
Cardiac index (CI)	2.5–4.0 L/min/M^2
Systemic vascular resistance (SVR)	8.0–15.0 units
Pulmonary vascular resistance (PVR)	0.2–1.12 units
Total pulmonary resistance (TPR)	1.0–3.0 units
Aortic valve area (AVA)	2.6–3.5 cm^2
Mitral valve area (MVA)	4.0–6.0 cm^2
Left ventricular (LV) end-diastolic volume	<90 ml/M^2
Ejection fraction	55–70%
His bundle electrogram AH interval	60–115 msec
HV interval	35–55 msec
Normal Pressures (mmHg)	
Right atrium (RA), mean	1–8
Right ventricle (RV) systolic	15–28
end-diastolic	0–8
Pulmonary artery (PA) systolic	15–28
diastolic	5–16
mean	10–22
Pulmonary artery wedge (PAW) mean	4–12
Left atrium (LA) mean	4–12
Left ventricle (LV) systolic	85–150
end-diastolic	4–12
Aortic (Ao) systolic	85–150
diastolic	60–90
mean	70–105

loplasty for severe aortic stenosis has markedly diminished because the restenosis rate is high and the natural history of the disease in most patients is unchanged (20).

A thorough review of the terminology and physiologic data derived from cardiac catheterization is beyond the scope of this text. However, a table of normal values is included for the reader's reference (Table 6.1).

References

1. American College of Cardiology/American Heart Association Ad Hoc Task Force on Cardiac Catheterization. ACC/AHA Guidelines for Cardiac Catheterization and Cardiac Catheterization Laboratories. Circulation 1991;84:2213.
2. Criley JM, French JW. Cardiac catheterization in adults with congenital heart disease. Cardiovasc Clin 1979;10:173.
3. Yang SS, Bentivoglio LG, Maranhoa V, et al. From cardiac catheterization data to hemodynamic parameters. 3rd ed. Philadelphia: FA Davis, 1988.
4. Landau C, Lange RA, Hillis LD. Percutaneous transluminal coronary angioplasty, N Engl J Med 1994;330:981.
5. Kuntz RE, Baim DS. Defining coronary restenosis. Newer clinical and angiographic paradigms. Circulation 1993;88:1310.
6. Fishman DT, Leon MB, Baim DS, et al. A randomized comparison of coronary stent placement and balloon angioplasty in the treatment of coronary artery disease. Stent Restenosis Study Investigators. N Engl J Med 1994;331:496.
7. Wong SC, Zidoc JB, Chuong YC, et al. Stents improve late clinical outcomes: results from the combined (I + II) Stent Restenosis Study. Circulation 1995;92(Suppl 1):1.
8. Macaya C, Serruys PW, Ruygrok P, et al. Combined benefits of coronary stenting versus balloon angioplasty: one year follow-up of BENESTENT trial. J Am Coll Cardiol 1996;27:255.
9. Douglas JS, Savage MP, Bailey ST, et al. Randomized trial of coronary stent and balloon angioplasty in the treatment of saphenous vein graft stenosis. J Am Coll Cardiol 1996;27(Suppl A):A-178.
10. Pepine CJ, Holmes DR. Coronary artery stents. J Am Coll Cardiol 1996;28:782.
11. Topol EJ, Teya F, Pinkerton CA, et al. A comparison of directional atherectomy with coronary angioplasty in patients with coronary artery disease. The CAVEAT Study Group. N Engl J Med 1993;329:221.
12. Baim DS, Cutlip D, Ho KK, et al. Acute results of directional coronary atherectomy in the Balloon versus Optimal Atherectomy Trial (BOAT) pilot phase. Coron Artery Dis 1996;7:290.
13. Dussaillant GR, Mintz GS, Popma JJ, et al. Intravascular ultrasound,

directional coronary atherectomy, and the Optimal Atherectomy Restenosis Study (OARS). Coron Artery Dis 1996;7:294.

14. Ellis SG, Popma JJ, Buchbinder M, et al. Relation of clinical presentation, stenosis morphology, and operator technique to the procedural results of rotational atherectomy-facilitated angioplasty. Circulation 1994;89:882.

15. Worth DC, Leon MB, O'Neill W, et al. Rotational atherectomy multicenter registry: acute results, complications and six-month angiographic follow-up in 709 patients. J Am Coll Cardiol 1994;24:641.

16. Safian RD, Grines CL, May MA, et al. Clinical and angiographic results of transluminal extraction coronary atherectomy in saphenous vein bypass grafts. Circulation 1994;89:302.

17. Bittl JA, Kuntz R, Estella P, et al. Analysis of late lumen narrowing after excimer laser-facilitated angioplasty. J Am Coll Cardiol 1994; 23:1314.

18. Rao PS, Fawzi ME, Solymar L, et al. Long term results of balloon pulmonary valvuloplasty of valvular pulmonary stenosis. Am Heart J 1989;115:1291.

19. Palacios IF, Block PC. Percutaneous mitral balloon valvulotomy. Update of immediate results and follow-up. Circulation 1988;78(Suppl II):II-490.

20. Bashore TM, Davidson CJ. Follow-up recatheterization after balloon aortic valvuloplasty. Mansfield Scientific Aortic Valvuloplasty Registry Investigators. J Am Coll Cardiol 1991;17:1188.

Chapter 7

Ischemic Heart Disease: Risk Factors and Prevention

Cardiovascular disease claims approximately 1 million American lives per year, half of which are caused by coronary artery disease (CAD). The CAD mortality rate remains higher in the United States than in other industrialized nations. According to the World Health Organization, 55 of 100,000 Americans die of CAD each year, as compared to 33 and 15 per 100,000 people in Switzerland and Japan, respectively. The ability to identify and manage CAD risk factors will profoundly affect efforts to maintain the trend of declining CAD mortality rates.

CAD is still our nation's number one killer, but there has been a dramatic reduction (more than 50%) in age-adjusted mortality rates during the last 20 years. The decline has been attributed to many causes, such as better emergency care and advances in hospital treatment and improved prehospital care, but the major credit goes to the reduction in coronary risk factors. The most impressive risk factor changes have been the decline in prevalence of smoking, more widespread treatment and control of hypertension, and a decrease in average serum cholesterol levels.

RISK FACTORS

A risk factor is an element that is associated with an increased likelihood that disease will develop at a later time. Risk factors can be categorized as modifiable or nonmodifiable. *Modifiable* risks, such as smoking, can be changed; *nonmodifiable* risks, such as age or gender, can not. Prevention of risk factors can be primary or secondary. *Primary prevention* involves intervention before the onset of disease. *Secondary prevention* involves intervention after the onset of disease. The risk of a coronary event in any individual rises exponentially when two or more major risk factors are present.

Modifiable risks include the following:

1. Cigarette smoking
2. Low-density lipoprotein cholesterol
3. Hypertension
4. Diabetes mellitus
5. Estrogen deficiency
6. Inactivity
7. Obesity

Nonmodifiable risks include the following:

1. Family history
2. Gender
3. Age

Modifiable Risk Factors

Cigarette Smoking

Tobacco smoking is the leading preventable cause of death in the United States (1); 46 million American adults are smokers (28% of adult American males and 22% of females). Cigarette smoking is estimated to have been responsible for 418,690 of the more than 2 million deaths in the United States in 1990, or one in every five deaths. Nearly 25% of the 418,690 deaths were caused by ischemic heart disease, and 43% were caused by all cardiovascular diseases (2). Research demonstrates that smoking causes transient and reversible prothrombotic increases in fibrinogen levels and platelet adhesion, increased blood carboxyhemoglobin levels, reduced high-density lipoprotein (HDL) cholesterol, and coronary artery vasoconstriction.

The percentage of Americans who smoke has declined 37% since 1965. Smoking cessation increased life expectancy; smokers who quit approach mortality rates of nonsmokers within 3 years of stopping (3,4). In a 10-year follow-up of patients in the Coronary Artery Surgery Study (CASS), smokers who quit had fewer hospitalizations, less angina, and less physical limitations than those who continue to smoke (5). We advise physicians to counsel any patient who smokes to quit, to set quit dates, to provide self-help material, and to have follow-up visits to assess compliance.

Low-Density Lipoprotein (LDL) Cholesterol

In the United States, the National Cholesterol Education Program (NCEP) Adult Treatment Panel II has stratified the risk of LDL levels as follows: LDL cholesterol >160 mg/dL is "high-risk LDL cholesterol;" 130–159 mg/dL is "borderline high-risk LDL cholesterol;" and <130 mg/dL is a "desirable LDL cholesterol" (6). Therapeutic lowering of LDL cholesterol levels is highly effective in secondary prevention. In the recently reported Scandinavian Simvastatin Survival Study (4S), LDL lowering induced by a 3-hydroxy-3-methylglutaryl coenzyme A (HMG-CoA) reductase inhibitor reduced coronary mortality by 42% and total mortality by 30% (7). This trial was the first to demonstrate convincingly that cholesterol-lowering therapy not only reduces coronary events but also prolongs life in patients with coronary disease. Clinical trials also demonstrate benefit from LDL lowering in primary prevention, as noted in the West of Scotland study. Pravastatin lowered the mean plasma LDL cholesterol level by 25%, and the relative risk of a definite coronary event (nonfatal myocardial infarction or death from coronary heart disease) was reduced by 31% (8). Several studies (STARS, SCRIP, REGRESS) have used serial arteriography to measure progression versus regression of coronary stenosis by using cholesterol-lowering therapies, each showing a reduction in coronary events (9–11).

Secondary prevention trials in the 1990s, such as the Scandinavian Simvastatin Survival Study (4S) in 1994 and the Cholesterol and Recurrent Events (CARE) trial, have shown a highly significant decline in all-cause mortality associated with LDL reduction with HMG-CoA reductase inhibitors.

Many angiographic studies have demonstrated that lipid-lowering therapy combined with low-fat diet can impede progression or bring about regression of atherosclerotic lesions. Lesion regression has been shown in three studies in the 1990s: the Familial Atherosclerosis Treatment Study (FATS), the St. Thomas Atherosclerosis Regression Study (STARS), and the Regression Growth Evaluation Statin Study (REGRESS). Early landmark studies such as the Framingham Heart Study reported in 1971 and the Multiple Risk Factor Intervention Trial (MRFIT) showed that high total cholesterol levels were strongly linked to an increased incidence of ischemic heart disease. In 1981, Brown and co-workers showed that the component of cholesterol designated LDL cholesterol is primarily responsible for atherogenesis.

It is estimated that 52 million American adults currently qualify for cholesterol-lowering intervention diets and/or drugs.

The major lipoprotein classes are chylomicrons, very low-density lipoproteins (VLDLs), intermediate-density lipoproteins (IDLs), LDLs, and HDLs. Each lipoprotein has an apoprotein content. Apoproteins are distinguished alphabetically and numerically as apo A-1 through apo E. Apo A-1 is associated with HDL and apo B-100 is associated with LDL. New factors that affect CAD have now been shown to be of clinical use and may change the course of treatment approach:

1. Some investigators have found that the concentration of apo A-1 and apo B-100 are better predictors of CAD than are measurements of total plasm lipids or lipoproteins. The greater the ratio of apo A-1 to apo B-100, the lesser the risk for development of CAD.
2. Lipoprotein-a or LP(a) has been established as an independent CAD risk factor. If serum levels of both LDL and LP(a) are elevated, the risk of CAD is markedly increased.
3. LDL cholesterol is further categorized into pattern A and pattern B, the latter being small and dense LDL and associated with a threefold increase of CAD risk. Of importance is the treatment: Gemfibrozil reduces small LDL in pattern B but not pattern A.

Medications used to treat hypercholesterolemia and their effects on the different lipoproteins are listed in Tables 7.1 and 7.2 (12).

THE SIMPLE APPROACH

1. Virtually all patients with atherosclerotic disease (if there are no contraindications) should be treated (usually with a statin).
2. Therapy should be implemented immediately rather than waiting for diet.

Table 7.1
Medications Used to Treat Hypercholesterolemia

Medication	Dosage range	Maintenance dosage	Cost of maintenance therapy[a]
Bile acid sequestrants: Colestipol (Colestid)	5 g twice daily to 30 g daily	5 g twice daily	$ 45.00[b]
		30 g per day, in divided doses	134.00
Cholestyramine (Questran, Questran Lite)	4 to 24 g per day	4 g twice daily	35.00[c]
		8 g twice daily	70.00
		12 g twice daily	104.00
Nicotinic acid	500 mg to 2 g three times daily	1.5 g in divided doses	3.00–7.00[d]
		2 g in divided doses	4.00–10.00
		3 g in divided doses	5.00–14.00
		4 g in divided doses	7.00–19.00
		5 g in divided doses	8.00–22.00
		6 g in divided doses	11.00–29.00

(continued)

Table 7.1 *(continued)*

Medication	Dosage range	Maintenance dosage	Cost of maintenance therapy[a]
Statins[e]:			
Fluvastatin (Lescol)	20 to 40 mg at bedtime	20 mg at bedtime	31.00
		20 mg twice daily	61.00
		40 mg at bedtime	34.00
Lovastatin (Mevacor)	20 to 80 mg with evening meal	20 mg with evening meal	60.00
		40 mg with evening meal	108.00
		80 mg with evening meal	216.00
Pravastatin (Pravachol)	10 to 40 mg at bedtime	10 mg at bedtime	50.00
		20 mg at bedtime	55.00
		40 mg at bedtime	92.00
Simvastin (Zocor)	5 to 40 mg at bedtime	5 mg at bedtime	53.00
		10 mg at bedtime	54.00
		20 mg at bedtime	98.00
		40 mg at bedtime	103.00
Fibric acid analogs			
Gemfibrozil (Lopid)	600 mg twice daily	600 mg twice daily	66.00[f]
Probucol (Lorelco)	500 mg with morning and evening meal	500 mg with morning and evening meal	70.00

[a] Costs represent average wholesale price for a 1-month supply, rounded to nearest dollar amount, in Red book. Montvale JJ. Medical Economics Date, 1995.

[b] Costs represent price of canister. Product is also available in packet form at higher cost.

[c] Costs represent price of canister. Product is also available in packet form at higher cost.

[d] Costs represent price range of generics.

[e] Statins are HMG CoA reductase inhibitors.

Table 7.2
Effects of Current Medications on Lipid Levels in the Management of Hypercholesterolemia

Medication	Total serum cholesterol level	LDL level	HDL level	Triglyceride level
Cholestryamine (Questran)	18% decrease	24% decrease	6% increase	10% increase
Colestipol (Colestid)	18% decrease	24% decrease	6% increase	10% increase
Gemfibrozil (Lopid)	11% decrease	12% decrease	15% increase	40% decrease
Lovastatin (Mevacor)	34% decrease	42% decrease	10% increase	24% decrease
Nicotinic acid (Lipo-Nicin, Nicolar)	20% decrease	25% decrease	10% increase	24% decrease
Pravastatin (Pravachol)	20% decrease	27% decrease	13% increase	7% decrease
Simvastatin (Zocor)	32% decrease	38% decrease	3% increase	15% decrease
Probucol (Lorelco)	10% decrease	10% decrease	23% decrease	3% decrease

Table 7.3
Classification of Blood Pressure for Adults 18 years and Older*

Category	Systolic blood pressure (mm Hg)	Diastolic blood pressure (mm Hg)
Normal	<130	<85
High normal	130–139	85–89
Hypertension†		
Stage 1 (mild)	140–159	90–99
Stage 2 (moderate)	160–179	100–109
Stage 3 (severe)	180–209	110–119
Stage 4 (very severe)	≥210	≥120

* Classification based on the average of two or more readings on two or more occasions in individuals who are not taking antihypertensive drugs and who are not acutely ill.

SBP = systolic blood pressure, DBP = diastolic BP. When systolic and diastolic pressures fall into different categories, the higher category should be selected to classify the individual's blood pressure status.

† Optimal blood pressure with respect to cardiovascular disease risk is <120 mm Hg systolic and <80 mm Hg diastolic. However, usually low readings should be evaluated for clinical significance.

Rationale for above:

- Lipid lowering reduces rate of myocardial infarction (MI) by 30% over 5 years. Benefits are also noted in decreasing frequency of angina and need for revascularization.
- Data suggests that lowering LDL-C to as low as 60 mg/dL should be of benefit.

DISORDERS FOR WHICH TREATMENT MUST GO BEYOND LDL CHOLESTEROL REDUCTION (13)

1. Familial heterozygous hypercholesterolemia.
2. Familial hyperlipidemia and hypoalphalipoproteinemia.
3. Hyperbetalipoproteinemia.
4. Homocystinemia.
5. Disorders of Lp(a).
6. ALP-LDL subclass pattern B.

Hypertension

Nearly 60 million American adults, roughly 30% of American adults, have hypertension (Table 7.3) (14). Both systolic and diastolic pressure are risk factors, even for the elderly. Blood pressure levels and end-organ damage are used as clinical markers in the estimation of hypertension severity. End-organ damage include the brain (strokes), eyes (retinopathy), heart (left ventricular hypertrophy), and kidneys (decreased renal function). A meta-analysis by MacMahon and colleagues of nine prospective studies showed a strongly positive relationship between both systolic and diastolic blood pressure and coronary heart disease (15). There is considerable evidence that reducing blood pressure decreases the development of cardiovascular disease events, including CAD, stroke, and congestive heart failure (14). Control of hypertension involves diet, exercise, and drug therapy. Many drugs are effective in treating hypertension in patients with coronary artery disease; the most notable classes are β blockers, calcium channel blockers, and the angiotensin-converting enzyme inhibitor drugs.

Diabetes Mellitus

The National Diabetes Data Group defines diabetes as a fasting blood sugar greater than 140 mg/dL. This abnormality is present in approximately 10% of adult Americans. Strong epidemiologic and clinical evidence indicates that diabetes mellitus (both insulin-dependent and non–insulin-dependent diabetes mellitus) is a major risk factor for CAD. Atherosclerosis accounts for 80% of diabetic mortality (16); CAD alone is responsible for 75% of total atherosclerotic death; the remainder results from stroke and peripheral vascular disease. It is estimated that 25% of all heart attacks in the United States occur in patients with diabetes.

Diabetes frequently exists in the presence of other risk factors. Hypertension and obesity are common in diabetics. The typical lipid disorder in diabetics is increased plasma triglyceride, decreased HDL cholesterol, and small, dense LDL particles. Resistance to insulin may play a role in the lipid disorder of diabetes.

Treatment of diabetes should emphasize maintenance of ideal body weight, appropriate diet, and a sensible exercise program. On the basis of the known adverse effects of prolonged hyperglycemia, strict glucose control may play a major role in reducing the risk of CAD.

Estrogen Deficiency

Women have a delay in onset of CAD of 10 years relative to men. MI and sudden death are delayed by 20 years and most commonly occur after 55 years of age in women. The fact that protection conferred upon women seems to be lost after natural menopause supports the concept that endogenous estrogen protects women against vascular injury. Several large prospective studies have yielded statistically significant protective effects of estrogen in postmenopausal women. Bush and colleagues noted that estrogen users had a higher mean HDL cholesterol level and significantly lower LDL cholesterol levels; it was noted that after 9 years, estrogen users had a 64% lower risk of CAD mortality than non users (17). Grady and colleagues reported a decrease in CAD (as well as a decrease in hip fractures) in women on hormone-replacement therapy (18). An increase in endometrial carcinoma is found among women on unopposed replacement therapy (estrogen without progesterone).

Obesity and Physical Inactivity

Approximately 34 million Americans are overweight, 12.4 million of which are severely overweight. Obesity itself predisposes hyperlipidemia, diabetes, and hypertension; therefore, the role of weight reduction in the treatment of these diseases makes it an obvious choice for an intervention (Table 7.4). Moreover, increased physical activity favorably influences lipoprotein levels, blood pressure, weight, glucose tolerance, and cardiovascular and pulmonary functional capacity.

Nonmodifiable Risks

Family History

Family history of heart disease is one of the most powerful determinants of CAD. The NCEP defines a family history of premature coronary heart disease as a definite MI or sudden death before 55 years of age in a father or other male first-degree relative or before 65 years of age in a mother or other female first-degree relative.

Age and Gender

CAD risk increases nearly linearly with age and is greater in men compared to women until approximately 75 years of age, when the prevalence is nearly equal. Before 55 years of age, the incidence of CAD among men is three to four times that in women.

Table 7.4
Guide to Comprehensive Risk Reduction for Patients With Coronary and Other Vascular Disease

Risk intervention	Recommendations
Smoking: Goal: Complete cessation	Strongly encourage patient and family to stop smoking. Provide counseling, nicotine replacement, and formal cessation programs as appropriate.
Lipid management: *Primary goal* LDL <100 mg/dL *Secondary goals* HDL >35 mg/dL TG <200 mg/dL	Start AHA Step II Diet in all patients: ≤30% fat, <7% saturated fat, <200 mg/dL cholesterol. Assess fasting lipid profile. In post-MI patients, lipid profile may take 4–6 weeks to stabilize. Add drug therapy according to the following guide: LDL <100 mg/dL — No drug therapy LDL 100 to 130 mg/dL — Consider adding drug therapy to diet, as follows: Suggested drug therapy TG <200 mg/dL — Statin, Resin, Niacin TG 200–400 mg/dL — Statin, Niacin TG >400 mg/dL — Consider combined drug therapy (niacin, fibrate, statin) If LDL goal not achieved, consider combination therapy. LDL >130 mg/dL — Add drug therapy to diet as follows: HDL <35 mg/dL — Emphasize weight management and physical activity. Advise smoking cessation. If needed to achieve LDL goals, consider niacin, statin, fibrate.

(continued)

Table 7.4 *(continued)*

Risk intervention	Recommendations
Physical activity: *Minimum goal:* 30 minutes 3–4 times per week	Assess risk, preferably with exercise test, to guide prescription. Encourage minimum of 30–60 minutes of moderate-intensity activity 3 or 4 times weekly (walking, jogging, cycling, or other aerobic activity) supplemented by an increase in daily life-style activities (e.g., walking breaks at work, using stairs, gardening, household work). Maximum benefit 5–6 hours per week. Advise medically supervised programs for moderate- to high-risk patients.
Weight management:	Start intensive diet and appropriate physical activity intervention, as outline above, in patients >120% of ideal weight for height. Particularly emphasize need for weight loss in patients with hypertension, elevated triglycerides or elevated glucose levels.
Antiplatelet agents anticoagulants:	Start aspirin 80–325 mg/dL if not contraindicated. Manage warfarin to international normalized ratio = 2–3.5 for post-MI patients not able to take aspirin.
ACE inhibitors post-MI:	Start early post-MI in stable high-risk patients (anterior MI, previous MI, Killip class II [S_3 gallop, rales, radiographic CHF]). Continue indefinitely for all with LV dysfunction (ejection fraction ≤40%) or symptoms of failure. Use as needed to manage blood pressure or symptoms in all other patients.
β blockers:	Start in high-risk post-MI patients (arrhythmia, LV dysfunction, inducible ischemia) at 5–28 days. Continue 6 months minimum. Observe usual contraindications. Use as needed to manage angina, rhythm or blood pressure in all other patients.
Estrogens:	Consider estrogen replacement in all postmenopausal women. Individualize recommendation consistent with other health risks.
Blood pressure control: *Goal* ≤140/90 mm Hg	Initiate life-style modification—weight control, physical activity, alcohol moderation, and moderate sodium restriction—in all patients with blood pressure >140 mm Hg systolic or 90 mm Hg diastolic. Add blood pressure medication, individualized to other patient requirements and characteristics (i.e., age, race, need for drugs with specific benefits) if blood pressure is not less than 140 mm Hg systolic or 90 mm Hg diastolic in 3 months or if *initial* blood pressure is >160 mm Hg systolic or 100 mm Hg diastolic.

After 55 years of age, the rate of increase with age in men declines and the rate of increase in women escalates. In the post-MI setting, older patients are at higher subsequent risk of death than younger patients, and the effects of age predominate over other risk factors (19).

Prevention

Preventive services are provided less often than experts recommend and less frequently than patients and their physicians prefer. For example, in a primary care setting, 75% of patients who smoke say they would attempt to stop smoking if their physician advised them to do so, but only 40–55% report that their physician provided such advice to them (20). Recent studies reveal that only 45–65% of patients with hypercholesterolemia had evidence of treatment (21). The following guide by Smith outlines the steps to risk reduction for patients with CAD (22).

References

1. Bartecchi CE, MacKenzie TK, Schriere RW. The human cost of tobacco use. N Engl J Med 1994;30:9097.

2. Rigotti NA, Pasternak RC. Cigarette smoking and coronary heart disease. Cardiol Clin 1996;14:51.

3. Rosenberg L, Palmer JR, Shapiro S. Decline in the risk of myocardial infarction among women who stop smoking. N Engl J Med 1990;322:213.

4. Rosenberg L, Kaufman DW, Helmrich SP, et al. The risk of myocardial infarction after quitting smoking in men under 55 years of age. N Engl J Med 1985;313:1511.

5. Cavender JB, Rogers WJ, Fisher LK, et al. Coronary artery surgery study (CASS): 10 year follow-up. J Am Coll Cardiol 1992;20:287.

6. Summary of The Second Report of the National Cholesterol Education Program (NCEP) Expert Panel of Detection, Evaluation, and Treatment of High Blood Cholesterol in Adults. JAMA 1993;269:3015.

7. The Scandinavian Simvastatin Survival Study (4S). Randomized trial of cholesterol lowering in 4444 patients with coronary heart disease. Lancet 1994;344:1383.

8. Shephard J, Cobbe SM, Ford I, et al. Prevention of coronary heart disease with Pravastatin in men with hypercholesterolemia. N Engl J Med 1995;333:1301.

9. Watts GF, Lewis B, Brunt JNH, et al. Effects on coronary artery disease of lipid-lowering diet, or diet plus cholestyramine. The St. Thomas' Atherosclerotic Regression Study (STARS). Lancet 1992;339:563.

10. Haskell WL, Alderman EL, Fair JM, et al. The Stanford Coronary Risk Intervention Project (SCRIP). Circulation 1994;89:975.

11. Jukema JE, Bruschke AVG, van Boven AJ, et al. The Regression Growth Evaluation Statin Study (REGRESS). Circulation 1995;9:2528.

12. Blake GH, Triplett LC. Management of hypercholesterolemia. Am Fam Physician 1995;51:1157.

13. Superko HR. Beyond LDL cholesterol reduction. Circulation 1996;94:2351.

14. The Fifth Report of the Joint National Committee on Detection, Evaluation, and Treatment of High Blood Pressure (JNC V), Arch Intern Med 153:154, 1993.

15. MacMahon S, Peto R, Cutler J, et al. Blood pressure, stroke and coronary heart disease. Part 1. Prolonged differences in blood pressure: prospective observational studies corrected for the regression dilution bias. Lancet 1990;335:765.

16. Schwartz CJ, Valente AJ, Sprague EA, et al. Pathogenesis of the atherosclerotic lesion. Implications for diabetes mellitus. Circulation 1992;15:1156.

17. Bush RL, Barrett-Conner E, Cowan LD, et al. Cardiovascular mortality and noncontraceptive use of estrogen in women: results from the Lipid Research Clinics Program Follow-up Study. Circulation 1987;75:1102.

18. Grady D, Rubin SM, Petitti DB, et al. Hormone therapy to prevent disease and prolong life in postmenopausal women. Ann Intern Med 1992;117:1016.

19. Pasternak RC. Task Force 3. Spectrum of risk factors for coronary heart disease. J Am Coll Cardiol 1996;27:978.

20. Anda RF. Are physicians advising smokers to quit? The patient's perspective. JAMA 1987;257:1916.

21. Kottke TE. The systematic practice of preventive cardiology. Am J Cardiol 1987;59:690.

22. Smith SC. Preventing heart disease and death in patients with coronary disease. Circulation 1995;92:2.

Angina Pectoris

Angina pectoris results from an imbalance between myocardial oxygen supply and demand and is most commonly caused by the inability of atherosclerotic coronary arteries to perfuse the heart under conditions of increased myocardial oxygen consumption (demand). Angina also occurs in patients with seemingly normal coronary arteries that are subjected to acute or chronic increases in myocardial work such as aortic stenosis, hypertension, or hypertrophic cardiomyopathy or decreases in supply such as anemia. An increase in coronary vasomotor tone or frank coronary artery spasm, superimposed upon normal or diseased arteries, can provoke pain in the absence of increased myocardial demands and has been shown to be responsible for variant (Prinzmetal's) angina and certain cases of unstable angina. Last, there is a sizable group of patients who have angina without evidence of coronary artery disease, with or without an increase in myocardial work. This latter syndrome has been termed "syndrome X" because of its enigmatic nature.

TYPICAL ANGINA

Description

Character

Most often described as a discomfort, pressure, heaviness, or squeezing sensation and not a pain. Less commonly described as burning or sharp.

Location

Most often in the substernal area, precordium, or epigastrium with radiation to the left arm, jaw, or neck. Less commonly felt only in radiation areas and not in the chest.

Precipitation

Often provoked by exertion, emotion, cold weather, eating, or smoking and relieved by rest, removal of provoking factors, or sublingual nitrates.

Duration

Usually lasts a few minutes, rarely more than 30 minutes.

Evaluation

History

The diagnosis of angina pectoris (AP) is established by obtaining a reliable description of the chest discomfort and its relationship to activity. The likelihood of underlying coronary artery disease is enhanced by a history of hypertension, diabetes mellitus, hyperlipidemia, or smoking or a family history of premature ischemic heart disease in first-degree relatives (age younger than 55 years).

Physical Examination

Although often normal, examination may yield important confirmatory information, i.e., hypertension, peripheral arterial disease, xanthelasma, tendinous xanthomata, tobacco-stained fingers or teeth, or diagonally creased earlobes. Episodic ischemia alters left ventricular compliance. Thus, a transient S_4, S_3, and/or apical systolic murmur (due to papillary muscle dysfunction) may be heard during an anginal chest pain episode.

Blood Chemistry

Basic screening is important to identify potentially treatable risk factors such as hypercholesterolemia and/or hyperglycemia. Hypertriglyceridemia is less well established as a risk factor. High low-density lipoprotein (LDL) is a risk factor, whereas elevated high-density lipoprotein (HDL) is protective against coronary heart disease. A complete blood count should be obtained to check for the presence of anemia. Thyroid function tests should be performed if hyperthyroidism is suspected.

Electrocardiogram

The electrocardiogram (ECG) is often normal in the absence of a myocardial infarction (MI) or a cause for left ventricular hypertrophy. An ECG during angina may show transient ST depression, T wave inversion, or ventricular arrhythmias. An ambulatory ECG (Holter) may demonstrate ischemic episodes with or without the patient having symptoms ("silent ischemia").

Exercise Stress Testing

Exercise stress testing (EST) (see Chapter 3) is invaluable in reproducing symptoms, documenting ischemic ECG changes, and assessing the level of disability. Patients with high-grade coronary artery disease may manifest inability to increase heart rate or blood pressure during exercise, angina may develop, or marked ST changes at low stress levels that persist after exercise may develop. Exercise-induced arrhythmias or left ventricular dysfunction provide diagnostic information with important therapeutic potential. **Radionuclide scintigraphy** (see Chapter 5) enhances the sensitivity and specificity of EST. In patients with significant coronary arterial obstructions, exercise-induced "cold spots" will usually develop on thallium or sestamibi perfusion scanning or left ventricular wall motion abnormalities will develop during nuclear scanning.

Coronary Arteriography

Although not necessary for the diagnosis of coronary artery disease in most instances, cardiac catheterization and coronary angiography permit localization and quantification of obstructive lesions, evaluation of left ventricular function, and assessment of any valvular or myocardial distal. The indications for these invasive studies vary widely in different centers. Widely accepted indications include the following:

• Angina refractory to medical management.
• Angina or MI in patients younger than 45 years of age.
• Unstable angina (after medical stabilization).
• Patients with persistent angina and/or low level EST abnormalities after MI.
• Marked (0.2 mV) ST changes at low-level exercise or persisting several minutes after cessation of EST.
• Suspected Prinzmetal's (variant) angina (coronary vasospasm).
• Preoperative evaluation of patients with valvular or congenital heart disease.

- Patients with life-threatening arrhythmias associated with ischemic heart disease.
- When needed for clarification of possible causes for recurrent chest pain when noninvasive testing has yielded negative or equivocal findings.

General Therapeutic Considerations

General Measures

Conditions that exacerbate or provoke angina should be sought in all patients. Treatment of anemia, arrhythmia, hyperthyroidism, and hypertension may relieve angina.

Risk Factor Reduction

Cessation of smoking, control of hypertension and diabetes, lowering cholesterol and lipids (initially by diet), and maintaining an ideal body weight are strongly advised.

Exercise

The role of exercise for patients with known ischemic heart disease remains controversial. It has been established that regular exercise can lower the heart rate and blood pressure at rest and, during submaximal workloads, favorably modify the blood lipid composition, consume calories, and provide psychological benefits. For certain patients, regular exercise may lessen cigarette smoking and result in more prudent eating habits. However, the widely held concepts that exercise causes regression of coronary atherosclerosis, increases collateral formation, improves ventricular performance, and prolongs life lack rigorous scientific proof. On the debit side, exercise causes an increase in the cardiac double product (heart rate × blood pressure), which increases myocardial oxygen demand. Exercise can threaten the supply/demand balance of the myocardium and can produce ischemic dysfunction and arrhythmias in certain patients with latent or overt coronary artery disease. Therefore, a "prescription" for exercise must be written carefully with the knowledge of each individual patient taken into consideration.

General Comments on Medical Therapy

Because the overall prognosis of stable angina is relatively good (annual mortality of 1.6–3.3%), many patients can be managed with medical therapy (1). The goal of drug therapy is to abolish or reduce angina and ischemia and to promote a normal life. The pharmacologic approach depends on the severity of the symptoms, side effect of the drugs, and the patient's response. Three major classes of drugs with different mechanisms of action are available and account for the improvement in medical therapy over the last decade. Optimal treatment with nitrates, β blockers, and calcium blockers will result in marked improvement or complete relief of symptoms in most patients (2).

Drug Therapy

Nitrates

The mechanism of action of nitrates in relieving angina is largely caused by a decrease in left ventricular work (by reducing venous return and preload, a determinant of myocardial oxygen demand) and a lesser extent by coronary vasodilatation and improved collateral flow (3). Other factors include decreased left ventricular end-diastolic pressure, which enhances subendocardial flow, and inhibition of coronary spasm. There is also some decrease in demand by decreasing systemic arterial compliance and lowering afterload.

Nitrates are safe and are considered to be the first line of therapy for stable angina pectoris. Short-acting nitrates are used for the relief of the acute attacks, whereas long-acting nitrates are used for antianginal prophylaxis (see Chapter 18 for individual nitrate drugs).

Nitrate Tolerance. It is not possible to provide continuous antianginal and anti-ischemic prophylaxis throughout the dosing interval with any of the nitrate preparations. With continuous application of the drug at a constant rate, tolerance can develop within 24 hours, and further therapy results in complete loss of the antianginal effect (4). The magnitude of tolerance varies with the nitrate preparation and the route of administration. Tolerance may be complete with constant dosing of patches or slow-release compounds or partial with the oral drugs that have peaks and valleys in plasma concentrations.

Providing a nitrate-free interval is the strategy for preventing tolerance. With oral isosorbide dinitrate, dosing at 7:00 am, 12:00 noon, and 5:00 pm seems to avoid tolerance problems.

With a patch-free interval of 10–12 hours, patches retain their effectiveness.

Contraindications. Contraindications are hypersensitivity, hypotension, and hypovolemia. A relative contraindication may be severe nitrate-induced headaches, although the severity of headaches usually decreases with continued use of the drug.

β-Adrenergic Blocking Agents

These agents competitively occupy β-receptor myocardial sites (β-1 receptors) and thus block the chronotropic and inotropic actions of catecholamines on the heart. In combination with nitrates, they can often prevent angina in a large percentage of patients with chronic stable angina (1). Noncardiac β receptors (β-2 receptors) in arterial walls and bronchial smooth muscle are also blocked by nonselective β blockers. Some β blockers have the capacity to activate the β-1 receptor and are referred to as having intrinsic sympathomimetic activity (ISA). Some newer agents also have a quinidine-like effect (referred to as membrane stabilizing effect). The principal mechanism of action with β-blocker therapy is β-1-receptor blockade, which results in a reduction of heart rate and myocardial contractility. Other beneficial effects include attenuating systolic blood pressure rise during exercise, lessening exercise-induced vasoconstriction, and increasing diastolic filling time. (See Chapter 18 for individual β-blocker drugs.)

All β blockers, irrespective of properties of cardioselectivity, ISA, and membrane stabilization, are effective for patients with stable angina who do not have other concomitant disease. Cardioselective agents are preferred for patients with angina and coexisting peripheral vascular disease, diabetes, or asthma. Some patients do not respond to β-blocker therapy because of the severity of their underlying CAD or because of congestive heart failure resulting from an excess in negative inotropic effect.

It is customary to adjust the dose of β blocker to secure a resting heart rate between 50 and 60 beats/min and an exercise heart rate less than 100 beats/min. β blockers should not be discontinued abruptly; if necessary, they should be tapered off gradually over a 10-day period.

Precautions and Contraindications. Overt congestive heart failure at rest is an absolute contraindication to the use of β blockers because of the dependence of the failing myocardium on intrinsic adrenergic mechanisms. Severe bronchospasm is an absolute contraindication to use of nonselective β blockers and a relative contraindication to the use of selective β-1 blockers. Insulin-dependent diabetes mellitus is a relative contraindication to all β blockers because the adrenergic response to hypoglycemia will be masked or blunted.

Many patients with chronic obstructive pulmonary disease (COPD; nonreversible airway obstruction due to emphysema) or well-controlled diabetes mellitus in combination with ischemic heart disease can tolerate and benefit greatly from β blockers administered cautiously with close follow-up observation. Similarly, patients with left ventricular dysfunction (ejection fraction 30–50%) that worsens with exercise can also benefit from cautious use of β blockers because the myocardial supply/demand imbalance during exercise may be substantially decreased.

Noncardioselective β blockers, by inhibiting β-mediated arteriolar dilation, may worsen chest pain in some patients with coronary vasospasm and may be poorly tolerated by patients with severe peripheral arterial disease. Systemic side effects in those patients at risk seem to be less with cardioselective blockers.

Calcium-Blocking Agents

Calcium channel blockers are a diverse group of compounds that inhibit calcium channel currents in cardiac and smooth muscle and have been shown to be effective for relief or prevention of angina (5). The mechanism of action is by afterload reduction, which decreases myocardial contractility and inhibits coronary vasoconstriction. (See Chapter 18 for individual calcium channel blocker drugs.)

Properties peculiar to each specific calcium blocker may be helpful in selecting a particular agent and depend on clinical circumstances. The hemodynamic effects of verapamil and diltiazem are similar to those of nonselective β blockers (decrease heart rate, decrease arterial pressure, decrease contractility). Nifedipine is a more potent arteriolar dilator than verapamil or diltiazem and thus is probably a preferable choice for patients with hypertension or congestive heart failure (CHF). Verapamil has the most negative inotropic effects and is not well tolerated in patients with moderate to severe left ventricular dysfunction.

Patients with recurrent, symptomatic reentrant supraventricular tachyarrhythmias are better treated with verapamil or diltiazem. For those with sick sinus syndrome, nifedipine would be the best choice.

Side effects from the vasodilatory properties of calcium channel blockers include palpitations, headache, flushing, hypotension, ankle edema, constipation, and abdominal discomfort. The negative inotropic effects may cause myocardial depression. The atrioventricular (AV) nodal delay may cause heart block.

Percutaneous Revascularization

Percutaneous transluminal coronary angioplasty (PTCA) is an effective treatment method for many patients with disabling symptoms and those with significantly jeopardized myocardium (6). PTCA was initially used mainly in the treatment of single and select cases of double-vessel disease but has been expanded to more complex cases with multivessel disease. PTCA is an attractive alternative to bypass surgery for many patients because of the decreased hospital time, major reduction in expense, minimal recovery time, and less operative insult. Relief of symptoms is usually seen in conjunction with objective improvement in exercise performance and improvement in ST changes. Restenosis continues to be a problem in approximately 30% of patients and is often heralded by recurrence of symptoms.

Coronary stenting and atherectomy techniques have greatly enhanced the ability to treat patients with angina and coronary artery disease and coronary graft disease.

Coronary Artery Bypass Grafting (CABG)

Coronary revascularization can provide significant relief from angina for more than 80% of patients with angina refractory to drug therapy and has a low operative mortality (1–2%) in patients with good left ventricular function. It continues to be a very common major operative procedure performed in the United States. Because it neither reverses the disease process nor ensures permanent revascularization, the use of the procedure should be limited to patients who cannot be managed medically (risk factor modification, nitrates, β blockers, and calcium channel blockers), patients who have failed angioplasty, or patients with significant obstruction of the main left coronary artery or significant obstruction (>70%) in all major arteries. Graft closure and recurrence of symptoms continues to be a problem with this form of therapy. The first-year saphenous vein graft closure rate is 10–15% and subsequently is 1–2% per year. The use of the internal mammary artery has markedly increased because of its superior long-term patency rates (90% in 10 years) and the unusual lack of atherosclerosis in this particular conduit.

UNSTABLE ANGINA

It is generally recognized that unstable angina pectoris (UAP) results from an interplay between fixed coronary artery disease and dynamic factors that contribute to intermittent coronary occlusion. UAP is probably not a single entity but a combination of syndromes. It is classified clinically into crescendo angina, non-Q-wave MI, new-onset angina with accelerating symptoms, and post-MI angina.

Description

The **character, location,** and **radiation** of chest discomfort may be similar to that of stable AP, although it is often more intense. UAP is distinguished from AP by the presence of one or more of the following criteria:

- **Precipitation.** May occur at rest or at a lower activity level compared with AP and may be less responsive to nitrates.
- **Duration.** May last longer than AP, up to several hours in some cases.
- **Frequency.** May occur more frequently than stable AP.
- **ECG changes.** More common than AP, UAP is often accompanied by reversible ECG changes of ischemia or injury. Such ECG changes may herald a poor long-term outcome (death due to a fatal cardiac event).

Clinical Manifestations

Unstable angina usually presents in one of the following ways:

- Abrupt onset of ischemic symptoms at rest or precipitated by effort in a patient without history of CAD.
- Intensification or change in pattern of ischemic symptoms in a patient with stable angina.

• Recurrence of ischemic symptoms soon (24 hours) after an acute MI.

Pathophysiology

Like chronic stable AP, UAP often represents an imbalance between supply and demand; however, in UAP, the level of demand is not always measurably increased. In contrast, patients with UAP develop symptoms due to a dynamic decrease in myocardial oxygen delivery. Angiographic studies have shown that patients with stable and unstable angina do not differ from each other when traditional indexes of the severity of CAD (number of significantly diseased vessels, percent of stenosis, and collaterals) are examined. However, antemortem angiographic investigations and postmortem studies show that at least 70% of patients with UAP have eccentric, irregular stenosis or hazy or radiolucent defects in the culprit lesion, whereas these features are infrequent (less than 20%) in patients with stable angina (7). These studies and information from coronary angioscopy have demonstrated the culprit lesion in UAP to be complex with fissures or cracks in the fibrous cap of the plaque. Whatever the mechanism of plaque fissure, it may result in increasing obstruction by triggering dynamic factors that contribute to intermittent coronary occlusion. These important factors include vasomotor tone, intermittent platelet aggregation, and intraluminal thrombus (8). When plaque fissure and these factors cause brief periods of coronary occlusion, the result is unstable angina.

Platelet aggregation has been shown to be an important factor in experimental studies in the setting of partially occluded coronary arteries. Pretreatment of experimental animals with aspirin before acute coronary occlusion has been shown to reduce the incidence of ventricular fibrillation and to increase collateral blood flow. Clinical evidence of platelet activation during UAP includes elevated levels of products of activation such as β-thromboglobulin, platelet factor 4, thromboxane metabolites, and prostaglandins. **Platelet microemboli** in the myocardial microvasculature downstream from the culprit coronary lesion as well as the protective effect of aspirin in UAP against MI underscore the importance of platelet aggregation in this setting.

Several angiographic studies have shown **intracoronary thrombosis** in a high percentage (50–80%) of UAP patients with recent symptoms. Histopathologic studies have confirmed the high prevalence of intraluminal thrombus at the site of the fissured plaque. In this regard, the effect of heparin on the development of transmural MI in randomized patients with unstable angina has been studied. Heparin significantly decreased the occurrence of acute MI, suggesting an important role of acute coronary thrombosis.

Coronary vasoconstriction superimposed on a fixed stenotic lesion may lead to total occlusion, infarction and cardiac death. It is unclear whether vasoconstriction alone can cause sufficiently severe ischemia to cause MI or if there is superimposed localized platelet aggregation with intimal injury and thrombus formation.

Evaluation

The evaluation of a patient with UAP should follow that described for stable angina, with the exception that EST should not be performed until the patient has been hospitalized and found to be clinically stable and free of pain for more than 24 hours. The presence of ECG changes of ischemia or injury during spontaneous UAP often precludes the necessity for EST. It is important to stratify patients with UAP into high-, intermediate-, or low-risk groups because this determines the subsequent therapeutic strategies. The three major determinants of this risk stratification are the likelihood of CAD, the tempo of recent clinical events (frequency, severity, duration, precipitating causes of chest pain), and the patient's likelihood of surviving a cardiac event (9) (see Tables 8.1 and 8.2).

Therapeutic Considerations

Patients with low-risk UAP may be managed as outpatients with early follow-up evaluations. Outpatient evaluation basically consists of stress testing. Hospitalization with imposition of bed rest and sedation in an ECG-monitored environment is absolutely indicated for patients with UAP classified as high and intermediate risk. Hypertension and other extra cardiac factors increasing demand or decreasing supply should be aggressively treated.

Nitrates

Sublingual nitroglycerin (0.4 mg) or isosorbide dinitrate (5 mg) should be administered for spontaneous episodes of pain with

Table 8.1
Likelihood of Significant CAD in Patients with Symptoms Suggesting UAP

High likelihood	Intermediate likelihood	Low likelihood
Any of the following features	Absence of high likelihood and features of any of the following:	Absence of high and intermediate features met may have:
Known history of CAD	Definite angina	Chest pain probably not angina
Definite angina pectoris	Probable angina	One risk factor not diabetes
Hemodynamic and ECG changes with pain	Probably not angina in diabetics or in nondiabetics with ≥ 2 other risk factors	
Variant angina	Extracardiac vascular disease	
ST segment increase or decrease ≥ 1 mm with pain	ST depression 0.5–1.0 mm	T wave flat or inverted ≤ 1 mm in dominant R wave leads
Marked symmetrical T wave inversion in multiple precordial leads	T wave inversion ≥ 1 mm in leads with dominant R waves	Normal ECG

monitoring of ECG and blood pressure changes with pain and after nitrates. For long-acting nitrate therapy, topical or oral nitrates may be used. Intravenous nitroglycerin may offer the most consistent relief of acute ischemic episodes and is often used in the more difficult cases. The starting dose is 5 μg/min and is then increased up to 200 μg/min as tolerated to control pain.

β Blockers

β blockers are administered in sufficient intravenous doses for high-risk patients and oral doses for intermediate- and low-risk patients to achieve a resting heart rate between 50 and 60 bpm.

Heparin

Heparin has been shown to reduce the risk of sudden cardiac death, MI, and recurrent ischemic events in the setting of UAP.

Table 8.2
Short-Term Risk of Death or Nonfatal MI in Patients with Symptoms Suggesting UAP

High risk	Intermediate risk	Low risk
At least one of the following features must be present:	No high-risk feature, but must have any of the following:	No high or intermediate risk feature but may have any of the following:
Prolonged ongoing (>20 min) rest pain	Rest angina now resolved, but not low likelihood or CAD	Increased angina frequency, severity, or duration
Pulmonary edema	Rest angina (>20 min or exertional angina relieved with rest or nitroglycerin)	Angina provoked at a lower threshold
Angina with new or worsening mitral regurgitation murmurs	Angina with dynamic T wave changes	New onset angina within 2 weeks to 2 months
Rest angina with dynamic ST changes ≥1 mm	Nocturnal angina	Normal or unchanged ECG
Angina with S3 or rales	New onset CCSC III or IV angina in past 2 weeks, but not low likelihood of CAD	
Angina with hypotension	Q waves or ST depression ≥1 mm in multiple leads	
	Age >65 years	

Unless there is a contraindication, full-dose heparin anticoagulation seems to be a logical therapy in the early coronary care unit (CCU) setting followed by chronic low-dose aspirin for patients with intermediate- or high-risk UAP.

Aspirin

Because platelet aggregation has been strongly implicated in the pathogenesis of unstable angina and MI, aspirin (a platelet inhibitor) was studied in a large Veterans Administration (VA) cooperative double-blind study to test whether endpoints of death and MI were altered. The data showed a 51% lower incidence of myocardial infarction and death in the aspirin group (324 mg/day) as compared to the placebo group (10). Aspirin causes irreversible acetylation of platelet cyclooxygenase, thereby preventing the formation of thromboxane A_2, an extremely potent vasoconstrictor and platelet activator. Even though the VA trial used 324 mg of aspirin, it is generally conceded that lower doses (1 mg/kg/day) work as well and are less inhibitory to the arterial endothelium's production of prostacyclin than higher doses.

Calcium Blockers

Calcium blockers are recommended to control ongoing pain, significant hypertension, or recurrent ischemia in patients who are unresponsive to aspirin, heparin, nitrates, and β blockers. Dihydropyridines may cause reflex tachycardia, with resultant worsening of angina. These agents should not be used in the absence of concurrent β blockade.

Thrombolytic Therapy

Because of the recognized role of thrombus formation in UAP, it would seem logical to assume that thrombolysis would be appropriate therapy. However, data from the TIMI IIIB randomized trial of 1473 patients showed no difference in the major outcomes (death or MI) or in the secondary outcomes (evidence of residual ischemia by Holter or exercise tests) between patients with UAP randomized into either a tissue-plasminogen activator (t-PA) or a placebo arm (11). Based on the absence of clinical benefit, a higher incidence of MI and risk of intracranial hemorrhage, it is recommended that thrombolytic therapy with t-PA not be used routinely in patients with UAP.

Clinical Course

Stable

Most patients with UAP will respond to the medical therapy outlined above and can then be evaluated for extent of disability with the diagnostic tests outlined for stable angina pectoris. The TIMI IIIB multicenter trial showed no significant difference in study end points (death, MI, a positive exercise test at 6 weeks) between patients randomized to early invasive therapy (cardiac catheterization within 18–48 hours) or to early conservative therapy. However, in the former, the average length of initial hospitalization, incidence of rehospitalization, and days of rehospitalization were significantly lower. A high percentage of patients underwent angiography and revascularization regardless of their randomization assignment. It is recommended that patients with UAP and without contraindications receive early invasive therapy if they have one or more of the following risk factors: prior revascularization, CHF or left ventricular ejection fraction <50%, malignant ventricular arrhythmias, persistent or recurrent ischemia, or other indicators of high risk. Elective cardiac catheterization is indicated for patients with UAP who experienced recurrent ischemic episodes while being managed as outpatients. Our interpretation of prospective randomized series of medical versus medical plus surgical management of patients stabilized after UAP indicates that there is no urgency to proceed with coronary arteriography for consideration of immediate bypass surgery. There is no significant difference in mortality or myocardial infarction rate between the two groups. However, more than 30% of the medically treated group eventually seeks other methods of treatment.

Unstable

A small percentage of patients with UAP will fail to respond to medical management and an MI will evolve. Another small percentage will remain unstable with unremitting pain. This latter group has a high incidence of eventual MI with a high mortality, and it is our opinion that aggressive management is indicated as outlined below.

- Use of intravenous nitroglycerin (5–200 μg) to control pain. The goal should be to lower the wedge pressure to 15–20 mm Hg without inducing arterial hypotension or an increase in heart rate.
- If aggressive medical therapy is ineffective, intra-aortic balloon counterpulsation (IABP) should be tried.
- Urgent coronary arteriography for consideration of angioplasty, coronary stenting, or coronary bypass surgery can be performed during IABP support.

Symptoms are relieved in most patients with UAP who undergo angioplasty. However, the rate of restenosis and MI is higher in patients undergoing angioplasty and directional coronary atherectomy acutely (12). The reason for the higher complication rate is unclear but probably relates to a stunned myocardium in patients with UAP. Glycoprotein IIB/IIIA platelet receptor blocker therapy has been shown to lower events of death, MI, and urgent CABG in patients with refractory angina undergoing PTCA or coronary stenting (13).

VARIANT ANGINA

Description

Variant angina pectoris (VAP) has also been termed Prinzmetal's angina and angina inversa because of its propensity to occur at rest and to be associated with ST segment elevation, which is the ECG inverse of typical AP. After the comprehensive clinical descriptions by Prinzmetal et al. in the late 1950s (14) and early 1960s, the first major breakthrough occurred in 1973 when Oliva et al demonstrated unequivocal coronary artery spasm associated with the pain and ST segment elevation of VAP (15). Subsequently, spasm has been seen in "normal" coronary arteries and those with fixed obstructions. Coronary artery spasm and VAP are probably not synonymous. Reversible spasm has been seen during unstable angina pectoris and early in the course of typical MIs; it can be provoked by ergonovine stimulation in patients with obstructive coronary artery disease and typical AP.

VAP is not a benign syndrome. MI can occur in the region affected by coronary artery spasm in approximately 25% of patients and either high-grade heart block or ventricular fibrillation can occur during an episode of spasm. Although collective knowledge of the degree of overlap between the coronary spasm in VAP and that seen in "typical" CAD (AP or UAP) is incomplete, advancing **a diagnosis of VAP should be limited to patients who fulfill two or more of the following criteria.**

- **Pain occurs principally at rest,** i.e., usually unprovoked. Because CAD may coexist, pain may also be provoked by exercise.
- **Pain may occur in a circadian manner,** i.e., recurrent episodes at a similar time of day, often during the early morning hours.
- **Pain is associated with ST segment elevation.** Often, subclinical (painless) episodes occur with "silent" ST segment elevations. Less commonly, **only ST segment depression** will occur (on a 12-lead, etc.) in a patient who otherwise has typical VAP.

- **Painful or "silent" episodes are often associated with arrhythmias,** usually heart block and/or ventricular tachyarrhythmias or bundle branch block (including fascicular blocks).

Evaluation

History

The history of chest pain is often so atypical of ischemic heart disease that it might be misconstrued by the physician as noncardiac in origin, particularly because VAP is frequently seen in patients who have a paucity of risk factors.

Electrocardiography

A 12-lead ECG during a spontaneous attack, demonstrating transient and reversible marked ST segment elevation, can establish the diagnosis with certainty. For patients with ST depression only, the diagnosis is less certain. Because the episodes are often short-lived and unpredictable, an ambulatory ECG (Holter) is statistically more likely to record the ECG changes; however, the limitation of conventional lead configurations may obscure the diagnostic features.

Coronary Arteriography

Coronary arteriography is indicated for severely symptomatic patients with established or suspected coronary artery disease. The following should be the goals of coronary arteriography:

- Establish the status of the coronary vessels in an asymptomatic state.
- Establish the extent of change in the coronary arteries during spontaneous or induced (ergonovine) spasm. A multilead ECG should be used to record simultaneous electrocardiographic and rhythm changes.
- Establish the response of spasm to sublingual nitrates.

Important Caveats in VAP

1. Because life-threatening arrhythmias, electromechanical dissociation, or profound spasm of major vessels unresponsive to sublingual nitrates after ergonovine provocation may develop in patients with VAP, it is **not** advisable to use ergonovine stimulation outside a closely monitored setting.

2. It is important to visualize both major coronary arteries during spontaneous or induced spasm because the surface ECG may reflect spasm of the more dominant artery (e.g., the right coronary artery) while another major artery branch (e.g., the left anterior descending coronary artery) is also in spasm.

Therapy
Nitrates

Sublingual nitrates (nitroglycerin 0.4 mg or isosorbide dinitrate 5 mg) usually reverse spasm within 30–60 sec, oral nitrates (isosorbide dinitrate 20–40 mg every 4 hours), or topical nitrates can reduce the frequency of attacks. Because nitrates are not always successful and abrupt withdrawal of nitrates can provoke spasm in patients with seemingly normal coronary arteries, it is important to taper nitrates and not stop them abruptly regardless of their seeming ineffectiveness.

Calcium Blockers

Calcium blockers are extremely effective in preventing spasm in patients with VAP; use of these agents will generally result in marked reduction in frequency of episodes and need for nitroglycerin.

β blockers are generally ineffective in VAP and have some theoretic disadvantages by blocking adrenergic coronary vasodilation.

Angioplasty or coronary bypass surgery is not effective for those patients with VAP without fixed lesions. Selected cases with fixed underlying stenosis may need revascularization along with medical therapy.

Syndrome X

As noted in the introduction to this chapter, there is a group of patients who have chest pain of seemingly ischemic origin but in whom neither CAD, VAP, nor other evident cause for pain can be established. Approximately 10% of patients with UAP and approximately 20% of patients believed to have typical AP have normal coronary arteriograms. These patients, for want of a better term, have been labeled as having **syndrome X.** It is not known whether the basis for the pain is a local metabolic imbalance, small-vessel disease undetected by conventional coronary angiography, or a vasoregulatory disorder.

References

1. Maseri A. Medical therapy of chronic stable angina pectoris. Circulation 1990;82:2258.

2. Ryden T, Malberg K. Calcium channel blockers of beta receptor antagonists for patients with ischemic heart disease. What is the best choice? Eur Heart J 1996;17:1.

3. Parker JO. Nitrates and angina pectoris. Am J Cardiol 1993;72:3C.

4. Mangione NJ, Glasser SP. Phenomenon of nitrate tolerance. Am Heart J 1994;128:137.

5. Opie LH. Calcium channel antagonists in the treatment of coronary artery disease: fundamental pharmacologic properties relevant to clinical use. Prog Cardiovasc Dis 1996;38:273.

6. Weintraub W, King SB, Douglas JS, et al. Percutaneous transluminal coronary angioplasty as a first revascularization procedure in single-double-, and triple-vessel coronary artery disease. J Am Coll Cardiol 1995;26:142.

7. Schwartz GG, Karliner JS. Pathophysiology of chronic stable angina. In: Atherosclerosis and coronary artery disease. Philadelphia: JB Lippincott, 1996:1389–1400.

8. Ribeiro PA, Shah PM. Unstable angina: new insights into pathophysiologic characteristics, prognosis, and management strategies. Curr Probl Cardiol 1996;21:669.

9. Braunwald E, Mark DB, Jones RH, et al. Unstable angina: diagnosis and management: Clinical Practice Guideline. AHCPR Publication No. 94-0602. Rockville, MD: Agency for Healthcare Policy and Research and the National Heart, Lung, and Blood Institute, Public Health Service, U.S. Department of Health and Human Services, 1994:154.

10. Lewis HD Jr, Davis JW, Archibald DG, et al. Protective effects of aspirin against acute myocardial infarction and death in men with unstable angina. Results of a Veterans Administration Cooperative Study. N Engl J Med 1983;309:396.

11. The TIMI IIIB Investigators. Effects of tissue plasminogen activator and a comparison of early invasive strategies in unstable angina and non-Q-wave myocardial infarction. Circulation 1994;89:1545.

12. Abdelmeguid AE, Ellis SG, Sapp SK, et al. Directional coronary atherectomy in unstable angina. J Am Coll Cardiol 1994;24:46–54.

13. Simoons ML, deBoer MJ, van den Brand MJ, et al. Randomized trial of GP IIb/IIIa platelet receptor blocker in refractory unstable angina. Circulation 1994;89:596.

14. Prinzmetal M, Kennamer R, Merliss R, et al. Angina pectoris. The variant form of angina pectoris. Am J Med 1959;27:375.

15. Oliva PB, Potts DE, Pluss RG. Coronary arterial spasm in Prinzmetal angina: documentation by coronary arteriography. N Engl J Med 1973;288:745.

Chapter 9

Myocardial Infarction

Coronary arteriography within 6 hours of myocardial infarction (MI) has demonstrated a thrombus occluding the infarct-related coronary artery in approximately 85% of cases. Although this thrombotic occlusion may be the result of multiple interacting factors (hemorrhage into a plaque, platelet aggregation with release of vasoconstrictive substances, and/or coronary spasm), it occurs in the setting of significant underlying coronary atherosclerosis in more than 90% of cases (1). The remaining small number of infarctions without coronary atherosclerosis has been attributed to coronary embolism, isolated coronary spasm, arteritis, trauma, congenital abnormalities, and hematologic disorders.

SYMPTOMS

The major symptom of an acute myocardial infarction (AMI) is chest pain, classically described as a substernal squeezing or pressure sensation, often radiating into the neck or down the arms (usually the left), lasting 15–30 min or longer. At times, the pain may be atypical and described as burning, dull aching, or sharp. It may even be localized just to the arms or neck without associated chest pain. Other symptoms may include shortness of breath, weakness, diaphoresis, and nausea (2). Studies have provided data regarding the relationship between the specific characteristics of the patient's symptoms and the likelihood of acute infarction (3). These data are summarized in Table 9.1.

Two important findings from the Framingham study deserve mention: *(a)* only 23% of first MIs were preceded by a history of angina; and *(b)* one out of every five MIs was clinically silent or unrecognized, i.e., the pain was atypical in nature or other complaints, such as fatigue or shortness of breath predominated so that the possibility of an MI was not considered (4). Unrecognized MI is more frequent in women, diabetic patients, and el-

Table 9.1
Pain Characteristics and Acute Myocardial Infarction

Characteristic	Probability of acute MI
Description of pain:	
pressure, tightness, crushing,	24%
burning, indigestion	23%
ache	13%
sharp, stabbing	5%
pleuritic or positional	1%
Radiation to jaw, neck, left arm, left shoulder	19%
Reproducibility with chest wall palpation	
partially	6%
fully	5%
Combination of variables	
sharp or stabbing; no diagnosis of angina or MI; pain pleuritic/positional or reproducible	0%

derly individuals (5–7). Certainly, some patients tend to deny or minimize their symptoms, leading to diagnostic difficulties.

Signs

Physical findings in patients with AMI vary; however, some generalizations can be made, assuming that pulmonary edema and/or cardiogenic shock is not present (2):

Appearance: Normal to diaphoretic, pale, anxious.

Vital Signs: Mild to moderate increase in heart rate (bradyarrhythmias commonly occur with inferior MI); blood pressure (BP) is usually elevated; respirations may be increased. Fever is common and rarely exceeds 103°F or persists beyond the eighth day post MI.

Lungs: If left ventricular (LV) dysfunction is present, rales or overt pulmonary edema may be seen. Otherwise, the lungs are clear.

Heart: S1 is usually of normal intensity but may be soft. New systolic murmurs may be heard (see below). The apical impulse may become diffuse and paradoxical (outward during systole). Paradoxical splitting of S2 may be heard due to a prolonged LV ejection time. An S4 is commonly noted, and occasionally, a soft S3 is present (due to ischemia-induced decrease in ventricular compliance).

A friction rub secondary to pericarditis (usually associated with a transmural MI) may be heard. A friction rub usually consists of two or three components (systolic, early and late diastolic) and may occur within hours of acute infarction. Generally, the rub is intermittent, transient, lasts hours to days, and can be heard in almost every patient with a transmural MI if listened for.

New systolic murmurs may occur and should be listened for carefully and documented accurately. Such murmurs are due to the following:

a. Mitral regurgitation secondary to transient ischemia or infarction of the base of the papillary muscle leading to papillary muscle dysfunction (8). This murmur can be early, mid, late or holosystolic in character. Pulmonary edema is a rare complication.

b. Mitral regurgitation secondary to papillary muscle rupture, as opposed to the murmur of papillary muscle dysfunction described above, is always hemodynamically significant and generally leads to pulmonary edema (8) (see section on complications).

c. Ventricular septal defect secondary to rupture of the septum (9) (see section on complications).

DIAGNOSTIC TESTS

Electrocardiogram

The electrocardiographic (ECG) diagnosis of an AMI depends on serial ECG tracings because it is not uncommon during the first few hours of an infarction to have absent or indeterminate ECG findings. Moreover, a classical history and a high index of suspicion should not be influenced by the initial lack of ECG findings. Patients with left bundle branch block or artificially paced rhythms present difficulties in electrocardiographic diagnosis due to secondary ST-T wave changes, but serial tracings may demonstrate changes (2).

Acute inferior, anterior, or lateral transmural myocardial ischemic injury is associated with ST segment elevation, i.e., a "subepicardial injury pattern," in those leads that reflect the affected area of the heart (see Chapter 1). The T wave in those leads initially is upright, may be very tall or peaked, and subsequently inverts as Q waves develop with infarction/necrosis.

A **posterior transmural MI** is represented by an ST segment vector that is directed posteriorly and reflected as **ST segment depression on the ECG in leads V1 and V2.** The T wave is initially inverted but usually becomes upright (positive) in these leads as a 40-msec R wave develops, representing unopposed anterior depolarization.

The T waves in a so-called **non-Q-wave myocardial infarction (NQMI)** or subendocardial MI become symmetrically inverted within minutes to hours after the acute event and remain inverted for at least 24–48 hours. They may remain inverted indefinitely but, on many occasions, eventually return to normal. The ST segment may be depressed within minutes to hours of the acute event and usually returns to baseline after several days. Q waves do not develop and there is no distinct change in the R wave. The persistence of the above changes for more than 24 hours distinguishes an NQMI from a prolonged ischemic episode without infarction.

Cardiac Enzymes

More than 12 muscle-associated proteins have been identified as potential markers for acute MI (10). Most are of limited value in the diagnosis of AMI due to lack of specificity, whereas some have proven difficult to assay reliably. Historically, the three serum enzymes most commonly used to diagnose AMI are creatine phosphokinase (CPK or CK) and its isoenzyme CK-MB, aspartate serum transaminase (AST or SGOT), and lactic dehydrogenase (LDH). AST and LDH are rarely used because of their limited specificity (these enzymes are found in many other tissues) and the ready availability of more specific serum markers. The efficacy of other markers, such as myoglobin, cardiac troponin T (cTnT), and cardiac troponin I (cTnI), are being studied. cTnI and cTnT may become the assay of choice in the near future for risk stratification of patients with chest pain and suspected acute cardiac ischemia (11,12). The following is a brief summary of the most frequently used enzymes in diagnosing acute MI (see Table 9.2).

CK

Creatine kinase is a ubiquitous enzyme and is released with skeletal or cardiac muscle injury or trauma. Three CK isoenzymes have

Table 9.2
Serum Markers in Acute MI

Serum marker	Earliest increase	Peak level	Normalize
Total CK	6 hours	24–30 hours	3–4 days
CK-MB	4–6 hours	18–24 hours	36–48 hours
Myoglobin	1–3 hours	8–12 hours	24–36 hours
Troponin I	4–8 hours	12–16 hours	7–10 days
Troponin T	3–4 hours	12–16 hours	7–14 days

been identified: CK-MM (specific for skeletal muscle), CK-BB (specific for brain tissue), and CK-MB (specific for cardiac muscle). Thus, the specificity of an elevated CK improves in myocardial injury by measuring the CK-MB isoenzyme. Detecting elevated levels of CK-MB in the serum has been the gold standard for the diagnosis of acute MI for many years (13). Elevated enzyme levels can occur, however, under a variety of circumstances. These include skeletal muscle crush injury, electrical injury, dermatomyositis, hypothyroidism, chronic renal failure (due to decreased excretion), rhabdomyolysis, strenuous exercise, cardiac surgery, and defibrillation/cardioversion. When both the CK-MB (ng/mL) and the CK (u/L) are elevated, a relative index is calculated (CK-MB/CK × 100); a value greater than 2.5 is suggestive of MI.

AST

AST lacks specificity, being found in high concentrations in liver and skeletal muscle. It has thus fallen out of favor as a marker for myocardial infarction.

LDH

Elevated in muscle, liver, and hematologic disorder, LDH is very nonspecific. The five isoenzymes of LDH provide a means of improving specificity over that of total LDH activity. Myocardium is the only tissue in which LDH1 is the most abundant isoenzyme; in normal serum and in tissue other than the heart, LDH2 activity exceeds that of LDH1. In cardiac injury, the normal LDH1:LDH2 ratio (usually less than 1.0) is ≥1. Elevated levels of LDH can remain elevated up to 7–10 days. The cardiac troponins are highly specific and remain elevated for >24 hours and will probably eliminate the measurement of LDH in diagnosing AMI when symptoms developed >24 hours before evaluation.

Myoglobin

Myoglobin is a heme protein that is ubiquitous in cardiac and skeletal muscle. It is abnormally elevated in the serum within 2 hours of an AMI and is cleared rapidly. Its rapid clearance explains the rising and falling (staccato pattern) values observed in some patients (14). Therefore, a solitary negative myoglobin level does not exclude acute infarction. It should not be used as a cardiac marker if the patient has suffered noncardiac trauma or has chronic renal or skeletal muscle disease.

Troponin

The newer markers such as cardiac troponin T(cTnT) and cardiac troponin I (cTnI) have very high specificity for cardiac injury, greater than that of CK-MB (15). However, cTnT is frequently elevated in uremic patients. Serum levels of the troponins increase about the same time after the onset of acute MI as CK-MB but remain elevated for a substantially longer period. If cTnI is performed serially at 0, 6, and 12 hours and levels do not rise above 0.4 ng/mL, it is unlikely that myocardial necrosis has occurred. A level between 0.4 and 1.5 ng/mL suggests MI, and a level greater than 1.5 ng/mL strongly suggests an AMI.

None of the current tests are perfect, and serial testing is still necessary to rule out MI. The sensitivity of a given marker in detecting acute MI is dependent upon the time it is measured after the onset of symptoms. It is imperative to understand that not even the most specific serum marker of myocardial damage can exempt the physician from careful clinical assessment of patients who presents with chest pain.

Radionuclide Scanning

In most AMIs, the clinical history, ECG , and pattern of enzyme changes will establish the diagnosis without difficulty, and radionuclide scanning will add little useful information. However, in certain situations in which the clinical history, ECG, and/or enzyme pattern is confusing or not available, a properly timed radio-nuclide scan can be helpful in establishing the diagnosis. Patients with left bundle branch block, patients who have delayed evaluation of their chest pain beyond the time range in which CK-MB determinations are useful, patients with non-Q wave infarctions, and patients who have had previous infarctions are particularly good candidates for radionuclide imaging. Several techniques using technetium pyrophosphate and thallium-201 are available (16,17) (see Chapter 5).

Echocardiography

Echocardiography may be valuable in evaluating patients with AMI and complications. Wall motion abnormalities such as hypo-kinesis, akinesis, and dyskinesis can be identified and help the clinician in determining the degree of functional impairment. Left ventricular ejection fraction can be calculated, which is useful in determining prognosis. Left ventricular thrombus formation can be detected; if the thrombus is large and "shaggy," anticoagulation may be indicated. Complications of mitral regurgitation with papillary muscle rupture, ventricular septal defect, right ventricular infarction, left ventricular aneurysm, and peri-cardial effusion can be identified (18).

PROGNOSTIC FACTORS

Infarct Size

The amount of damaged myocardium and resultant left ventricular dysfunction is the principal determinant of outcome following MI. Infarct size varies from minimal loss of myocardial muscle mass (less than 5% in-hospital mortality) to loss of approximately 40% of the LV muscle mass and resultant cardiogenic shock (in-hospital mortality often >80%). No perfect method of infarct size assessment is available; however, clinicians make general estimates based on clinical status, enzyme values, ECGs, nuclear ventriculography, two-dimensional echocardiography, and abnormalities during invasive hemodynamic monitoring (19–21). Limiting infarct size has been attempted using agents that decrease the oxygen demands of the myocardium (nitroglycerin, β blockers, calcium blockers, etc.) and/or by increasing supply (thrombolytic therapy, angioplasty, and coronary bypass surgery)

(22). Studies assessing benefit of interventions designed to limit infarct size must be interpreted cautiously in view of the imprecise methods of quantitation. Research techniques using positron emission tomography and magnetic resonance imaging (MRI) may prove to be of value.

Infarct Site

The site of the infarct is an important variable in determining outcome. Anterior MIs generally result from occlusion of the left anterior descending coronary artery. They tend to be larger infarcts and therefore are associated with a higher mortality. These infarcts are more prone to expansion, rupture, mural thrombus, and aneurysm formation. Occlusion of the circumflex coronary artery results in lateral infarction. When the circumflex is a dominant artery (10% of cases), the infarct may involve the posterior and inferior walls.

Right coronary artery occlusion may result in inferior or inferoposterior infarction. Although right coronary occlusion usually causes less loss of critical myocardium than obstruction of the left anterior descending branch, the spectrum of clinical presentation varies widely from a "benign" event to major hemodynamic consequences (right ventricular infarction, rupture of the posteromedial papillary muscle) and significant arrhythmias (bradycardia, heart block, and ventricular fibrillation).

Severity of Coronary Artery Disease

Another factor affecting outcome of MI is the presence of coexistent coronary artery disease in vessels supplying noninfarcted myocardium. Seventy-five percent of patients with AMI have at least two major vessels with critical lesions and 50% have triple vessel disease. It thus follows that angina may develop early after infarct (within 7–10 days) in approximately 25% of patients with acute MI and is often associated with poor prognosis. Patients with angina from "ischemia at a distance" (outside the zone of infarct) are now recognized as having a high mortality at 6 months (75%).

ACUTE INTERVENTION-REPERFUSION THERAPY

Prior to 1980, treatment of AMI was largely expectant or prophylactic in character or directed toward the management of complications. Overwhelming evidence now exists that reperfusion in the setting of AMI improves survival, decreases symptoms of heart failure, and increases left ventricular function. There are two primary methods available to achieve reperfusion: thrombolytic therapy or primary (direct) coronary angioplasty.

Intravenous Thrombolytic Therapy

Intravenous thrombolytic therapy is the most accepted interventional strategy for treatment of patients with acute myocardial infarction (23,24). The intravenous thrombolytic agents presently used and available in the United States are streptokinase (SK), recombinant tissue plasminogen activator (tPA), anistreplase (APSAC), and urokinase (UK). All have demonstrated a remarkable capacity to establish blood flow by dissolving occlusive thrombi especially when given within the first 6 hours of AMI. Each agent has been shown to reduce in-hospital mortality and improve left ventricular function when compared to placebo.

It is believed that thrombolytic therapy is underused and that only approximately 30–50% of eligible patients actually receive lytic therapy. Because of published exclusion criteria in many large, highly publicized trials, there has been confusion about who should or should not be treated. Several strategies have been implemented to increase the number of patients who receive therapy. These strategies include raising the upper age limit of therapy, treating patients beyond 4 hours after the onset of symptoms, and disregarding the site of the infarct. Support for widening inclusion criteria has been provided via a meta-analysis of large thrombolytic trials (25).

Eligibility for thrombolytic therapy in AMI have been simplified:

- Ischemic chest pain of >30 min and <12 hours in duration.
- ST segment elevation of ≥1.0 mV in two continuous ECG leads indicative of acute MI.
- New left bundle branch pattern on ECG.

Exclusion criteria include the following:

- Systolic BP > 180 mm Hg and diastolic BP > 110 mm Hg.
- History of bleeding disorder.
- Significant gastrointestinal bleeding within preceding 5 months.

- Major surgery, organ biopsy, or significant trauma within preceding 3 months.
- History of central nervous system (CNS) malignancy or arteriovenous malformation.
- History of stroke or transient ischemic attack (TIA).
- Warfarin therapy with an International Normalized Ratio (INR) >1.4 (PT >14 sec).
- Cardiopulmonary resuscitation (CPR) >10 min duration.

Many trials have studied the various thrombolytic agents in an attempt to define which is the best. There have been a number of trials looking at different end-points, such as early patency rates, late patency rates, and early survival, and trials comparing different thrombolytic agents, various regimens of anticoagulation, and adjunctive therapy (e.g., angiotensin-converting enzyme [ACE] inhibitors). This has led to enormous confusion for the clinician in translating trial results to clinical practice. Other studies such as the GISSI-II, ISIS-3, and GUSTO-1 trials have simpler designs and less rigid entry criteria and focus on end points of mortality and morbidity. In these statistically powerful studies, there was no advantage of one lytic agent over another when comparing mortality rates. In the ISIS-3 trial, all three agents (SK, t-PA, and APSAC) had a 10% mortality rate. In the GISSI-II and GUSTO-1 trials, there was no difference in mortality between SK and t-PA (26–28).

The GUSTO trial did show an advantage for accelerated t-PA over streptokinase in addition to conventionally used concomitant treatment. The 30-day mortality was 6.3% with t-PA and 7.3% with streptokinase (28). Analysis of subgroups in this study showed that those who benefited most from t-PA were patients with large infarctions, patients with anterior MI, patients presenting within 6 hours, and patients younger than 75 years of age. Because of this, it has been recommended that patients with late treatment (>6 hours after pain onset), patients with small MIs, and patients with increasing risk of stroke (age >75, female, and low body weight) be treated with streptokinase. An important observation of the GUSTO trial is that survival after infarction even as early as the first day is critically limited to the establishment of complete antegrade flow (TIMI grade 3 flow) in the infarct related vessel.

There are several limitations of thrombolytic therapy for acute myocardial infarction:

- Less than one-half of patients with acute MI actually receive thrombolytic therapy.
- Regardless of agent or dose, maximal patency rate is 80%, and only 55% of vessels achieve normal flow.
- Patients who receive thrombolytic therapy have a 15–30% incidence of recurrent ischemic events and there is a 0.5–2.0% incidence of intracranial bleeding.
- There are no clinical markers that accurately predict clot lysis and reperfusion.

Angioplasty in Acute MI

Primary (Direct) Percutaneous Transluminal Coronary Angioplasty (PTCA)

Primary (direct) angioplasty refers to the use of PTCA without prior thrombolytic therapy. Primary angioplasty during AMI was first applied in 1982 and has subsequently been used with increasing frequency during the last 15 years. One limiting factor of this approach has been that only 20% of U.S. hospitals have catheterization facilities; therefore, the main nationwide strategy has been to administer immediate intravenous thrombolytic therapy. Other limiting factors include setup time, cost, and need for skilled personnel. Despite these factors, primary angioplasty has been shown to be a remarkably valuable therapy for patients with MI (29). It is the most effective method of confirming the diagnosis and establishing high-risk subsets by obtaining coronary artery anatomy and left ventricular function data. Opening of the infarct-related artery is angiographically confirmed; this a major advantage over having to estimate vessel patency with the intravenous lytic approach. Another benefit is that adjunctive therapies such as intra-aortic balloon counterpulsation (IABP), pacing, and hemodynamic monitoring can be applied at the time of the procedure. The direct PTCA approach is applicable to nearly all patients with MI, including those that have been excluded in most thrombolytic trials (elderly, previous coronary artery bypass grafting [CABG], recent surgery or trauma, cerebrovascular accident [CVA] or CNS damage, active bleeding, etc.). Direct PTCA approaches a 99% success rate (30) and there is a decreased incidence of recurrent ischemic events and risk of hemorrhagic stroke.

The first randomized trial comparing direct angioplasty to

thrombolytic therapy was not available until 1993 (31). Patients were randomized to rt-PA (200 patients) or to primary PTCA (195 patients) with both groups having closely matched baseline characteristics. All patients were treated with ASA (aspirin) 325 mg/day, intravenous heparin for 3–5 days, and intravenous NTG (nitroglycerin) for 24 hours. The in-hospital mortality rate was 2.6% for the direct PTCA group and 6.5% for the rt-PA group. At 6 months, reinfarction or death had occurred in 16.8% of the rt-PA group and only 8.5% of the PTCA group. Recurrent ischemia occurred in 10% of the PTCA group versus 28% of the rt-PA group.

Two other randomized single center trials were published in 1993 (32,33). Meta-analysis of the three randomized trials has shown an in-hospital death rate for PTCA of 2.2% versus 5.8% for the thrombolytic group. In-hospital reinfarction rate was 1.9% for the PTCA group and 7.6% for the thrombolytic group. In patients randomized to PTCA, there was less recurrent ischemia and early and late patency rates were greater with lower residual stenosis. More than 90% of the PTCA groups showed TIMI-3 flow, which is the strongest predictor of improved ejection fraction and survival at 30 days.

Several subsets of infarct patients are particularly well served by direct angioplasty. Those patients with cardiogenic shock who are successfully treated with direct PTCA and IABP have a much better survival rate (>70%) than those treated with thrombolytics or conventional medications (<25%) (34). Patients with MI who have had prior CABG are usually better treated with mechanical intervention than thrombolytic treatment. Contemporary thrombolytic agents are less efficacious in saphenous vein grafts than in native occlusions. Thrombus-laden saphenous vein grafts are associated with the risk of distal embolization regardless of the method of reperfusion (34).

Despite the large-scale development of thrombolytic agents during the last decade and expanded indications for their use, a large percentage of thrombolytic ineligible patients (estimated 35–65% of all infarcts) still present to large community hospitals throughout the country (35). This high-risk subset (usually older with more chronic diseases) have an 18% mortality risk and are best treated with direct PTCA (36).

Advantages of Primary PTCA in AMI

- Patients who are ineligible for intravenous thrombolytic agents can be treated.

- Early and sustained high percentage of TIMI grade 3 flow.
- Lower incidence of recurrent ischemia.
- Lower incidence of intracranial hemorrhage.
- Better LV function.
- Less expensive when compared to accelerated t-TPA regimens.
- Immediate availability of coronary anatomy with catheterization.

Immediate Angioplasty

Immediate angioplasty in acute MI refers to the use of PTCA immediately after thrombolysis. The theoretic advantages of combining thrombolysis with immediate PTCA include achieving a higher reperfusion rate than lytic agents alone, addressing the underlying residual stenosis, which is not affected by lysis alone, and potentially eliminating flow-limiting stenosis and improving function and recovery. This combination of medical and mechanical intervention has been the subject of several clinical trials, including the Thrombolysis and Angioplasty in Myocardial Infarction study (TAMI) (37), the Thrombolysis in Myocardial Infarction study (TIMI 2A) (38), and the European Cooperative Study Group trial (ECSG) (39). Each tested the strategy of immediate angiography and PTCA after thrombolytic therapy versus the alternative strategy of deferred angiography and PTCA after 48 hours to 10 days or indefinitely if stress testing showed no provocable ischemia. When the end point of left ventricular function was evaluated, no benefit was shown with immediate PTCA over the deferred strategy. In-hospital mortality was higher and emergency CABG surgery was required more commonly with the immediate strategy. There was also a substantially higher incidence of bleeding complications and blood transfusions with the immediate strategy.

Rescue Angioplasty

Rescue (salvage) angioplasty refers to PTCA after failed thrombolysis. Patients with an occluded infarct artery (TIMI 0–1 flow) 90 minutes after thrombolytic therapy have worse LV function and an increased early mortality (40). Rescue PTCA is indicated in this group to establish reperfusion, salvage myocardium, and improve healing. Patients requiring rescue PTCA to achieve patency had an increased reocclusion rate in several trials (41).

With new understanding of the importance of aspirin, heparin, and ACT monitoring, reocclusion rates in the GUSTO angiographic substudy appear to be decreasing (42). Unfortunately, the mortality rate in patients who fail rescue PTCA is high (>30%).

Deferred Angioplasty

Delayed angioplasty refers to angioplasty performed electively 1–7 days after thrombolysis. PTCA has been commonly used for post-MI angina or ischemia after thrombolytic therapy. The DA-NAMI study enrolled 1008 patients who had post-MI angina or an abnormal exercise test after thrombolysis (43). Patients were randomized to receive a mechanical intervention ($n = 503$) versus conservative therapy ($n = 505$). Major events with the interventional approach were diminished (MI, 5.6%; death, 3.6%). It is recommended that patients with post-MI angina or ischemia should undergo catheterization and mechanical revascularization if indicated.

Emergency Bypass Surgery

Emergency coronary bypass has the potential value of myocardial salvage if difficult logistics can be overcome within the first 4 hours of MI. Surgery should be considered for patients whose coronary anatomy has been previously assessed with angiography and who develop ischemia while in the hospital awaiting surgery or for patients who develop the onset of MI while undergoing routine angiography or coronary angioplasty. Bypass of diseased, but non–infarct-related, arteries at the time of surgery could have additional value. However, the usual delay in clinical presentation of the patient who develops MI out of the hospital and the time required for clinical evaluation, angiography, assembling the surgical team, and placing the patient on cardiopulmonary bypass will generally preclude this intervention in most patients.

PHARMACOLOGIC ADJUNCTS TO REPERFUSION THERAPY

Multiple pharmacologic adjuncts to reperfusion have been studied. These generally fall into two categories: those that stabilize platelet-fibrin plaques, such as aspirin and heparin, and those that promote tissue recovery, such as nitrates and β blockers, by improving the myocardial oxygen supply:demand ratio.

Antiplatelet/Antithrombin Agents

Platelet activation is a key step in acute arterial thrombosis. **Aspirin** irreversibly inhibits the cyclo-oxygenase enzyme responsible for the synthesis of eicosanoids. In platelets, aspirin prevents the formation of thromboxane A_2, a substance that induces platelet aggregation. Because platelets are unable to generate new cyclo-oxygenase, inhibition of the enzyme lasts for the lifetime of the cell (about 10 days). In vascular endothelial cells, aspirin prevents the synthesis of prostacyclin, which inhibits platelet aggregation. However, because endothelial cells can recover cyclo-oxygenase synthesis, this inhibitory effect of aspirin may be of shorter duration. Aspirin is rapidly absorbed in the stomach and upper gastrointestinal tract, causing platelet inhibition in approximately 60 min (44). The different effects of various doses of aspirin (20–1500 mg/day) on platelet and vessel-wall eicosanoid synthesis have been extensively investigated. Doses of 80–325 mg/day are most commonly used in the management of coronary artery disease.

Antiplatelet therapy is effective in secondary prevention of myocardial infarction. A meta-analysis of data from six randomized, placebo-controlled, double-blind trials of patients surviving MI demonstrated that platelet inhibitors reduces vascular mortality rate by 13%, the nonfatal reinfarction rate by 31%, and the nonfatal stroke rate by 42%. No statistically significant differences among the various antiplatelet regimens used were found (45). It is currently recommended that all survivors of acute MI be treated indefinitely with aspirin at a dosage of 160–325 mg/day (46).

The importance of aspirin therapy early in the course of acute myocardial infarction was highlighted by the ISIS-2 trial (47). In this study, the clinical efficacy of streptokinase alone, aspirin alone, or the combination of both agents was assessed. The mortality rate for patients treated with aspirin alone was 21% lower than that for the placebo group. This reduction was only slightly less than that achieved with streptokinase alone. However, when both aspirin and streptokinase were administered, the reduction on mortality was dramatically increased. Aspirin (160–325 mg) should be administered as soon as the diagnosis of acute MI (or unstable angina) is considered, regardless of whether a thrombolytic agent is used.

Ticlopidine (Ticlid) is a more potent antiplatelet agent than aspirin. It inhibits binding of fibrinogen to the platelet GP IIb/IIIa receptor. Combined ASA and ticlopidine has a synergistic effect in reducing coronary platelet deposition (48). Due to cost, ticlopidine is generally used as a substitute for aspirin in patients who are unable to take aspirin or for whom aspirin therapy has failed. The standard dosage is 250 mg twice a day. When direct PTCA results in dissection treated with stenting, 250 mg twice daily for 2 weeks post intervention may prevent reocclusion (49).

Glycoprotein IIb/IIIa receptor antagonists are new agents that block the GP IIb/IIIa receptor and lead to a dose-dependent inhibition of platelet aggregation (50). Reports of reduced acute and 6-month ischemic events in the EPIC trial using c7E3, a monoclonal antibody, are promising, but the beneficial effects must be weighed against the increased risk of major bleeding (14% versus 7% control) and the high cost ($1300/dose) (51). The TAMI 8 pilot study reported improved coronary artery patency and a trend to fewer ischemic events with 7E3 (added to aspirin and heparin) following thrombolytic therapy for myocardial infarction (52).

Commercial **heparin** is a heterogenous mixture of polysaccharides, not all of which are active in inhibiting the coagulation cascade. Heparin requires the plasma protein cofactor antithrombin III to express anticoagulant activity. This occurs by heparin binding both antithrombin III and activated coagulation proteases, such as thrombin, to catalyze the protease inhibition by antithrombin III (53). Despite numerous clinical trials, the role of heparin after reperfusion is still debated (54). Early administration of heparin combined with a lytic agent does not appear to hasten reperfusion, but heparin may play an important role in preventing reocclusion, especially when used in conjunction with rt-PA (55,56). Several large-scale trials have used subcutaneous heparin combined with thrombolytic therapy, which has led to considerable confusion in defining the role of heparin in acute myocardial infarction. The GISSI-2 and the ISIS trials (collectively involving >20,000 patients) failed to show a clinical or survival benefit associated with delayed subcutaneous heparin (57). The GUSTO trial demonstrated the importance of systemic intravenous heparinization when tPA is used as the thrombolytic agent and intravenous heparin is strongly recommended for patients receiving tPA (46) with the continuous infusion rate being guided by determination of PTT (45–75 sec). With direct PTCA, high-dose heparin to achieve an ACT between 350 and 400 sec is often used. Little is known about the optimal dose and duration of heparin infusion after PTCA for AMI. There are no data to support intravenous heparin use for more than 24–48 hours. Several studies have suggested that intravenous heparin should not be stopped abruptly because of the risk of a rebound hypercoagulable state and increased risk of reinfarction (58,59). Based on these data, tapering the heparin infusion rate to one-half of the therapeutic dose for 12 hours before discontinuation seems prudent.

Direct thrombin inhibitors, such as hirudin and hirulog, are not dependent on antithrombin III, are better specific inhibitors of fibrin-bound thrombin than heparin, and are actively being investigated in the management of acute ischemic heart disease (53).

β-Adrenergic Blockade

β blocker therapy reduces heart rate, blood pressure, and myocardial contractility, which results in a decrease in myocardial oxygen consumption. Experimental models have shown that β blockers decrease myocardial ischemia and reduce infarct size. These observations provided the rationale for clinical studies, which can be divided into two main categories: "early" administration (beginning at the time of acute presentation) and "late entry" (after the evolution of the infarct is complete which is usually after four days). Most of the "late entry" trials were completed before the widespread use of thrombolytic therapy.

Five large, multicenter, prospective randomized trials with a total of >11,500 patients have evaluated late β blocker therapy in myocardial infarction. Included in this group are the Norwegian Multicenter Study Group (timolol, 20 mg/day) (60), the Beta Blocker Heart Attack Trial (propanolol, 180–240 mg/day) (61), and the Goteborg Trial (metoprolol, 200 mg/day) (62). These studies have demonstrated that β blocker therapy reduces mortality by approximately 25% when compared to placebo controls (63). It is postulated that much of the benefit in the patients treated with β blockers is due to a reduction in the risk of sudden cardiac death, i.e., an antiarrhythmic effect resulting from inhibition of adrenergic stimulation. It is difficult to separate this effect from the anti-ischemic effect.

A meta-analysis of data from 32 randomized trials, which included a total of approximately 29,000 patients, showed a 13% relative reduction in overall mortality among patients receiving intravenous β-blocker therapy initiated within 24 hours of signs and symptoms of myocardial infarction (64). In the TIMI-IIB trial, patients who received early intravenous metoprolol combined with TPA, had a lower incidence of nonfatal reinfarction (2.3% versus 4.5%) and recurrent ischemic events (15.4% versus 21.2%) when compared to patients receiving delayed administration of oral metoprolol (65). Because of contraindications such as hypotension, bradycardia, and reactive airway disease, only approximately 30–40% of patients receiving intravenous thrombolytics will be eligible for β-blocker therapy. The ultrashort-acting β blocker esmolol has been shown to be effective in lowering heart rate and blood pressure in acute ischemia and its ability to be titrated may broaden its clinical usefulness in the current era of reperfusion therapy. It is currently recommended that all patients without a contraindication to β-blocker therapy receive these such drugs within 12 hours of onset of infarction, irrespective of administration of concomitant thrombolytic therapy (46).

Contraindications to β-blocker therapy include (66):

- Heart rate <50 beats/min.
- Systolic blood pressure <90 mm Hg.
- Severe left ventricular failure.
- Signs of peripheral hypoperfusion.
- Atrioventricular (AV) conduction abnormalities: PR interval >0.22 sec, 2° AV block, or complete heart block.
- Severe chronic obstructive pulmonary disease.

Nitrates

Nitrates have been shown in both clinical and experimental infarction to improve left ventricular function, increase cardiac output, and reduce filling pressures. Nitrates also reduce peripheral resistance and relieve coronary spasm. Nitrates have the potential for adverse effects if hypotension or reflex tachycardia increase myocardial oxygen consumption.

The clinical efficacy of intravenous nitroglycerin in AMI has been the subject of at least seven randomized trials. Taken separately, these individual trials have been too small to provide a reliable estimate of the effects of treatment on mortality, but collectively, they show evidence of benefit. The mortality for the pooled group allocated to intravenous nitroglycerin was 12% (51/426) versus 20.5% (86/425) in the controls (67). Intravenous nitroglycerin is currently recommended for the first 24–48 hours in patients with acute MI and congestive heart failure, large anterior infarction, persistent ischemia, or hypertension. Its use in other patients with MI is not well established (46). Intravenous nitroglycerin is usually started at an infusion rate of 10 μg/min and increased by 10 μg/min at 10-minute intervals to achieve relief of chest pain, a 10% reduction in systolic pressure, a systolic pressure of 95 mm Hg, or a maximal dose of 200 μg/min. After 2 days, a decision regarding a long-term therapy should be made, depending on left ventricular function and residual ischemia.

Calcium Channel Blockers

As a group, the **calcium channel blockers** have failed to demonstrate significant benefits in patients with Q-wave infarctions. Nifedipine and verapamil have been shown to be of no benefit or deleterious in this setting (68–71). Coadministration of lytic agents and calcium channel blockers has yet to demonstrate any benefit but will be the subject of further trials. Diltiazem has been shown to reduce cardiac events after non-Q-wave MI in the absence of pulmonary congestion (72). Verapamil or diltiazem may be given to patients in whom β blockers are ineffective or contraindicated for relief of continuing ischemia or for rapid control of ventricular response rate if atrial fibrillation complicates acute MI (46).

Angiotensin Converting Enzyme (ACE) Inhibitors

ACE inhibitors have both cardioprotective properties and vasculoprotective properties that are unrelated to their blood-pressure-lowering effect. ACE inhibitors seem to have a role in reducing myocardial and vascular hypertrophy, progression of atherosclerosis, plaque rupture, and thrombosis.

The combined results of the CONSENSUS II, ISIS-4, GISSI-III, and the Chinese Cardiac Study, in addition to 11 small trials show that ACE inhibitors started early in acute MI will save 5 lives per 1000 treated in the first month (73–76). The ISIS-4 trial demonstrated that the benefit of only 1 month of early ACE-inhibitor treatment seemed to persist for at least 1 year and the benefit was greater in patients at higher risk (74). The acute MI trials have generally shown ACE-inhibitor therapy to be very safe even when added to other agents that lower blood pressure. There also seems to be a benefit of long-term ACE inhibitor treatment started days to weeks post MI and for patients with LV dysfunction with or without overt heart failure. In the SOLVD and SAVE trials, an additional 2 lives per 1000 were saved during each later month of treatment (77–80). It is currently recommended that ACE inhibitor therapy be initiated within 24 hours in patients with suspected acute MI who meet ST-segment elevation criteria or in those patients with clinical heart failure in the absence of significant hypotension or known contraindications to use of ACE inhibitors. Patients with MI and a left ventricular ejection fraction <40% or patients with symptomatic heart failure on the basis of systolic pump dysfunction are most likely to benefit from such therapy (46). In patients without complications and no evidence of symptomatic or asymptomatic left ventricular dysfunction at 6 weeks post MI, ACE inhibitors can be discontinued.

THE 10 COMMANDMENTS OF MI TREATMENT

I. Reperfusion therapy should be given to as many patients as possible with MI (including those with left bundle/branch block [LBBB]); benefits exist up to 12 hours from the onset of symptoms.

II. If thrombolysis is chosen for reperfusion, accelerated tPA should be given when the time frame is 0–4 hours, with an anterior MI, and when the patient is younger than 75 years of age. Streptokinase is preferred if the patient is older than 75 years of age, when the MI is smaller, and when there is an increased risk of hemorrhagic stroke.

III. Primary angioplasty is superior to thrombolytic therapy.

IV. Aspirin and β blockers should be given at the onset of treatment. ACE inhibitors should be given early (within first 24 hours) especially in those with larger infarcts.

V. Nitrates are not necessary in the ongoing therapy of acute MI. There is no effect on mortality, left ventricular function, or infarct size.

VI. Intravenous heparin should be given to those who are treated with tPA; there is no evidence of improved outcome if intravenous heparin is used with streptokinase.

VII. There is evidence to support tapering heparin as opposed to abruptly stopping heparin.

VIII. Avoid prophylactic lidocaine (see below).

IX. Avoid calcium channel blockers.

X. Cardiac catheterization should be performed for patients with post-MI ischemia.

COMPLICATIONS OF ACUTE MYOCARDIAL INFARCTION

Cardiac Rhythm Disturbances

Prompt recognition and treatment of arrhythmias is important to minimize their deleterious hemodynamic effects (reduced cardiac output and increased myocardial oxygen demand—MVO_2) and their tendency to lead to more serious electrical instability. Recognition and management of common arrhythmias is discussed in Chapter 2. This section is limited to selected rhythm disturbances and management issues in the setting of acute myocardial infarction.

Supraventricular Arrhythmias

1. **Sinus tachycardia:** This rhythm is detrimental in the setting of myocardial ischemia because of the increase in MVO_2 in the presence of a fixed blood supply. With adequate pain control, appropriate sedation, no fever, and no clinical evidence of LV failure, sinus rates higher than 110 may require investigation with a pulmonary artery flotation catheter to determine the underlying etiology: hypovolemia, subclinical LV failure, or hyperadrenergic state. Therapy should be directed at correcting the underlying abnormality. β blockers may be used for the control of sinus tachycardia in isolated hyperadrenergic states (normal pulmonary capillary wedge pressure [PCWP], increased cardiac output, increased heart rate). Decreased preload (low PCWP) can be corrected with volume infusions using normal saline or a colloid solution.

2. **Sinus bradycardia:** Bradycardia may be transient or persistent and may be associated with hypotension. The combination of hypotension and bradycardia usually represents a vasovagal

reaction (Bezold-Jarisch reflex) and is a common occurrence in acute inferior MI. This is not required unless the patient is symptomatic or the bradycardia is accompanied by premature ventricular contractions (PVCs) or escape rhythms.

3. **Atrial fibrillation:** Atrial fibrillation complicates the clinical course of acute MI in approximately 10% of patients and is associated with a higher early mortality. In the setting of acute MI, it is usually encountered in patients with extensive infarction resulting in LV failure, atrial infarction, or, occasionally, is seen in patients with post-MI pericarditis. Approximately 90% of episodes will occur within the first 48 hours and usually persist for less than 24 hours. Electrical cardioversion is for patients with severe hemodynamic compromise or intractable ischemia. Intravenous β blockers can be used to control ventricular response rate in patients without contraindications to their use. Intravenous diltiazem or verapamil can be used to slow the ventricular response rate if β blockers are contraindicated.

Ventricular Arrhythmias

Before 1992, prophylactic lidocaine was in widespread use due to its ability to reduce the incidence of primary ventricular fibrillation in limited clinical studies (81). However, randomized control trials have not demonstrated any significant mortality effect with prophylactic lidocaine (82). In addition, lidocaine may be harmful to some patients who are treated prophylactically but who later are found not to have suffered AMI. Meta-analysis of 14 randomized control trials with lidocaine suggests that there may be some negative mortality effect, as well as reports of several life-threatening lidocaine-related events (sinus arrest, marked bradycardia, and seizures) (83). Based on these data, routine use of lidocaine for PVC suppression is no longer recommended in the setting of acute MI.

1. **Premature ventricular contractions:** PVCs are usually treated if they are frequent (>6/min), multiform (multifocal) in character, occur in pairs or in "runs" (≥3 consecutive PVCs) or are closely coupled (R on T). Lidocaine is usually the first drug administered. The loading dose is 1.0–1.5 mg/kg intravenously. Additional doses of 0.5–0.75 mg/kg can be given at 5- to 10-min intervals to a maximum of 3 mg/kg total

loading dose. A constant infusion (with an infusion pump) of 2 mg/min should be started with the first dose. The maximum infusion rate is 4 mg/min. The loading dose and infusion rate should be reduced by half in the presence of congestive heart failure (CHF), shock, liver disease, or age older than 70 years. The infusion can be stopped (not tapered) at 36 hours in the absence of ventricular arrhythmias. If ventricular ectopy develops with cessation of the infusion, lidocaine should be restarted and continued for another 24–36 hours. If complex ventricular ectopy, i.e., multiform, runs or pairs, or frequent PVCs (>5/min), develops when the infusion is stopped, oral antiarrhythmics may be necessary. Almost all patients will have PVCs during the acute phase of MI. Complete or nearly complete suppression of ventricular ectopy in the acute phase of an infarction is the goal of therapy. If lidocaine is not effective consider:

a. **Procainamide:** 20–30 mg/min loading infusion up to 12–17 mg/kg is recommended. Monitor BP and ECG closely because hypotension and conduction disturbances (prolonged QRS and QT interval) can occur if dose is given too rapidly. After loading is completed, a constant infusion at 1–4 mg/min should be started.

b. **A combination of procainamide and lidocaine** may be used but can result in neurotoxicity (altered mental status, seizures) because the two drugs have additive central nervous system (CNS) effects; combined infusion rate should not exceed 5 mg/min.

c. **Bretylium:** 5–10 mg/kg can be administered intravenously over 10 minutes, followed by a constant infusion of a rate of 1–2 mg/min. After an initial increase in blood pressure, hypotension may occur due to the blocking of the efferent limb of the baroreceptor reflex. Initial sinus tachycardia may be caused by catecholamine release. Bretylium should not be used for patients with a fixed cardiac output, e.g., severe aortic stenosis. Postural hypotension is a common complication.

d. **Amiodarone:** 150 mg infused over 10 min followed by a constant infusion at 1.0 mg/min for 6 hours and then a maintenance infusion of 0.5 mg/min (46).

The management of PVCs after AMI has been the subject of intense interest and clinical trials. At present, no strong data show a benefit from treating asymptomatic complex ventricular ectopy after AMI. The highly publicized CAST study has shown a twofold to threefold increase in mortality when the class 1C agents flecainide and encainide were tested in comparison to placebo controls (84). Pooled data with class 1A and 1B agents also show a higher mortality in the treated group (85). These data have underscored the need for caution when using any oral antiarrhythmic after AMI. Patients with ejection fractions less than 40%, late potentials on signal-averaged ECGs, and complex ventricular ectopy may benefit from suppression of the PVCs if the drug is well tolerated (see Chapter 15, Sudden Cardiac Death).

2. **Ventricular tachycardia:** This rhythm is defined as more than 3 consecutive PVCs at a rate of 120/min or greater. Therapy is dictated by the clinical status of the patient. If transient or sustained without clinical evidence of hypoperfusion, intravenous lidocaine may be used (see above). Synchronized countershock at 50–400 W/sec should be used if the rhythm is sustained and associated with hemodynamic deterioration.

3. **Accelerated idioventricular rhythm:** This rhythm may be the result of enhanced automaticity of an ectopic ventricular pacemaker or the result of variable exit block of a focus of ventricular tachycardia. The wide ectopic QRS complexes occur at regular intervals, resulting in atrioventricular dissociation when the prevailing supraventricular rhythm slows below the intrinsic rate of the idioventricular pacemaker (60–90/min). It is usually benign and does not result in ventricular fibrillation. Close monitoring for 24 hours is advisable because of rare association with ventricular tachycardia. If the rhythm is not hemodynamically tolerated, suppression with lidocaine, procainamide, or atropine (by increasing the sinus rate) can be used. Overdrive atrial pacing is also effective. Treatment is infrequently necessary.

AV Block and MI

The incidence of progression to high-degree AV block, without previous ECG evidence of conduction disturbance, is approximately 6%. The onset of complete heart block (CHB) is different, depending on the site of infarction:

Inferior MI. Complete heart block is the result of increased vagal tone or ischemia of the AV node. CHB rarely occurs suddenly. Progression from first-degree block to various degrees of second-degree AV block usually precedes CHB. During CHB, the heart rate is generally 50 beats/min, and QRS is commonly narrow. Treatment ranges from observation of the stable patient to using intravenous atropine in the hemodynamically unstable patient (dosage of 0.5 mg intravenously up to 2 mg intravenously).

Anterior MI. Caused by ischemia or infarction of the His bundle or both bundle branches, CHB frequently develops suddenly and results in wide, bizarre QRS complexes and bradycardia. Pacemaker therapy may be necessary. A permanent pacemaker should be implanted in any patient who develops permanent or transient high-degree AV block associated with bundle branch block during an MI.

Indications for temporary pacing (transcutaneous or transvenous) in acute MI:

- Symptomatic bradycardia (sinus bradycardia or type I second-degree AV block) unresponsive to atropine.
- Type II second-degree AV block or complete heart block.
- Bilateral bundle branch block (BBB), alternating BBB, or RBBB and alternating left anterior superior hemiblock (LASH), left posterior inferior hemiblock (LPIH).
- Newly acquired or age-indeterminate LBBB or RBBB with LASH or LPIH
- RBBB or LBBB and first-degree AV block.

Recurrent Chest Pain

Recurrent chest pain during and after the first 24 hours is not unusual and is often relieved with nitrates alone. Nitroglycerin should be used in small doses (0.4 mg sublingual) in normotensive patients. If chest pain persists or recurs, consider the following:

1. A combination of sublingual nitroglycerin tablets and parenteral morphine (in incremental 2-mg intravenous doses). Adequate sedation is usually achieved with morphine.
2. If the pain persists or recurs and hypotension is not present, start topical nitroglycerin ointment at $\frac{1}{2}$ inch every 4 hours

with rapid stepwise increase to 2 inches every 4 hours if necessary.

3. If the above are ineffective, start intravenous nitroglycerin—40 mg in 250 mL of 5% dextrose in water at 5 mL/hr. Intravenous nitroglycerin can be safely administered to hemodynamically stable patients without pulmonary artery (PA) pressure monitoring. The usual range of nitroglycerin needed for pain control is 10 μg to 200 μg/min. In invasively monitored patients, fluids should be administered if PCWP falls below 15 mm Hg and is associated with a significant drop in blood pressure or cardiac output. If clinical evidence of hypoperfusion occurs in a patient without PA pressure monitoring in the low-dose range, fluids should be given judiciously and a PA catheter should be inserted. Intravenous nitroglycerin is an arterial vasodilator as well as a venodilator; therefore, attempts to maintain blood pressure by volume challenge may not always be successful. The rationale of intravenous nitroglycerin therapy is reduction of MVO_2, coronary vasodilation, promotion of collateral supply, and reversal of any coronary spasm.

4. If pain recurs or persists despite maximal intravenous nitroglycerin, intravenous propranolol or metoprolol may be used if PCWP is less than 18 and cardiac index is greater than 2.4 L/min/M^2. Invasive pressure monitoring is recommended. Propanolol can be given in 1-mg doses every 10–15 min to a total dose of 0.05–0.1 mg/kg. Metoprolol can be given in 5-mg boluses at 5-min intervals to a total dose of 15 mg. In the setting of an AMI, β-blocking agents may affect the myocardium unpredictably and their use must be monitored closely. If acutely effective and tolerated, β blockers can then be given orally—propanolol 20–80 mg every 6 hours or metoprolol 50–100 mg every 12 hours.

5. Calcium channel blockers should be used with caution in the setting of acute MI (see above) but may be of value if recurrent or persistent chest pain is unresponsive to nitrates and β blockers.

6. Recurrent chest pain may not be due to ongoing myocardial ischemia. Postinfarction pericarditis should be considered and can be treated with additional aspirin or nonsteroidal anti-inflammatory drugs.

7. If low BP, low cardiac index, or a high PCWP prohibit the

use of β blockers or calcium channel blockers or they are not effective, intra-aortic balloon pumping (IABP) (see below) and continued intravenous nitroglycerin may result in pain relief.

Coronary arteriography and coronary revascularization (PTCA or bypass surgery) should be considered if the above measures fail to control symptoms.

Hemodynamic Dysfunction

An acute myocardial infarction almost always causes some degree of acute LV dysfunction. Whether this dysfunction becomes clinically apparent or important depends on the amount of myocardium damaged; a loss of myocardium greater than 40% generally leads to cardiogenic shock. Several classifications have been developed that correlate LV dysfunction during an AMI to in-hospital mortality. The Killip Classification is one of the most frequently quoted and is based entirely on clinical findings (86) (see Table 9.3).

A clinical, noninvasive evaluation of the patient with an AMI has significant limitations in that it will overestimate cardiac index in 25% of patients and it will underestimate PCWP in 15% of patients. Therefore, in high-risk mortality groups (Killip classes III and IV) or in a patient with a confusing clinical picture, a PA catheter should be inserted so that therapeutic decisions can be based on hemodynamic findings.

Indications for balloon flotation right heart monitoring in acute MI (46):

Table 9.3
Killip Classification

	Incidence	Mortality
I. No heart failure	33%	6%
II. Mild failure (bibasilar rales)	38%	17%
III. Frank pulmonary edema	10%	38%
IV. Cardiogenic shock (hypotension with BP of <90 mm Hg, peripheral vasoconstriction, oliguria, and pulmonary vascular congestion)	19%	81%

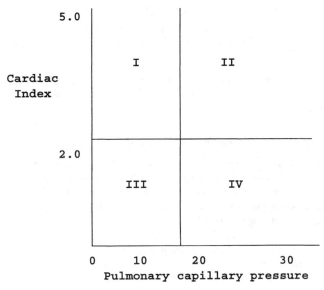

Figure 9.1. Hemodynamic Subsets in Acute Myocardial Infarction.

- Severe or progressive CHF or pulmonary edema.
- Cardiogenic shock or progressive hypotension.
- Suspected mechanical complications (see below).
- Hypotension that does not respond promptly to fluid administration in a patient without pulmonary congestion.

It should be noted, however, that the value of right heart monitoring in acute MI and in other critically ill patients has not been well established (87).

A classification that correlates clinical signs with invasive hemodynamic data and that is helpful in planning treatment is that of Forrester et al (88), which is shown in Figure 9.1. Subsets or groups of patients (noted by roman numerals) are defined based on the measurement of PCWP (mm Hg) and cardiac index (L/min/M^2).

Subset I. Uncomplicated. No specific therapy indicated. Mortality is approximate 3%.

Subset II. Mild to moderate CHF. Major problem is elevated PCWP. Treatment involves reduction of preload with either diuretics or nitrates. In evaluating therapeutic response, it should be remembered that there is a "lag period" between normalization of PCWP and disappearance of rales and radiographic resolution. Mortality is approximately 9%.

Subset III. Low cardiac output in the setting of a "normal" PCWP. This group would include patients with an inappropriately low wedge pressure in the setting of acute infarction (optimal in acute MI is 14–18 mm Hg) and those patients with right ventricular infarction (see below). Management should be directed toward optimizing preload with fluid administration. Mortality is approximately 20%.

Subset IV. Cardiogenic shock. The major problem is a markedly reduced confidence interval (CI), usually <2.2 L/min/M^2 and an elevated pulmonary pressure. Mortality is approximately 60–80%.

The systolic pressure will primarily dictate the therapeutic approach:

1. If the systolic pressure is higher than 100 mm Hg, increase cardiac index through afterload reduction with very cautious vasodilator therapy.
2. With moderately severe hypotension (systolic BP, 75–90 mm Hg), dobutamine may improve CI and BP. Dopamine may be added to increase BP if dobutamine alone fails to do so.
3. With significant hypotension (systolic pressure lower than 75 mm Hg), use a pressor agent (e.g., dopamine) because rapid attainment and maintenance of an adequate BP (systolic, 90–100) is of prime importance in treating cardiogenic shock. Dobutamine may be added for its effect on cardiac output, but usually it will not raise the BP enough to be used without a pressor. A combination of dobutamine and dopamine may be most effective (89).

IABP in Cardiogenic Shock

Ideal candidate criteria for IABP include early in course (less than 6 hours post infarction), younger patients, first MI, absence of any terminal disease, and no aortic insufficiency.

Indications for intra-aortic balloon counterpulsation (46):

• Cardiogenic shock not quickly reversed with pharmacologic therapy as a stabilizing measure for angiography and prompt revascularization.

- Acute mitral regurgitation or ventricular septal defect complicating MI as a stabilizing intervention before angiography and repair/revascularization.
- Recurrent intractable ventricular arrhythmias with hemodynamic instability.
- Refractory post-MI angina as a bridge to angiography and revascularization.
- Signs or hemodynamic instability, poor left heart function, or persistent ischemia in patients with large areas of myocardium at risk

Hemodynamic Effects of IABP. Afterload is reduced and diastolic pressure is increased, thereby improving coronary perfusion pressure and cardiac output. Overall effect is to improve myocardial metabolism and decrease LV size.

Course. Twenty percent of patients with AMI and cardiogenic shock recover to be weaned off IABP and discharged to their homes. The remainder usually improve but continue to be IABP dependent. Heart catheterization and cardiac surgery may be beneficial. Surgery is most successful in patients with a correctable mechanical defect (i.e., ventricular septal defect [VSD], aneurysm, or ruptured papillary muscle) in addition to bypassable coronary artery obstructions (90).

Complications of IABP

There is a 15–30% incidence of complications. These include: *(a)* rupture of balloon; *(b)* emboli from balloon to kidneys or lower extremities; *(c)* dissection of the aorta; *(d)* leg ischemia resulting in neuropathy, myopathy or amputation; *(e)* groin infections; *(f)* thrombocytopenia and anemia; and *(g)* leg claudication. Embolic phenomena are markedly decreased by the use of anticoagulation with heparin during IABP therapy.

Right Ventricular Infarction

This complication is almost exclusively associated with acute inferior infarction. Nineteen to 43% of inferior infarctions are complicated by right ventricular (RV) involvement, but only 3–8% of these have clinical findings suggestive of right ventricular dysfunction, such as neck vein distention or arterial hypotension (91). The syndrome of hypotension and low cardiac output associated with a right ventricular infarction is attributed to the inability of the infarcted right ventricle to maintain adequate left ventricular filling. Confirm the diagnosis by the following:

ECG: An ECG sign of RV infarct is the presence of ST elevation in the right precordial leads, especially V4R (92).

Swan-Ganz catheter: Elevated mean right atrial pressures (12–20 mm Hg), which is equal to or greater than the PCWP (91).

Gated cardiac blood pool scan: Poor right ventricular function (91).

Therapy includes **(a)** plasma expanders to increase the filling pressure in the right heart, favoring increased passive flow through the lungs to the left heart (follow PCWP as a guide to fluid therapy), and **(b)** afterload reduction of the left heart to increase cardiac output and decrease left atrial pressure, encouraging passive filling from the right heart (91).

Cardiogenic shock due to predominant RV dysfunction is uncommon; however, this is an important entity to recognize because it represents a treatable subset of cardiogenic shock with a survival of better than 50% compared to 10–15% survival in shock due to anterior LV wall infarction.

MECHANICAL DEFECTS CAUSING DECOMPENSATION (93,94)

1. **Ruptured papillary muscle.**

    Clinical picture: Sudden appearance of an apical systolic murmur associated with abrupt clinical LV failure. Course may be less severe if only papillary head and not the entire body of the muscle is ruptured.

    Incidence: 1–5% among patients dying of an acute myocardial infarction. Occurs 2–10 days post MI, primarily involves the posterior side of the papillary muscle and is associated with inferior-posterior MI.

    Mortality: 70% within 24 hours; 90% within 2 weeks.

    Diagnosis: Large V waves on PCWP tracing. Two-dimensional ECG may show the ruptured papillary muscle. Doppler echocardiography will demonstrate severe mitral regurgitation.

    Therapy:

a) Afterload reduction and inotropic support; if ineffective, consider IABP.

b) If stabilized medically, surgery in weeks to months. If unstable and in need of IABP, cardiac catheterization is indicated and possibly immediate surgery.

2. **Ventricular septal rupture.**

   Clinical picture: Very similar to ruptured papillary muscle. Sudden onset of harsh systolic murmur along the left sternal border associated with hemodynamic deterioration.

   Incidence: Incidence is 0.5–1%, accounting for approximately 2% of deaths after an infarction. Usually associated with an anteroseptal infarction occurring 9–10 days post infarction. Rupture commonly involves the apical anterior muscular septum.

   Mortality: 24% within 24 hours; 87% within 2 months.

   Diagnosis: Oxygen saturation step-up in the pulmonary artery as compared to right atrium in blood samples drawn from the Swan-Ganz catheter. ECG may demonstrate the defect in the interventricular septum. Doppler echocardiography will show flow from left to right across the defect.

   Therapy: Same as for ruptured papillary muscle.

EMBOLIC COMPLICATIONS

Pulmonary Embolism

With the advent of early ambulation in patients with AMI, incidence of pulmonary embolism has seemingly decreased. Predisposing factors include LV failure, arrhythmias, old age, obesity, and varicose veins. Low-dose heparin (5000 units subcutaneously two times a day) markedly reduces the incidence of deep vein thrombosis (DVT) in patients with AMI and should, therefore, reduce the incidence of pulmonary emboli.

Arterial Embolism

Older studies (before 1973) quoted a 2.5–4.9% incidence of arterial emboli to the brain, kidneys or limbs, supposedly from intraventricular mural thrombus overlying the infarction. There are no current figures; clinically, the incidence seems less. Recommendations regarding the use of prophylactic anticoagulation therapy vary among institutions. Therapeutic recommendations include anticoagulation in patients with echo or nuclear scan documented new ventricular aneurysms or mural clots.

HYPERTENSION

Hypertension is not uncommon in the early phase of an acute myocardial infarction. It has many possible causes, including underlying essential hypertension, CHF, or elevated catecholamines secondary to chest pain or anxiety. Hypertension causes an increase in intraventricular pressure, which results in an increased MVO_2 via LaPlace's Law. This may worsen ischemia and even cause extension of the MI. If the patient is seen early in the infarction period (less than 6 hours after the onset of pain) or has evidence of ongoing ischemia (recurrent chest pain), cautious but aggressive management of hypertension is recommended in hopes of modifying infarct size. Attempt to adequately control chest pain with nitrates and/or morphine.

Sedation is recommended if the patient is anxious. If BP remains elevated, continue the use of nitrates and β blockers and consider the cautious use of low doses of diuretics. If the BP remains significantly elevated, the use of intravenous medication is warranted. With mild cases, intravenous nitroglycerin is recommended, but with a markedly elevated BP, intravenous antihypertensive agents in the form of β blockers (labetalol) or ACE inhibitors should be given. Intra-arterial pressure monitoring will facilitate dose titration.

NON–Q-WAVE MYOCARDIAL INFARCTION (NQMI)

Historically, two types of myocardial infarction have been described: nontransmural and transmural. Other terms used to make this distinction are subendocardial and intramural. These older terms have been replaced by the new terms non–Q-wave MI and Q-wave MI. However, it should be understood that there is no absolute relationship between the extent of necrosis into the thickness of the ventricular wall and the presence or absence of Q wave. Strictly speaking, nontransmural MI may include Q waves and transmural MI may not have Q waves. Pathologic studies have shown that true subendocardial MIs were associated with a low percentage of new Q waves (10%) and true transmural MIs with a high percentage of new Q waves (70%). Some MIs are mixed, appearing nontransmural on gross examination but histologically transmural at one point. Despite these considerations, it is still valid to make the differentiation between

NQMI and QMI on prognostic, pathophysiologic, and therapeutic grounds (95).

NQMI can be diagnosed when two of the following three criteria are present: *(a)* prolonged anginal chest pain, *(b)* significant elevation of cardiac enzymes, and *(c)* persistent ST or T changes without Q waves. Multiple reports have compared the differences in QMI and NQMI. One MI out of three or four is NQMI. NQMI affects a slightly older population with a slightly higher proportion of women. The size of the NQMI is more limited than that of the QMI when analyzing enzymatic, angiographic, scintigraphic, and echocardiographic data. However, noninvasive stress testing has shown that residual myocardial ischemia is more frequent in the NQMI. Coronary angiography has demonstrated a lower incidence of complete occlusion but the same degree of coronary disease. Pathologic studies have shown a smaller number of coronary thrombi in the necrotic area in the NQMI and a high proportion of contraction band necrosis; this pattern is typical of reperfusion and is characteristic of the pathology seen with thrombolytic therapy. This finding has led to the speculation that early spontaneous reperfusion may be the underlying pathophysiologic mechanism in NQMI. Despite a low incidence of acute complications, patients with NQMI have a significantly higher rate of reinfarction and subsequent angina. One study has shown a 43% incidence of extension in NQMI versus 8% in QMI. Reinfarction most often occurs in the same area as the initial event, which is most commonly the anterior myocardium. Gibson found more frequent unstable angina post NQMI (36%) than in the QMI (22%) and the incidence of bypass operation or angioplasty was 33% versus 19%. Reinfarction and angina are more frequent because of a peri-infarction zone of ischemia maintained by a high-grade coronary stenosis and inadequate collateral circulation.

These observations have led to the emerging concept that NQMI is a limited but unstable event. Because myocardial ischemia is potentially reversible, its presence should be energetically sought in the NQMI setting. Along with medical therapy of aspirin and nitrates, evidence from the Multicenter Diltiazem Post-Infarction Trial (MDPIT) and the Diltiazem Reinfarction Study (DRS) shows a substantial reduction (48%) in myocardial events for diltiazem-treated patients compared to placebo. Therefore, diltiazem may be given to patients with NQMI without pulmonary congestion unless there is some contraindication. After stabilization with medication, strong consideration should be given to early angiography in search of lesions to be treated by PTCA or CABG.

REINFARCTION

Recurrent chest pain and sudden deterioration of functional status, as well as secondary elevation of plasma CPK-MB, are the clues that reinfarction has occurred. Eighty-five percent of reinfarctions occur during the initial hospitalization (between the third and tenth hospital day). The overall incidence is 25% of cases, with an incidence of 10% in transmural MIs and 42% in subendocardial MIs. In addition to recurrent chest pain and the clinical setting of subendocardial MI, other predictors of extension of MI include female gender and obesity. Early reinfarction carries a high mortality (25%) during first 3 weeks.

LOW-LEVEL EXERCISE TESTING

Under close supervision of trained personnel, a slow, gradual increase in activity levels is started in the coronary care unit (CCU) and then continued throughout the hospital course. A low-level stress test may be performed just before discharge to: *(a)* determine a safe level of home activity and a safe exercise prescription for outpatient cardiac rehabilitation and *(b)* to identify patients at high risk for future cardiac events. Patients with a positive low-level stress test have a significant risk of cardiac-related mortality during the subsequent year (66,96). This subgroup of patients should have close observation and possibly early heart catheterization and bypass surgery, PTCA, or other interventional procedure.

CARDIAC REHABILITATION

One of the goals of a comprehensive rehabilitation program is to encourage risk factor modification, such as cessation of smoking, dietary counseling, and treatment of hypertension and diabetes. Exercise training is also a significant component of cardiac rehabilitation and should focus on improving work capacity and reducing symptoms. The positive training effects of a lower heart rate and BP reduce myocardial oxygen consumption and thus help relieve symptoms. Attention should also be given to vocational status and psychosocial manifestations of the illness. Unfortunately, cardiac rehabilitation patients have not been shown to have significant reduction in mortality after myocardial infarction.

References

1. Fuster V, Badimon L, Badimon JJ, et al. The pathogenesis of coronary artery disease and the acute coronary syndromes. N Engl J Med 1992; 326:310.
2. Reeder GS, Gersh BJ. Modern management of acute myocardial infarction. Curr Probl Cardiol 1996;21:591.
3. Gaspoz JM, Lee TH, Goldman L. Emergency room evaluation and triage strategies for patients with acute chest pain: lessons from the pre-thrombolytic era. In: Califf RM, Mark DB, Wagner GS, eds. Acute coronary care. 2nd ed. Philadelphia: Mosby-Year Book, 1995: 255–263.
4. Kannel WB, Feinleib M. Natural history of angina pectoris in the Framingham study. Am J Cardiol 1972;29:154.
5. Kannel WB, Abbott RD. Incidence and prognosis of unrecognized myocardial infarction. An update on the Framingham study. N Engl J Med 1984;311:1144.
6. Chiariello M, Indolfi C. Silent myocardial ischemia in patients with diabetes mellitus. Circulation 1996;93:2089.
7. Duncan AK, Vittone J, Fleming KC, et al. Cardiovascular disease in elderly patients. Mayo Clin Proc 1996;71:184.
8. Tcheng JE, Jackman JD, Nelson CL, et al. Outcome of patients sustaining acute ischemic mitral regurgitation during myocardial infarction. Ann Intern Med 1992;117:18.
9. Pohjola-Sintonen S, Muller JE, Stone PH, et al. Ventricular septal and free wall rupture complicating acute myocardial infarction: experience in the Multicenter Investigation of Limitation of Infarct Size. Am Heart J 1989;117:809.
10. Puleo PR, Roberts R. An update on cardiac enzymes. Cardiol Clin 1988;6:97.
11. Ohman EM, Armstrong PW, Christenson RH, et al. Cardiac troponin T levels for risk stratification in acute myocardial ischemia. N Engl J Med 1996;335:1333.
12. Antman EM, Tanasijevic MJ, Thompson B, et al. Cardiac-specific troponin I levels to predict the risk of mortality in patients with acute coronary syndromes. N Engl J Med 1996;335:1342.
13. Adams JE, Abendschein DR, Jaffee AS. Biochemical markers of myocardial injury: is MB creatine kinase the choice for the 1990's? Circulation 1993;88:750.

14. Guest TM, Jaffee AS. Rapid diagnosis of acute myocardial infarction. Cardiol Clin 1995;13:283.

15. Keffer J. Myocardial markers of injury. Evolution and insights. Clin Chem 1996;105:305.

16. Zaret BL, Wackers FJ. Nuclear cardiology (Part 1). N Engl J Med 1993;329:775.

17. Gersh BJ. Noninvasive imaging in acute coronary disease. A clinical perspective. Circulation 1991;84(Suppl I):I-140.

18. Feigenbaum H. Role of echocardiography in acute myocardial infarction. Am J Cardiol 1990;66:17H.

19. Moss AJ, Benhorin J. Prognosis and management after a first myocardial infarction. N Engl J Med 1990;322:743.

20. O'Rourke RA. Risk stratification after myocardial infarction. Clinical overview. Circulation 1991;84 (Suppl I):I-177.

21. Reeder GS, Gibbons RJ. Acute myocardial infarction: risk stratification in the thrombolytic era. Mayo Clin Proc 1995;70:87.

22. Mehta JL. Emerging options in the management of myocardial ischemia. Am J Cardiol 1994;73:18A.

23. Anderson HV, Willerson JT. Thrombolysis in acute myocardial infarction. N Engl J Med 1993;329:703.

24. Gossage JR. Acute myocardial infarction. Reperfusion strategies. Chest 1994;106:1851.

25. Fibrinolytic Therapy Trialists' (FTT) Collaborative Group. Indications for fibrinolytic therapy in suspected acute myocardial infarction: collaborative overview of early mortality and major morbidity results from all randomized trials of more than 1000 patients. Lancet 1994; 343:311.

26. Gruppo Italiano per lo Studio della soprovvivenza nell'Infarcto Miocardico: GISSI-2: a factorial randomized trial of alteplase versus streptokinase and heparin versus no heparin among 12,490 patients with acute myocardial infarction. Lancet 1990;336:65.

27. ISIS-3 (Third International Study of Infarct Survival) Collaborative Group. ISIS-3: a randomized trial of streptokinase vs tissue plasminogen activator vs anistreplase and of aspirin plus heparin vs aspirin alone among 41, 299 cases of suspect acute myocardial infarction. Lancet 1992;339:753.

28. The GUSTO Investigators. An international randomized trial comparing four thrombolytic strategies for acute myocardial infarction. N Engl J Med 1993;329:673.

29. O'Keefe JH Jr, Rutherford BD, McConahay DR, et al. Early and late results of coronary angioplasty without antecedent thrombolytic therapy for acute myocardial infarction. Am J Cardiol 1989;64:1221.

30. Horrigan MCG, Ellis SG. Primary angioplasty for myocardial infarction. J Invasive Cardiol 1995;7(Suppl F):47.

31. Grines CL, Browne KF, Marco J, et al. A comparison of immediate

angioplasty with thrombolytic therapy for acute myocardial infarction. N Engl J Med 1993;328:673.

32. Gibbons RJ, Holmes DR, Reeder GS, et al. Immediate angioplasty compared with the administration of a thrombolytic agent followed by conservative treatment for acute myocardial infarction. N Engl J Med 1993;328:685.

33. Zijlstra F, de Boer MJ, Hoorntje JCA, et al. A comparison of immediate coronary angioplasty with intravenous streptokinase in acute myocardial infarction. N Engl J Med 1993;328:680.

34. Belli G, Topol E. Coronary angioplasty in acute MI. Adv Cardiovasc Med 1994;1(2):1–8.

35. Rodgers WJ, Bowlby LJ, Chandra NC, et al. Treatment of myocardial infarction in the United States (1990 to 1993). Observations from the National Registry of Myocardial Infarction. Circulation 1994;90:2103.

36. Fan T, Mueller HS. Recent trends in thrombolytic therapy. Adv Cardiovasc Med 1995;2:1.

37. Topol EJ, Califf RM, George BS, et al. A randomized trial of immediate versus delayed elective angioplasty after intravenous tissue plasminogen activator in acute myocardial infarction. N Engl J Med 1987;317:581.

38. Rodgers WJ, Baim DS, Gore JM, et al. Comparison of immediate invasive, delayed invasive, and conservative strategies after tissue-type plasminogen activator. Results of the Thrombolysis in Myocardial Infarction (TIMI) Phase II-A Trial. Circulation 1990;81:1457.

39. Simoons ML, Arnold AER, Betriu A, et al. Thrombolysis with tissue plasminogen activator in acute myocardial infarction: no additional benefit from immediate percutaneous coronary angioplasty. Lancet 1988;1:197.

40. Ellis SG, Vande Weft F, DaSilva ER, et al. Present status of rescue angioplasty: current polarizations of opinion and randomized trials. J Am Coll Cardiol 1992;19:681.

41. Gibson CM, Cannon CP, Piana RN, et al. Rescue PTCA in the TIMI 4 trial. J Am Coll Cardiol 1994;1A:225A.

42. Ross AM, Reiner JS, Thompson MA, et al. Immediate and follow-up procedural outcome of 214 patients undergoing rescue PTCA in the GUSTO trial: no effect of the lytic agent. Circulation 1993;88(Suppl I):I–410.

43. Grande P, Madsen JK, Saunamaki K, et al. The Danish multicenter randomized study of invasive vs. conservative treatment in patients with inducible ischemia following thrombolysis in acute myocardial infarction (DANAMI). A multivariate analysis. Circulation 1996;94(Suppl I):I–29.

44. Fuster V, Dyken ML, Vokonas PS, et al. Aspirin as therapeutic agent in cardiovascular disease. Circulation 1993;87:659.

45. Antiplatelet Trialists' Collaboration. Secondary prevention of vascular disease by prolonged antiplatelet treatment. BMJ 1988;296:320.

46. ACC/AHA. ACC/AHA guidelines for the management of patients with acute myocardial infarction: executive summary. Circulation 1996;94:2341.

47. ISIS-2 Collaborative Group. Randomized trial of intravenous streptokinase, oral aspirin, both, or neither among 17,187 cases of suspected acute myocardial infarction (ISIS-2). Lancet 1988;2:349.

48. Turpie A. Anticoagulant therapy after acute myocardial infarction. Am J Cardiol 1990;65:20C.

49. Jeong M, Owen W, Staab ME, et al. Does ticlopidine effect platelet deposition and acute stent thrombosis? Circulation 1995;92(Suppl I):I-489.

50. Schafer AI. Antiplatelet therapy. Am J Med 1996;101:199.

51. The EPIC Investigators. Use of a monoclonal antibody directed against the platelet glycoprotein IIb/IIIa receptor in high risk coronary angioplasty. N Engl J Med 1994;330:956.

52. Kleiman NS, Ohman ME, Califf RM, et al. Profound inhibition of platelet aggregation with monoclonal antibody 7E3 Fab following thrombolytic therapy: results of the TAMI 8 pilot study. J Am Coll Cardiol 1993;22:381.

53. Rodgers GM. Novel antithrombotic therapy. West J Med 1993;159:670.

54. Ridker PM, Hebert PR, Fuster V, et al. Are both aspirin and heparin justified as adjuncts to thrombolytic therapy for acute myocardial infarction? Lancet 1993;341:1574.

55. Prins MH, Hirsh J. Heparin as an adjunctive treatment after thrombolytic therapy for acute myocardial infarction. Am J Cardiol 1991;67:3A.

56. Hsia J, Hamilton WP, Kleiman N, et al. A comparison between heparin and low-dose aspirin as adjunctive therapy with tissue plasminogen activator for acute myocardial infarction. N Engl J Med 1990;323:1433.

57. Delanty N, Fitzgerald DJ. Subcutaneous heparin during coronary thrombolysis. Too little, too late. Circulation 1992;86:1636.

58. Granger C, Miller, Bovell E, et al. Rebound increase in thrombin generation and activity after cessation of intravenous heparin in patients with acute coronary syndromes. Circulation 1995;91:1929.

59. Flather M, Weitz J, Campeau J, et al. Evidence for rebound activation of the coagulation system after cessation of intravenous anticoagulant therapy for acute MI. Circulation 1995;92(Suppl I):I-485.

60. Norwegian Multicenter Study Group. Timolol-induced reduction in mortality and reinfarction in patients surviving acute myocardial infarction. N Engl J Med 1981;304:801.

61. Beta Blocker Heart Attack Trial Research Group. A randomized trial

of propranolol in patients with acute myocardial infarction. I: Mortality results. JAMA 1982;247:1707.

62. Hjalmarson A, Elmfeldt D, Herlitz J, et al. Effect on mortality of metoprolol in acute myocardial infarction: a double-blind randomized trial. Lancet 1981;2:823.

63. Koch-Weser J. Beta-adrenergic blockade for survivors of acute myocardial infarction. N Engl J Med 1984;310:830.

64. Held PH, Yusuf S. Effects of beta-blockers and calcium channel blockers in acute myocardial infarction. Eur Heart J 1993;14(Suppl F):18.

65. Roberts R, Rodgers WJ, Mueller HS, et al. Immediate versus deferred beta-blockade following thrombolytic therapy in patients with acute myocardial infarction. Results of the Thrombolysis in Myocardial Infarction (TIMI) II-B study. Circulation 1991;83:422.

66. Gunnar RM, Bourdillon PDV, Dixon D, et al. ACC/AHA guidelines for the early management of patients with acute myocardial infarction. Circulation 1990;82:664.

67. Yusuf S, Collins R, MacMahon S, et al. Effect of intravenous nitrates on mortality in acute myocardial infarction: an overview of the randomized trials. Lancet 1988;1:1088.

68. Muller JE, Morrison J, Stone PH, et al. Nifedipine therapy for patients with threatened and acute myocardial infarction: a randomized double-blind, placebo-controlled comparison. Circulation 1984;69:740.

69. Wilcox RG, Hampton JR, Banks DC, et al. Trial of early nifedipine in acute myocardial infarction: the TRENT study. BMJ 1986;293:1204.

70. Danish Multicenter Study Group on Verapamil in Myocardial Infarction. Verapamil in acute myocardial infarction. Am J Cardiol 1984; 54:24E.

71. The Multicenter Diltiazem Postinfarction Trial Research Group. The effect of diltiazem on mortality and reinfarction after myocardial infarction. N Engl J Med 1988;319:385.

72. Gibson RS, Boden WE, Theroux P, et al. Diltiazem and reinfarction in patients with non-Q wave myocardial infarction. Results of a double-blind, randomized, multicenter trial. N Engl J Med 1986;315:423.

73. Swedberg K, Held P, Kjekshus J, et al. Effects of the early administration of enalapril on mortality in patients with acute myocardial infarction. Results of the Cooperative New Scandinavian Enalapril Survival Study II (CONSENSUS II). N Engl J Med 1992;327:678.

74. ISIS-4 (Fourth International Study of Infarct Survival) Collaborative Group. ISIS-4: a randomized factorial trial assessing early oral captopril, oral mononitrate, and intravenous magnesium sulphate in 58,050 patients with suspected acute myocardial infarction. Lancet 1995;345:669.

75. Gruppo Italiano per lo Studio della Soprovvivenza nell'Infarto Miocardico. GISSI-3: effects of lisinopril and transdermal glyceryl trini-

trate singly and together on 6-week mortality and ventricular function after acute myocardial infarction. Lancet 1994;343:1115.

76. Chinese Cardiac Study Collaborative Group. Oral captopril versus placebo among 13,634 patients with suspected acute myocardial infarction: interim report from the Chinese Cardiac Study (CCS-1). Lancet 1995;345:686.

77. The SOLVD Investigators. Effect of enalapril on survival in patients with reduced left ventricular ejection fractions and congestive heart failure. N Engl J Med 1991;293:641.

78. The SOLVD Investigators. Effect of enalapril on mortality and the development of heart failure in asymptomatic patients with reduced left ventricular ejection fractions. N Engl J Med 1991;327:685.

79. Pfeffer MA, Braunwald E, Moye LA, et al. Effect of captopril on mortality and morbidity in patients with left ventricular dysfunction after myocardial infarction: results of the Survival and Ventricular Enlargement Trial. N Engl J Med 1992;327:669.

80. Rutherford JD, Pfeffer MA, Moye LA, et al. Effects of captopril on ischemic events after myocardial infarction. Results of the Survival and Ventricular Enlargement Trial. Circulation 1994;90:1731.

81. Harrison DC. Should lidocaine be administered routinely to all patients after acute myocardial infarction? Circulation 1978;58:581.

82. MacMahon S, Collins R, Peto R, et al. Effects of prophylactic lidocaine in suspected acute myocardial infarction. An overview of results from the randomized, controlled trials. JAMA 1988;260:1910.

83. Hine LK, Laird N, Hewitt P, et al. Meta-analytic evidence against prophylactic use of lidocaine in acute myocardial infarction. Arch Intern Med 1989;149:2694, 1989.

84. Echt DS, Liebson PR, Mitchell B, et al. Mortality and morbidity in patients receiving encainide, flecainide, or placebo. The Cardiac Arrhythmia Suppression Trial. N Engl J Med 1991;324:781.

85. Teo KK, Yusuf S, Furberg CD. Effects of prophylactic antiarrhythmic drug therapy in acute myocardial infarction. An overview of results from randomized controlled trials. JAMA 1993;270:1589.

86. Killip T III, Kimball JT. Treatment of myocardial infarction in a coronary care unit: a two-year experience with 250 patients. Am J Cardiol 1967;20:457.

87. Connors AF, Speroff T, Dawson NV, et al. The effectiveness of right heart catheterization in the initial care of critically ill patients. JAMA 1996;276:889.

88. Forrester JS, Diamond G, Chatterjee K, et al. Medical therapy of acute myocardial infarction by application of hemodynamic subsets. Part 1. N Engl J Med 1976;295:1356.

89. Richard C, Ricome JL, Rimailho A, et al. Combined hemodynamic effects of dopamine and dobutamine in cardiogenic shock. Circulation 1983;67:620.

90. Goldenberg IF. Nonpharmacologic management of cardiac arrest and cardiogenic shock. Chest 1992;102(Suppl 2):596S.

91. Kinch JW, Ryan TJ. Right ventricular infarction. N Engl J Med 1994; 330:1211.

92. Robalino BD, Whitlow PL, Underwood DA, et al. Electrocardiographic manifestations of right ventricular infarction. Am Heart J 1989;118:138.

93. Lavie CJ, Gersh BJ. Mechanical and electrical complications of acute myocardial infarction. Mayo Clin Proc 1990;65:709.

94. Chatterjee K. Complications of acute myocardial infarction. Curr Probl Cardiol 1993;18:7.

95. Gibson RS. Non-Q-wave myocardial infarction: pathophysiology, prognosis, and therapeutic strategy. Annu Rev Med 1989;40:395.

96. Pitt B. Evaluation of the postinfarct patient. Circulation 1995;91:1855.

Chapter 10

Congestive Heart Failure

DEFINITION

Congestive heart failure (CHF) is not a single disease but a symptom complex with many different presentations and etiologies. CHF can be defined in hemodynamic terms as a pathophysiologic state in which impaired cardiac performance is responsible for the inability of the heart, at normal filling pressures, to increase cardiac output (CO) in proportion to the metabolic demands placed upon the circulation. In clinical terms, CHF is a pathophysiologic condition in which ventricular dysfunction is accompanied by reduced exercise capacity. The latter definition incorporates less severe forms of ventricular dysfunction (1).

PATHOPHYSIOLOGY

Because CO = stroke volume (SV) × heart rate (HR), the variables that regulate these determinants play a role in the etiology and therapy of CHF. Heart rate is a reflection of the interaction between sympathetic and parasympathetic tone. Stroke volume is determined by three factors: preload, contractility, and afterload. These factors actually relate to isolated muscle strip performance and, therefore, cannot be measured accurately in the clinical setting. However, the terms are widely used in clinical practice in the following context (2):

1. **Preload:** This term refers to the passive stretch of myocardial fibers and is approximated by the left ventricular end-diastolic volume. **Clinically, it is often equated with the pulmonary capillary wedge pressure (PCWP).** It is important to recognize that **the left ventricular end-diastolic pressure (LVEDP) or PCWP is inversely related to the compliance of**

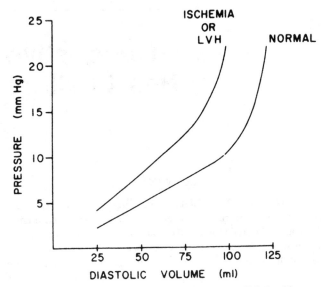

Figure 10.1. Left Ventricular Pressure-Volume Relationship

the ventricle. As shown in Figure 10.1, the ventricle becomes stiffer (less compliant) with ischemia or hypertrophy; therefore, a rise or fall in PCWP in a given patient may reflect changes in volume or compliance or both.

2. **Contractility:** Contractility refers to a reflection of the force-velocity-length relationship of the myocardium, independent of ventricular load or volume. It is often **equated with the rate of rise of ventricular pressure (dp/dt).**

3. **Afterload.** This term refers to the load or resistance encountered by the contracting myocardium, often **clinically approximated by the aortic pressure or the systemic vascular resistance.** It should be recognized that *(a)* afterload is directly related to the left ventricular wall tension and is, therefore, higher in a larger ventricle and *(b)* preload directly alters afterload. A stenotic aortic valve or systemic hypertension greatly increases left ventricular afterload.

When added work is imposed on the heart (i.e., hypertension, valvular disease, the three principal **compensatory mechanisms** may function to help maintain CO (3,4):

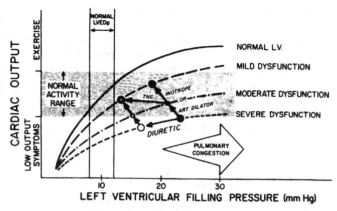

Figure 10.2. Frank-Starling Curves

1. **The Frank-Starling curve:** A myocardial muscle strip will contract with greater force if stretched to a greater resting or presystolic length. Clinical application of this principle requires substituting left ventricular end-diastolic volume (LVEDV) or LVEDP (approximated by PCWP) for fiber length and stroke work, SV, or CO for force. Frank-Starling curves relating preload (LVEDP) to force CO in the normal heart and in progressive left ventricular (LV) dysfunction are shown in Figure 10.2. **An impaired or failing left ventricle requires a higher filling volume or pressure to perform the same work as a normal ventricle.** It can be appreciated from Figure 10.2 that as the need for increased cardiac work occurs, the rise in filling pressure may exceed the pulmonary capillary oncotic pressure (approximately 25 mm Hg) and pulmonary edema may ensue. Diuretics, nitrates (TNG), arterial vasodilators, and inotropic agents (digoxin, dopamine) alter the LVEDP-CO relationship and are useful in the acute and chronic management of CHF (see below).

2. **Ventricular hypertrophy:** Hypertrophy, or an increased muscle mass, is stimulated by both pressure and volume overload states. Although hypertrophy potentially provides a beneficial increase in contractile elements, the benefits are counterbalanced by decreasing ventricular compliance, which is fur-

ther reduced by ischemia when the oxygen demand exceeds supply (2).
3. **Sympathetic nervous system:** The heart is richly innervated by sympathetic fibers and the increased release of endogenous catecholamines increases contractility and heart rate.

CLINICAL SIGNS AND SYMPTOMS

The major clinical manifestations of CHF can be arbitrarily divided into two categories: those due to fluid retention (right heart failure) and those due to pulmonary vascular congestion (left heart failure) (5,6). This division is clinically useful but can be misleading because the right and left heart are intimately associated with each other; moreover, the most common cause of right heart failure (RHF) is left heart failure (LHF).

Left Heart Failure

Basic abnormality: Increased left atrial pressure, resulting from an elevation in LVEDP or from mitral valve disease, is transmitted to the pulmonary vascular bed and is reflected clinically by an increased PCWP. If this pressure elevation exceeds the colloid osmotic pressure of the pulmonary vascular bed, fluid accumulation within the interstitial spaces (seen as Kerley A and B lines on the chest radiograph) will result. Progression of this pathologic process will subsequently result in the accumulation of fluid within the alveolar spaces (pulmonary edema), leading to poor oxygen exchange and hypoxia.

Symptoms: Decreased exercise tolerance, dyspnea, cough, orthopnea, and/or paroxysmal nocturnal dyspnea.

Signs: Tachycardia and inspiratory rales (beginning at the base of the lungs and heard progressively higher as the severity of LHF increases). Expiratory wheezes caused by bronchospasm (cardiac asthma) are not infrequent.

Laboratory: Arterial blood gas analysis may reveal hypoxemia and hypocarbia. Chest radiograph may demonstrate prominent upper lobe vessels ("reversal of flow"), Kerley's lines, the classic "butterfly" pattern of alveolar pulmonary edema, and/or pleural effusions (see below).

Right Heart Failure

Basic abnormality: Physiologic hormonal and renal responses occur to compensate for chronically decreased CO. These adaptive mechanisms lead to sodium and water retention in an effort to increase intravascular volume and (by means of the Starling mechanism) CO.

Symptoms: Dyspnea on exertion and fluid retention.

Signs: Increased central venous pressure, hepatojugular reflux, hepatomegaly, ascites, and peripheral or sacral edema may be seen.

Laboratory: Abnormal liver function tests may occur (elevated transaminases, elevated bilirubin, prolonged prothrombin time). Pleural and pericardial effusions are not uncommon. Hyponatremia with a low urinary sodium (<20 mEq/L) ("dilutional hyponatremia") and an elevated blood urea nitrogen (BUN) are frequent and reflect a decrease in renal perfusion.

RADIOGRAPHY OF CONGESTIVE HEART FAILURE

Irrespective of the underlying cause of CHF in an individual patient, the diagnosis of CHF must be confirmed before the initiation of any therapy. The physical examination may be very helpful, especially in RHF, but may be less helpful in diagnosing LHF because inspiratory rales may be associated with chronic lung abnormalities. Thus, the chest radiograph then becomes of clinical importance in diagnosing CHF.

Different **radiographic stages** reflecting the severity of CHF have been described, but the classical radiographic progression is not always seen. Moreover, the appearance and resolution rates of CHF on the chest x-ray are variable. The chest radiograph may not correlate temporally with the patient's immediate condition, i.e., there may be as much as a 12-hour diagnostic lag with the onset of CHF and a post therapeutic lag of up to 4 days after the clinical resolution of CHF.

1. **Pulmonary venous congestion and redistribution of flow.** Normally, more blood flow occurs to the dependent portions of the lungs. When the PCWP is elevated from 12 to 18 mm Hg, flow to the lower lung fields is reduced because of vasoconstriction whereas flow to the upper lung fields is increased. Recognition of flow distribution depend on the quality of the upright chest radiograph and is usually seen only in cases of chronic elevation of the PCW, such as in mitral stenosis.

2. **Interstitial pulmonary edema:** This is probably the most com-

mon radiographic sign of LHF. Fluid that accumulates in the interstitial spaces within the lung is seen as Kerley B lines (found in the lower lung fields peripherally and usually extending to the pleural surface). Fluid can also accumulate in the lobular septa, which form the framework of support for the lung and are seen as Kerley A lines (found emanating from the hila outward to the lung parenchyma). The pulmonary vessels typically are somewhat enlarged and their radiographic shadows are blurred. A PCWP of 18–25 mm Hg is usually present.

3. **Alveolar edema:** As the severity of the LHF increases and the PCWP rises acutely above 25 mm Hg, actual filling of the alveolar spaces with fluid can occur, i.e., pulmonary edema. This is recognized by the classic butterfly pattern of bilateral perihilar infiltrates.

IMPORTANT QUESTIONS IN CHF ASSESSMENT

What is the Underlying Cardiac Disorder?

CHF itself is not a diagnosis but only a symptom complex. Two different classifications of the etiology of CHF follow.

Functional Classification of CHF

1. Disorders of contractility (e.g., ischemic heart disease, cardiomyopathy).
2. Diastolic mechanical inhibition of cardiac performance (e.g., mitral stenosis, left atrial myxoma, pericardial tamponade); abnormalities of left ventricular relaxation (due to hypertrophy, fibrosis, ischemia, infiltrative disorders).
3. Systolic mechanical ventricular overload (pressure: aortic stenosis, hypertension; volume: aortic insufficiency, mitral regurgitation).

Anatomical Classification of CHF

1. Valvular.
2. Systemic hypertension.
3. Pulmonary hypertension.
4. Pericardial disease.
5. Myocardial disease.
6. Congenital.

7. High output states.
8. Traumatic (acute aortic insufficiency).

What is the Precipitating Cause of the CHF?

Knowing the precipitating cause(s) of CHF may greatly aid in the management of the disorder. Common precipitating factors include the following:

1. Infection.
2. Pulmonary embolus.
3. Lack of medications.
4. Arrhythmias.
5. Myocardial infarction.
6. Physical stress.
7. Increased sodium intake.
8. Sodium-retaining drugs.
9. Anemia.
10. Thyroid diseases.
11. Bacterial endocarditis.

PULMONARY EDEMA

Clinical Presentation

The end result of LHF may be acute pulmonary edema, which is associated with considerable morbidity and mortality if not recognized quickly and treated appropriately. Because the identification of the underlying abnormality producing CHF is just as important as making the clinical diagnosis of CHF, some comments on the physical examination, electrocardiogram (ECG), and chest radiograph in regard to this end in a typical patient may be helpful.

1. **Feel the carotid arteries carefully:** The quality of the upstroke may be helpful in identifying pathologic conditions (i.e., aortic stenosis) because its rate of rise is related to left ventricular function. The carotid pulse also serves as an invaluable tool in helping to correctly identify and time any murmurs heard on auscultation of the heart.

2. **Auscultate the heart.** Do not let the presence of adventitious breath sounds limit your attempt to correctly identify heart sounds and murmurs. Listen for signs of mitral stenosis (a

loud first heart sound, an opening snap best heard at the apex, and an apical diastolic rumble). Appreciation of these findings may be hindered by atrial fibrillation with a rapid ventricular response rate. A loud mid-diastolic crescendo-decrescendo murmur should alert one to the possibility of acute aortic insufficiency. This murmur, at times, is so loud that house staff consistently call it a systolic murmur, failing to properly time it with the carotid upstroke. A midsystolic murmur and loud S4 gallop in the presence of sinus rhythm should alert one to the possibility of acute mitral regurgitation.

3. **Examine the ECG:** Evidence of an old or new myocardial infarction may be present. Atrial fibrillation in combination with large fibrillatory waves in the anterior precordial leads (V1) suggests mitral valvular disease with left atrial enlargement.

4. **Examine the chest radiograph.** This is used to confirm a clinical diagnosis. Clear lung fields in the presence of a large cardiac silhouette in a dyspneic patient suggests pericardial tamponade (see Chapter 14).

Therapy of Acute Pulmonary Edema (6)

1. **Identify and eliminate any aggravating factors.**

2. **High-flow oxygen:** Best tolerated if administered by nasal prongs. Pulse oximetry may be helpful in determining the response to supplemental oxygen administration.

3. **Morphine sulfate:** Use in doses of 3- to 5-mg slow intravenous push. This drug is beneficial in several ways:
   Venous dilatation rapidly decreases preload.
   Sedative effect relieves extreme anxiety.
   Hyperventilation is decreased by directly depressing the respiratory center.
   The venodilatation does not become prominent until higher doses are reached. At high doses, respiratory depression may occur before venodilatation. Intravenous Lasix and the nitrates are more potent venodilators and should be used initially.

4. **Diuretics:** Rapidly acting loop diuretics (furosemides) are usually effective in doses of 40- to 80-mg intravenous push. Venous dilatation ensues quickly and decreases preload. An

increase in urinary output will occur later (7). If no clinical response is noted after 15–30 min, double the diuretic dose and administer again.

5. **Bronchodilators:** Useful if substantial bronchospasm is present (cardiac asthma). $\beta 2$ selective inhaled bronchodilators such as albuterol sulfate can be administered via a handheld nebulizer. Aminophylline has been used in the past but may precipitate arrhythmias, nausea, and vomiting. Bronchospasm is usually brief and will frequently diminish or resolve with the use of oxygen and diuretics.

6. **Endotracheal intubation:** Indications for intubation and artificial airway control include uncontrollable and excessive secretions, marked hypoxemia, excessive work of breathing, and/or severe respiratory acidosis.

7. **Inotropic agents: Dopamine** and **dobutamine** are potent cardiac inotropes that can be given intravenously and titrated to clinical response in the acute setting. Usual effective dose range is 5–15 mg/kg/min. These agents are also chronotropes and may produce arrhythmias. **Digitalis** does not produce consistent beneficial hemodynamic effects in acute CHF. It is a weaker inotropic agent compared with dopamine or dobutamine, and thus it is not the drug of choice for inotropic support in pump failure complicating acute myocardial infarction. Digitalis therapy, because of its late onset of action (6–8 hours), is also of limited value in the acute setting for the control of atrial fibrillation with a rapid ventricular response. **Amrinone** and **milrinone** are phosphodiesterase inhibitors and are additional potent inotropic drugs with a different hemodynamic profile. Both agents increase cardiac cyclic adenosine monophosphate (AMP) and increase contractility while producing vasodilation (decreased afterload). Amrinone is used at an initial dose of 0.75 mg/kg followed by a maintenance infusion of 5–20 μg/kg/min. Milrinone is approximately 15 times more potent than amrinone but has fewer side effects.

8. **Nitrates:** Pulmonary venous pressure decreases promptly with acute nitrate administration; sublingual nitrates can be very effective in relieving congestive symptoms in the immediate treatment of pulmonary edema. With **intravenous nitroglycerin,** the arterial pressure decreases slightly, the heart rate remains unchanged, and there may be a modest increase

in cardiac output. These beneficial effects progressively decline with continuous use. After 24 hours, most of the hemodynamics return to control levels; this appears to be caused by nitrate tolerance.

9. **Nitroprusside:** Nitroprusside (10–200 μg/min) can be used for hypertensive patients or patients with aortic or mitral regurgitation who do not respond to diuretics and nitroglycerine. Caution must be used because of reflex tachycardia, which can exacerbate ischemia. With prolonged use and in the setting of renal dysfunction, thiocyanate, a metabolite of nitroprusside, may accumulate and cause lactic acidosis.

10. **Intra-aortic balloon counterpulsation:** In the setting of acute myocardial infarction, acute mitral regurgitation, or acute rupture of the interventricular septum following infarction, intra-aortic balloon counterpulsation augments diastolic coronary blood flow and helps decrease afterload. This device is usually placed in the cardiac catheterization laboratory but can be inserted at the bedside if the patient is being treated at a facility without catheterization facilities. Contraindications include aortic regurgitation and aortic dissection, which, if suspected, can be diagnosed by transesophageal echocardiography.

11. **Pulmonary artery catheterization:** Placement of a pulmonary artery balloon catheter can be useful for patients who are in cardiogenic shock or pulmonary edema and who are not responding to pharmacologic therapy. Additionally, this is a valuable diagnostic tool in determining whether pulmonary edema is of noncardiac origin. The optimal pulmonary capillary wedge pressure is 14–18 mm Hg.

We have found the pneumonic **"UNLOAD ME"** to be helpful in the treatment of acute pulmonary edema:

U— head of the bed upright
N— nitrates (sublingual or intravenous)
L— Lasix
O— oxygen
A— albuterol (if needed for bronchospasm)
D— dopamine or dobutamine
M— morphine
E— electrical cardioversion for tachyarrhythmias (atrial fibrillation or ventricular tachycardia)

MANAGEMENT OF CHRONIC CHF

The treatment of CHF is best guided by knowledge of the etiology and pathophysiology of the underlying cardiac abnormality. The most common cause of both acute and chronic heart failure is systolic dysfunction, usually due to ischemic heart disease, hypertension, and idiopathic dilated cardiomyopathy (a diagnosis of exclusion). However, up to 30% of patients with heart failure have normal systolic function, defined as an ejection fraction of >55%, and have evidence of diastolic dysfunction echocardiographically (see Chapter 4). Diastolic dysfunction can precede and commonly occurs together with systolic dysfunction. Common causes for diastolic dysfunction include ischemic heart disease, ventricular hypertrophy (usually secondary to systemic hypertension or aortic stenosis), diabetes, and the aging process. Echocardiography is the noninvasive diagnostic test of choice in defining ventricular function. The importance of a correct diagnosis is emphasized by the differing treatments (7–9).

Treatment of Patients with CHF and Systolic Dysfunction

In patients with signs and symptoms of chronic CHF, medical therapy is necessary to maintain a near optimal LVEDP (15–20 mm Hg) to maximize CO, thereby preventing pulmonary vascular congestion. The mainstays of medical therapy consist of the following (10).

1. **Restriction of physical activity:** Bed rest may sometimes be required in patients with decompensated heart failure (American Heart Association [AHA] class IV). In stable compensated patients, skeletal muscle conditioning may play a role in the exercise capacity of patients with heart failure. Although mild to moderate dynamic exercise may be beneficial, isometric exercise (such as weight training) can cause an acute increase in afterload and may be detrimental (11).

2. **Low-sodium diet:** For patients on an extremely low-sodium diet (1 g), free water restriction may also be necessary to prevent symptomatic hyponatremia. Low-sodium diets are difficult to comply with and extensive dietary counseling is often required (11).

3. **Diuretics:** The **loop diuretics** (furosemide, ethacrynic acid, bumetanide, torsemide) are most effective in doses titrated

to the desired clinical effort without inducing hypotension or azotemia. For patients who do not respond to a loop diuretic alone, the addition of a **thiazide** diuretic (hydrochlorothiazide or metolazone), which works at a different nephron site (the early distal tubule), may be helpful (12). After the initiation of diuretic therapy, serum electrolyte monitoring should be performed because clinically significant electrolyte abnormalities may occur, specifically hypokalemia. If hypokalemia becomes a chronic problem, the use of **potassium-sparing diuretics** such as triamterene, spironolactone, or amiloride may be helpful. Magnesium depletion commonly occurs with chronic diuretic therapy and can worsen potassium loss. Nonsteroidal anti-inflammatory drugs (NSAIDs), because of their effects on prostaglandin metabolism, can block the effectiveness of diuretics as well as promote fluid retention.

4. **Digoxin:** Digoxin therapy is unlikely to be of benefit in all patients with chronic CHF (13–15). Minimal or no benefit is seen in patients with mild heart failure and relatively well preserved left ventricular systolic function. For patients with more severe heart failure with significantly reduced left ventricular ejection fraction, digoxin therapy combined with diuretics and vasodilators should be considered. Clinical studies indicate that digoxin can increase ejection fraction, increase exercise tolerance, and decrease the compensatory sympathetic activity that accompanies a chronic decrease in CO. However, digoxin has not been shown to improve 5-year mortality in patients with CHF. A reduced daily dose of digoxin is usually required in patients with renal failure. Digitalis toxicity is more likely to occur in: (a) elderly patients, (b) renal failure, (c) small body size, (d) chronic obstructive pulmonary disease (COPD), (e) hypokalemia, or (f) digoxin in combination with quinidine, verapamil, or the macrolide antibiotics. The most frequent symptoms of digitalis toxicity are anorexia and nausea. Serum digoxin levels may be helpful in documenting toxicity but should not be overused and should be drawn at least 6 hours after the last dose. Patients with chronic atrial fibrillation may require higher than normal "therapeutic levels" to control the ventricular rate but may not be clinically toxic. Digoxin-specific Fab antibody fragments are the recommended therapy in the management of life-threatening digitalis toxicity. Approximately 75% of

patients will exhibit a clinical response within 60 min of anti-body administration (16).

5. **Vasodilator therapy:** One often assumes that reflex compensatory mechanisms for maintaining CO and BP in the face of acute or chronic CHF will produce a favorable effect. Unfortunately, this is not always true. The increase in systemic vascular resistance (SVR), which usually occurs when CO decreases, may have a deleterious effect on the heart by increasing the afterload or wall tension of the left ventricle. Vasodilator drugs can frequently alter the vicious circle of increasing SVR leading to decreased CO by decreasing total peripheral vascular resistance (TPVR) and impedance to left ventricular ejection. Hemodynamic improvement is the result of the following:

Improved ejection fraction, which decreases LVEDP and pulmonary congestion.

Decreased pressure work of the failing ventricle.

Reduced wall tension, decreasing myocardial oxygen demand.

Mechanism of Action

Nitrates: These drugs have their most pronounced effect on venous capacitance (venodilatation leading to a decrease in preload) and a variable effect on arterial resistance (decreased afterload). Nitrates may also produce dilatation of the coronary arteries and possible redistribution of blood flow to the subendocardium in ischemic heart disease. Nitrates have no direct effect on myocardial contractility. Sublingual, oral, and topical preparations may be used. Long-term therapy is frequently complicated by nitrate tolerance, which can be minimized by appropriate dosing (usually three times daily) (17).

Hydralazine: An effective arterial vasodilator, hydralazine is usually administered orally in combination with diuretics and/or long-acting nitrates. Used alone, hydralazine has little effect on preload; it is predominantly an arteriolar vasodilator and increases cardiac output. The combined regimen of hydralazine and nitrates provides substantial advantage in CHF by combining the increase in cardiac output with a decrease in pulmonary capillary wedge pressure. In the Veterans Administration Cooperative Study, the combination of hydralazine (300 mg per day) and isosorbide dinitrate (160 mg per day) was shown to decrease mortality of patients with mild to moderately severe CHF by approximately 25% compared to the placebo group, who received digitalis and diuretics. This combination has been effective in improving symptoms and improving exercise tolerance (18). Lower doses of hydralazine and nitrates do not improve mortality. The combination of hydralazine and oral nitrates is most commonly reserved for those patients who are unable to tolerate ACE inhibitor therapy.

ACE inhibitors: It has been shown that the renin-angiotensin system (RAS) is stimulated in patients with CHF, resulting in elevated levels of angiotensin II, plasma renin, and aldosterone (19). Angiotensin-mediated vasoconstriction results in increased systemic vascular resistance, and the increased renin and aldosterone contribute to sodium and water retention. Local autocrine-paracrine RASs have been described in many tissues, including blood vessels, heart, kidney, and adrenals. These may participate in the pathophysiology of CHF.

The principal action of the ACE inhibitors is the blockade of the conversion of angiotensin I to angiotensin II in the serum as well as at local tissues. Data suggest that the acute effect of ACE inhibitors occurs in the circulation and the chronic effect is related to the inhibition at the tissue level (19).

ACE inhibitors have been shown to improve hemodynamics, enhance diuresis, reduce symptoms, improve exercise capacity, and prolong survival of patients with CHF. The main hemodynamic effects include systemic vasodilation, reduction in blood pressure, increased cardiac output, and reduced filling pressures. A total of 70–80% of patients report symptomatic improvement, compared to 25% of placebo controls. The most compelling case for the use of ACE inhibitors is the data on improved survival (20). The Cooperative North Scandinavian Enalapril Survival Study (CONSENSUS) showed that enalapril significantly reduced mortality (by 31%) compared to placebo at the end of 1 year (21). Similar positive results were reported in the Captopril Multicenter Research Group study (22). Presently, ACE inhibitors should be given preference to other vasodilators in the management of chronic CHF. These drugs have emerged as the most important advance in CHF therapy in recent years.

Asymptomatic patients with left ventricular systolic dysfunction also benefit from ACE inhibitors. In the Studies of Left Ventricular Dysfunction Trial (SOLVD), enalapril reduced the incidence of symptomatic heart failure and rate of hospitalization for heart failure compared with a placebo group. There was also an overall trend toward decreased cardiovascular mortality in the enalapril treatment group (23). In the Survival and Ventricular Enlargement Trial (SAVE), patients with asymptomatic left ventricular dysfunction (LVEF <40%) who received captopril after myocardial infarction had an improvement in survival and a reduction in morbidity and due to cardiovascular events (24). Two other large, multicenter controlled trials, GISSI-3 and ISIS 4, also support the use of ACE inhibitors in patients with and without heart failure after myocardial infarction (25,26). However, intravenous administration of enalapril followed by oral therapy after infarction has not been shown to improve survival (27). All patients who have an ejection fraction <35–40% should receive an ACE inhibitor, if tolerated, after myocardial infarction.

Captopril (Capoten) inhibits angiotensin-converting enzyme and thus attenuates the vasoconstrictor properties of the active metabolite angiotensin II. The reduction in systemic vascular resistance in patients with CHF taking captopril is not entirely due to the inhibition of angiotensin II. The drug also seems to inhibit degradation of bradykinin as well as decreasing sympathetic activity (reducing circulating catecholamines). Captopril is a balanced vasodilator with actions on both the arteriolar and venous beds. There is usually no increase in heart rate associated with the decrease in SVR.

Captopril was the first ACE inhibitor to be approved for hypertension and CHF. It has a unique chemical structure in that it contains a sulfhydryl (-SH) group. The initial dose of captopril is 6.25–25 mg. The lower beginning dose is used for patients who are prone to first-dose hypotension, such as those who are volume-depleted, hyponatremic, or likely to have high plasma renin activity. Maintenance dosage ranges from 25 to 150 mg two or three times a day. The dose that has been shown to decrease mortality in clinical trials is 50 mg three times a day.

Enalapril (Vasotec) has properties similar to captopril. The initial dose is 2.5–5 mg. The maintenance dose ranges from 5 to 40 mg once or two times a day. The dose that has been shown to reduce mortality in clinical trials is 10 mg twice a day. Intravenous enalapril can be given at a starting dose of 0.625 mg every 6–8 hours up to 1.25 mg every 6–8 hours.

Lisinopril (Prinivil, Zestril) is initially given in a dose of 2.5–5 mg with the maintenance dose ranging from 20 to 80 mg in a single daily dose. Lisinopril has been shown to improve exercise tolerance and symptoms in patients with symptomatic heart failure.

Quinapril (Accupril) given in doses of 5 mg two times a day has also been approved for the treatment of CHF.

Ramipril (Altace) at 5 mg two times a day has been shown to decrease mortality when given between 3 and 10 days after myocardial infarction in patients with heart failure.

Other ACE inhibitors that have not been approved for use in CHF include benazepril (Lotensin), fosinopril (Monopril), moexipril (Univasc), and trandolapril (Mavik).

Adverse effects of ACE inhibitors include marked hypotension, bradycardia, skin rash, impaired renal function, and occasional cases of immune complex glomerulonephritis. Cough occurs in 1–5% of patients. Taste disturbance occurs in approximately 5% of patients. Proteinuria occurs in 1% of all patients but is more common in patients with azotemia (2.1–2.5%). Hypotension is usually encountered only with the first several doses, and the drug seldom needs to be withdrawn because of hypotension (0–6%). Attenuation of this hypotensive effect occurs rapidly and clinical symptoms of hypotension during maintenance therapy are rare. Hydralazine and isosorbide dinitrate should be considered for patients who cannot tolerate ACE inhibitors.

ADDITIONAL CONSIDERATIONS IN THE TREATMENT OF HEART FAILURE

Calcium channel blockers: These drugs should not be used to treat heart failure due to systolic dysfunction because of their negative inotropic properties. However, some patients have angina and/or hypertension as well as CHF. Preliminary data from the PRAISE trial (Prospective Randomized Amlodipine Survival Evaluation) suggest that amlodipine does not adversely affect morbidity or mortality in patients with CHF and may confer survival benefit in patients with nonischemic dilated cardiomyopathy.

β-adrenergic blockers: Because of the activation of the sympathetic nervous system in patients with dilated cardiomyopathy and CHF, β blockers have been investigated for use in treating this population (28). Metoprolol has been shown to be effective in reducing the need for heart transplantation and mortality in patients with dilated cardiomyopathy (29). Because β blockers are known to decrease mortality after myocardial infarction, patients who develop left ventricular dysfunction and CHF after infarction would be good candidates for this therapy. Newer β blockers that have both vasodilating and β-blocking activity, such as bucindolol and carvedilol, are being evaluated for use in such patients with CHF. Carvedilol has been shown to reduce morbidity and mortality in patients with heart failure who are receiving digoxin, diuretics, and ACE inhibitors (30). However, β-blocker therapy for the treatment of CHF is still considered investigational.

Warfarin: Anticoagulation with warfarin to prevent systemic emboli from a LV thrombus in patients with CHF has not been proven effective in randomized clinical trials. However, patients with atrial fibrillation, left ventricular thrombus after acute myocardial infarction, or prior documented embolism should be anticoagulated (31).

Home (outpatient) dobutamine/dopamine/milrinone: In patients with recurrent admissions for refractory CHF, home or outpatient clinic inotropic therapy may ameliorate symptoms but has not been shown to decrease mortality. Low-dose dobutamine ($2-5$ $\mu g/kg/min$) can be given in the outpatient setting with a percutaneous intravenous central catheter (32).

Cardiac transplantation: In patients with disabling symptoms of CHF or unacceptable risk of cardiac death and no contraindications to the procedure, heart transplantation remains an option. Unfortunately, there are far too many patients who need transplants compared to the number of donor hearts available. LV assist devices are experimental but provide a bridge to transplantation in selected patients. Contraindications include excessive age, active infection, active peptic ulcer disease, chronic seizure disorder, severe peripheral vascular disease, insulin-dependent diabetes, renal failure, liver failure, severely elevated pulmonary vascular resistance (unless a combined heart-lung transplant is considered), alcoholism or drug abuse, psychiatric instability, or risk of medical noncompliance.

TREATMENT OF PATIENTS WITH DIASTOLIC HEART FAILURE

Patients with diastolic dysfunction have abnormal LV relaxation due to a noncompliant left ventricle. This discussion will exclude the diastolic abnormalities seen in mitral stenosis, pericardial constriction, and hypertrophic cardiomyopathy. Symptoms are usually related to elevated filling pressures with pulmonary congestion and dyspnea. The goal of therapy is to reduce filling pressures without lowering cardiac output (7–9). Diuretics and nitrates are the mainstay of therapy, although calcium channel blockers and β blockers have been used with the intention of increasing the diastolic filling period and relaxing the ventricle. However, studies have not shown these agents to be effective. There is no role for digoxin in diastolic heart failure. ACE inhibitors may help if the patient has diastolic heart failure due to LV hypertrophy from untreated hypertension. Coronary revascularization may be beneficial for patients who have a noncompliant LV due to ischemic heart disease.

References

1. Ventura HO, Murgo JP, Smart FW, et al. Current issue in advanced heart failure. Med Clin North Am 1992;76:1057.
2. Arai AE, Greenberg BH. Medical management of congestive heart failure. West J Med 1990;153:406.
3. Burkart F, Kiowski W. Circulatory abnormalities and compensatory mechanisms in heart failure. Am J Med 1994;90(Suppl 5B):19S.
4. LeJemtel TH, Sonnenblick EH. Heart failure: adaptive and maladaptive processes Circulation 1993;87(Suppl VII):VII–1.
5. Karon BL. Diagnosis and outpatient management of congestive heart failure. Mayo Clin Proc 1995;70:1080.
6. American College of Cardiology/American Heart Association Task Force on Practice Guidelines (Committee on Evaluation and Management of Heart Failure). Guidelines for the evaluation and management of heart failure. Circulation 1995;92:2764.
7. Bonow RO, Udelson JE. Left ventricular diastolic dysfunction as a cause of congestive heart failure. Mechanisms and management. Ann Intern Med 1992;117:502.
8. Goldsmith SR, Dick C. Differentiating systolic from diastolic heart failure: pathophysiologic and therapeutic considerations. Am J Med 1993;95:645.
9. Vasan RS, Benjamin EJ, Levy D. Congestive heart failure with normal left ventricular systolic function. Clinical approaches to the diagnosis and treatment of diastolic heart failure. Arch Intern Med 1996;156:146.

10. Cohn JN. The management of chronic heart failure. N Engl J Med 1996;335:490.

11. Dracup K, Baker DW, Dunbar SB, et al. Management of heart failure. II. Counseling, education, and lifestyle modifications. JAMA 1994; 272:1442.

12. Cody RJ, Kubo SH, Pickworth KK. Diuretic treatment for the sodium retention of congestive heart failure. Arch Intern Med 1994;154:1905.

13. Jaeschke R, Oxman AD, Guyatt GH. To what extent do congestive heart failure patients in sinus rhythm benefit from digoxin-therapy? A systematic overview and meta-analysis. Am J Med 1990;88:279.

14. Smith TW. Digoxin in heart failure. N Engl J Med 1993;329:51.

15. The Digitalis Investigation Group. The effect of digoxin on mortality and morbidity in patients with heart failure. N Engl J Med 1997;336: 525.

16. Antman EM, Wenger TL, Butler VP, et al. Treatment of 150 cases of life-threatening digitalis intoxication with digoxin-specific Fab antibody fragments. Final report of a multicenter study. Circulation 1990; 81:1744.

17. Abrams J, ed. A symposium: Third North American Conference on Nitroglycerin Therapy. Am J Cardiol 1992;70:1B.

18. Cohn JN, Archibald DG, Ziesche S, et al. Effect of vasodilator therapy on mortality in chronic congestive heart failure. Results of a Veterans Administration Cooperative Study (V-HeFT). N Engl J Med 1986; 314:1547.

19. Gavras H. Angiotensin-converting enzyme inhibition and the heart. Hypertension 1994;23:813.

20. The SOLVD (Studies of Left Ventricular Dysfunction) Investigators. Effect of enalapril on survival in patients with reduced left ventricular ejection fractions and congestive heart failure. N Engl J Med 1991; 325:293.

21. The CONSENSUS Trial Study Group. Effects of enalapril on mortality in severe congestive heart failure. N Engl J Med 1987;316:1429.

22. Captopril Multicenter Research Group. A placebo-controlled trial of captopril in refractory congestive heart failure. J Am Coll Cardiol 1983;2:755.

23. The SOLVD Investigators. Effect of enalapril on mortality and the development of heart failure in asymptomatic patients with reduced left ventricular ejection fractions. N Engl J Med 1992;327:685.

24. Pfeffer MA, Braunwald E, Moye LA, et al. Effect of captopril on mortality and morbidity in patients with left ventricular dysfunction after myocardial infarction. Results of the Survival and Ventricular Enlargement Trial. N Engl J Med 1992;327:669.

25. GISSI-3. Effects of lisinopril and transdermal glyceryl trinitrate singly and together on 6-week mortality and ventricular function after acute myocardial infarction. Lancet 1994;343:1115.

26. ISIS-4. A randomised factorial trial assessing early oral captopril, oral mononitrate, and intravenous magnesium sulphate in 58,050 patients with suspected acute myocardial infarction. Lancet 1995;345:669.

27. Swedberg K, Held P, Kjekshus J, et al. Effects of the early administration of enalapril on mortality in patients with acute myocardial infarction. Results of the Cooperative New Scandinavian Enalapril Survival Study II (Consensus II). N Engl J Med 1992;327:678.

28. Sackner-Bernstein JD, Mancini DM. Rationale for treatment of patients with chronic heart failure with adrenergic blockade. JAMA 1995;274:1462.

29. Waagstein F, Bristow MR, Swedberg K, et al. Beneficial effects of metoprolol in idiopathic dilated cardiomyopathy. Metoprolol in Dilated Cardiomyopathy (MDC) Trial Study Group. Lancet 1993;342:1441.

30. Packer M, Bristow MR, Cohn JN, et al. The effect of carvedilol on morbidity and mortality in patients with chronic heart failure. N Engl J Med 1996;334:1349.

31. Baker DW, Wright RF. Management of heart failure. IV. Anticoagulation for patients with heart failure due to left ventricular systolic dysfunction. JAMA 1994;272:1614.

32. Miller LW, Mirkle EJ, Hermann V. Outpatient dobutamine for end-stage congestive heart failure. Crit Care Med 1990;18:530.

Chapter 11

Valvar Heart Disease

NORMAL VALVE FUNCTION

The efficiency of the heart as a pump is heavily dependent on the integrity of the cardiac valves. In health, cardiac valves ensure unimpeded anterograde flow when opened and prevent retrograde flow when closed. In this section, the functional anatomy of the normal cardiac valves will be reviewed and correlated with the hemodynamic events, heart sounds, and echo-Doppler ultrasonography to provide a basis for understanding the alterations that result from valvar disease. Although only the left heart valves are depicted, the same events occur in the right heart, at lower pressure and a fraction of a second later (Figs. 11.1–11.4).

It is possible to calculate mitral and aortic valve flow rates by dividing the cardiac output by the period of time that the valve is open as follows:

Mitral Valve Flow in mL/sec

$$= \frac{\text{Cardiac Output in mL/min}}{\text{Diastolic Filling Time in sec/min}}$$

Aortic Valve Flow in mL/sec

$$= \frac{\text{Cardiac Output in mL/min}}{\text{Systolic Ejection Time in sec/min}}$$

The subject depicted in Figure 11.5 has a cardiac output of 7.5 L/min (7500 mL/min). Blood only traverses the mitral valve during the diastolic filling period and the aortic valve during the systolic ejection period. These periods are separated by brief intervals during which both valves are closed and there is no flow. The isovolumic contraction period occurs during the ventricular systolic upstroke, and the isovolumic relaxation period occurs during the ventricular pressure downstroke.

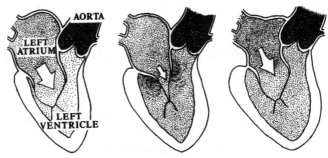

Figure 11.1. The Left-Sided Cardiac Valves During Diastole. Pressures in the chambers are denoted by the density of the shading; the darkest shading represents pressures above 80 mm Hg. Rapid (passive) inflow (on the left) follows mitral valve opening. The valve opens when the ventricular pressure falls below that in the left atrium, and up to 80% of the diastolic inflow volume (large white arrow) enters the ventricle. Diastasis (center) occurs when the pressures in the atrium and ventricle equilibrate and inflow is reduced or ceases as the valve leaflets float toward apposition. Next, atrial systole adds approximately 20% of the diastolic inflow volume, followed by a wake that initiates valve closure.

The diastolic filling time, in sec/min, is determined by measuring the time from mitral valve opening to mitral valve closure (the diastolic filling period) and multiplying that time by the heart rate. Similarly, the systolic filling time is the systolic ejection period, between the opening and closing of the aortic valve, multiplied by the heart rate. The heart rate can be calculated by dividing the number of seconds in a minute (60) by the interval between repeated events, e.g., the R-R interval. Using the above formulae, the mitral valve flow and aortic valve flow, in mL/sec can be calculated.

$$\text{Diastolic filling period} = 0.40 \text{ sec/cycle}$$

$$\text{Systolic ejection period} = 0.30 \text{ sec/cycle}$$

$$\text{Heart rate} = \frac{60 \text{ sec/min}}{\text{R-R interval} = .08 \text{ sec}} = 75/\text{min}$$

$$\text{Diastolic filling time} = 30 \text{ sec/min}$$

$$\text{Systolic ejection time} = 22.5 \text{ sec/min}$$

$$\text{Mitral valve flow} = 250 \text{ mL/sec}$$

$$\text{Aortic valve flow} = 333.3 \text{ mL/sec}$$

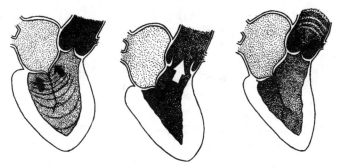

Figure 11.2. Left Heart During Systole. Mitral valve closure (left) initiated by the wake trailing the atrial systolic flow bolus is completed by a systolic rise in ventricular pressure. The black arrows denote the abrupt deceleration of the blood propelled toward the low-pressure left atrium, which affects the tensing mitral leaflets, resulting in a "shock wave," which results in the first heart sound at the ventricular apex. Ventricular ejection (white arrow, center) ensues when the intracavitary pressure exceeds the aortic diastolic pressure, opening the aortic valve and propelling a column of blood anterograde in the aortic root. Aortic valve closure (right) occurs as pressure in the left ventricle falls, resulting in flow reversal in the aortic root. The black arrows represent the abrupt impact of the retrograde surge of blood on the tensed aortic valve leaflets; the shock wave, the second heart sound (aortic valve closure sound) resulting from this collision, emanates in an anterograde fashion.

Normal atrioventricular (mitral and tricuspid) valves are capable of remarkable performance. At rest, the diastolic inflow rate across the atrioventricular valves averages approximately 200 mL/sec, and the systolic pressure difference between the left ventricle and left atrium—the back pressure on the closed mitral valve—is higher than 100 mm Hg. During exercise, cardiac output often triples, whereas tachycardia markedly reduces diastolic filling time. When the heart is beating rapidly, disproportionately more time per minute is used by the increased number of systoles. As a result, the diastolic flow rate through atrioventricular valves may approach 1000 mL/sec. Left ventricular systolic pressure nearly doubles during exercise; therefore, the back pressure on the mitral valve may be 200 mm Hg or more.

The diastolic filling time is the time that is available each minute after all of the systoles and all of the isovolumic times have been expended. The length of systole shortens somewhat

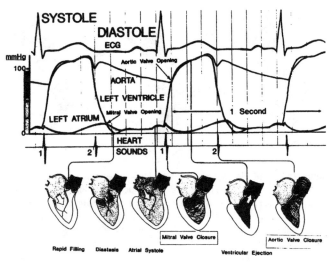

Figure 11.3. The Pressures and Heart Sounds in the Left Heart Correlated with Valve Function. Mitral valve opening occurs as ventricular pressure approaches its nadir; rapid inflow produces rapid filling waves. Atrial and ventricular pressures equilibrate during diastasis. Atrial contraction causes an *a* wave in the atrium and ventricle. Mitral valve closure is completed as the systolic rise in ventricular pressure begins. The first sound (1) and the sharp left atrial *c* wave are analogous to valve closure. Aortic valve opening begins as ventricular pressure exceeds aortic. Ventricular ejection ensues, continuing until ventricular relaxation causes a pressure decline. The atrium has no outlet during ventricular systole and increases in volume from venous inflow. The *v* wave in the left atrial pressure reflects filling. Aortic valve closure, the second heart sound (2), and the aortic dicrotic notch are synchronous.

with increasing heart rate and each isovolumic contraction; relaxation times also shorten slightly. Nevertheless, tachycardia progressively shortens the diastolic filling times, because systole and the isovolumic periods occupy more time per minute as the heart rate increases. These relationships can be seen in the Table 11.1.

LABORATORY ASSESSMENT OF VALVAR FUNCTION

Laboratory procedures that aid in the assessment and characterization of valvar function are listed below.

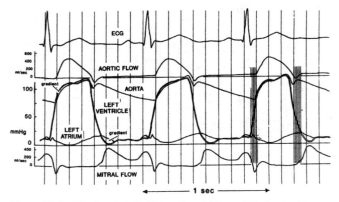

Figure 11.4. Mitral and Aortic Valve Flow Patterns. Mitral valve flow, as recorded with a flow transducer, occurs during the time that the mitral valve is open, termed the diastolic filling period. The flow pattern is bimodal with an early peak during the rapid filling phase and a lesser peak during atrial systole. During the high flow phases, small pressure differences, called gradients, can be recorded between the upstream (left atrium) and downstream (left ventricle) chamber, and the magnitude of the gradient is proportional to the flow rate across the valve. Aortic valve flow is confined to the systolic ejection period, reaches an early peak, and then declines progressively before actually reversing, when aortic valve closure interrupts the backflow. A small pressure gradient can be seen during the rapid outflow phases between the upstream (left ventricle) and downstream (aorta) compartments. Later in systole, the gradient reverses as reflecting waves return from peripheral reflecting sites in the arterial tree. Isovolumic contraction and relaxation are indicated by shading on the third cardiac cycle.

Noninvasive
    Routinely performed
        Electrocardiogram
        Chest radiography
        Cardiac echo-Doppler
    Selected cases
        Chest fluoroscopy
        Computed axial tomography
        Radionuclide angiography
Invasive
    Cardiac catheterization
    Cineangiography

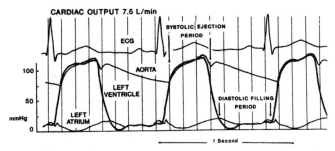

Figure 11.5.   The Systolic Ejection Period and Diastolic Filling Period. These tracings are used for the calculation of mitral and aortic valve flow rates (see text).

Table 11.1
Increasing Heart Rate with Constant Cardiac Output
(Cardiac Output 7.5 L/min)

Heart rate (beats/min)	Systolic ejection period (sec/beat)	Systolic ejection time (sec/min)	Isovolumic contract and relax (sec/min)	Systolic ejection time and isovolumic time (min)	Diastolic filling time (min)	Mitral valve flow (mL/sec)
50	0.320	16	6	22	38	197
75	0.300	22.5	7.5	30	30	250
100	0.240	24	10	34	26	288
150	0.200	30	12	42	18	417
175	0.194	34	14	48	12	625

It can be seen that an increase in heart rate, without any increase in output, markedly increases the mitral valve flow.

Electrocardiography (ECG)

Ventricular enlargement or hypertrophy usually causes ECG changes manifested by a frontal plane axis shift toward the affected ventricle and increased regional precordial-lead QRS voltage. Right ventricular hypertrophy may cause a rightward shift in the frontal plane and increased voltage or duration of R waves in the right precordial leads V1–V3. Left ventricular enlargement or hypertrophy shifts the axis leftward and increases the R-wave voltage in the left precordial leads V5–V6.

Severe or rapidly progressive ventricular hypertrophy may be manifest by T-wave inversion in leads with tall R waves ("strain" pattern). P-wave abnormalities may be seen when the atria are enlarged; tall P waves ("P pulmonale") suggest right atrial enlargement, and broad P waves (>110 msec) with terminal inversion in V1 ("P mitrale") indicate left atrial enlargement. Atrial fibrillation or frequent atrial premature beats are commonly associated with left atrial enlargement due to mitral valve disease.

Chest Radiography

Chest radiographs provide better depiction of overall cardiac size and pulmonary vascular distribution than any laboratory test. Valvar regurgitation usually increases the overall cardiac size on a chest radiograph because one or more chambers have dilated to compensate for the volume overload. Valvar stenosis may cause little if any cardiac enlargement, particularly if the stenosis affects the aortic or pulmonic valve. The ventricles usually compensate for obstructed outflow by developing concentric ("ingrowth") hypertrophy with decreased chamber size.

Lesions that elevate left atrial pressure and size (e.g., mitral stenosis) often cause a shift in the pulmonary vascular pattern, with increased filling of the upper lobe pulmonary veins and arteries in upright radiographs. The upper lung vessels are nearly collapsed when left atrial pressure is normal. As left atrial pressures rise, there is a shift away from the dependent lower lobe vessels to those in the upper lobes. When left atrial pressures acutely exceed the pulmonary oncotic pressure (approximately 25 mm Hg), the pulmonary vascular pattern may become blurred by edema in a butterfly pattern. Kerley B lines, fine horizontal lines extending to the pleura at the lung bases, are caused by edema-thickened interlobular septa and indicate chronic elevation of left atrial pressure.

Valvar calcification may be appreciated on chest radiographs, but can best be seen by cardiac fluoroscopy. Calcification is rarely seen in right-sided valves and is almost universally present in adult aortic stenosis. The location and pattern of motion of diseased valves enable the fluoroscopist to make an accurate prediction of valve pathology (Fig. 11.6).

Echocardiography (see Chapter 4) encompasses a number of related procedures that use ultrasound to provide two-dimensional images of the cardiac chambers and valves in motion, accu-

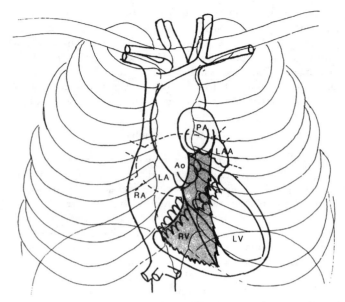

Figure 11.6. The Location of the Cardiac Chambers and Valves on a Frontal Chest Radiograph. Note that the right atrium (RA) forms the right heart border. The right ventricle (RV, shaded) is substernal and left parasternal; it is not a border-forming structure. The left atrium (LA) is a central, basal, and dorsal chamber; only the left auricular appendage (LAA) forms a border of the cardiac silhouette. The left ventricle forms the cardiac apex, which is in the fifth left intercostal space in the midclavicular line, and most of the left heart border.

rate dimensions of these structures, and flow–velocity profiles. All of these modalities are integrated in time and space, so it is possible to depict diseased valves, abnormal chamber dimensions, altered wall motion, and abnormal flow–velocity patterns simultaneously. These noninvasive procedures do not use ionizing radiation and are, therefore, invaluable in the initial assessment of patients with suspected cardiac valve disease as well as in serial examinations in long-term follow-up.

Noninvasive estimation of intracardiac pressure is dependent on the ability to measure accurately high-velocity flow across valves, which is possible in most patients.

INVASIVE LABORATORY STUDIES—CARDIAC CATHETERIZATION

Cardiac catheterization—the insertion of flexible catheters through veins and arteries to record intracardiac pressures and flow—is almost always combined with cineangiography. Injections of radiopaque contrast media into the cardiac chambers render them momentarily opaque so that their size, contour, and wall motion can be recorded by an image intensifier coupled to a motion picture or video camera. Injections downstream from a diseased valve will record valvar regurgitation; for example, an injection into the left ventricle will record mitral regurgitation. An injection upstream will depict the narrow jet of valvar stenosis. Without contrast media in the cardiac chambers, the myocardium, valves, and blood have the same radiodensity, so the operator monitors the passage of the catheter by observing the intracardiac pressure as well as the general location by the fluoroscopic image.

The combined study of catheterization and cineangiography provides quantitative as well as qualitative assessment of the severity and extent of heart disease. Quantitative data from the study include the magnitude of pressure, flow, and derived indexes: vascular resistance and valve orifice areas. Qualitative data include magnitude of valvar regurgitation, valve thickness and mobility, and ventricular wall motion. Ventricular volumetric measurements—diastolic volume, systolic volume, and ejection fraction—can be measured reasonably accurately, but the measurements are time-consuming and subject to considerable error.

Because there are risks associated with cardiac catheterization, this invasive procedure is usually reserved for patients who are considered candidates for valve surgery. When catheterization is performed on potential operative candidates, coronary arteriography is performed to assess the status of the coronary arteries by selective injections of contrast media into the coronary ostia. It can be legitimately argued that cardiac catheterization has been rendered almost obsolete by echo-Doppler ultrasonography, but noninvasive tests do not provide images of the coronary arteries in enough detail to rule out obstructions (Fig. 11.7).

STRUCTURAL AND FUNCTIONAL ABNORMALITIES

Abnormal valve function can result from structural as well as functional alterations. Structural valvar disease can be congenital

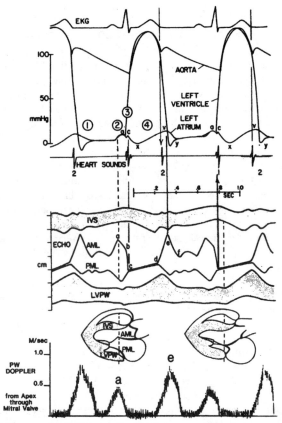

Figure 11.7. Echo-Doppler Ultrasonography Correlated with Left Heart Pressures and Heart Sounds. The circled numbers denote (1) rapid filling, (2) diastasis, (3) atrial systole, and (4) ventricular ejection. The pressure events are aligned with the apical heart sounds, M-mode echocardiogram, two-dimensional echocardiogram, and the mitral valve Doppler flow. The M-mode echocardiographic (*d-e*) represents the mitral valve opening motion, which is completed at *e*. The Doppler signal reveals a surge of flow toward the apical transducer (inflow), also labeled *e*. A second opening of the mitral valve, *a*, caused by atrial systole, is accompanied by a second surge in trans-mitral flow on the Doppler signal, also labeled *a*. Mitral valve closure (*a-b-c*), ends in *c;* note that *c* coincides with the first heart sound as well as the *c* wave of the left atrial pressure pulse. Note also that the mitral M-mode configuration and the Doppler waveforms closely resemble the mitral valve flow pattern illustrated in Figure 11.4, because they represent analogous events depicted by different recording modalities. During the periods of high-volume transvalvar flow, the mitral valve is forced open. During diastasis, when the inflow declines, the valve leaflets float back toward closure, *e-f*.

or acquired and can result in obstruction, backflow, or a combination of stenosis and regurgitation. Complete obstruction, or atresia, of a valve may occur as a result of faulty development of the fetal heart. Functional abnormalities or valve function can occur in structurally normal valves subjected to elevated pressures or distorted chamber anatomy caused by either underfilling or overfilling of the affected ventricle.

Surgically implanted prosthetic heart valves are intrinsically stenotic and may acquire more severe stenosis and/or develop regurgitation as a result of partial dehiscence, pannus ingrowth, thrombus, and/or wear and tear.

PRESSURE AND VOLUME OVERLOAD—COMPENSATORY MECHANISMS

Valvar lesions that cause obstruction to ventricular outflow cause a pressure overload, which results in hypertrophy greater than dilation of the affected ventricle. Regurgitant lesions of either the inflow or outflow valves primarily result in a volume overload, in which the ventricle dilates to accommodate the mandatory increase in stroke volume and, to a lesser extent, develops hypertrophy. Both hypertrophy and dilation are compensatory mechanisms that may allow the heart to continue to function reasonably well despite the burdens of valvar disease. Hypertrophy maintains a more favorable Laplace relationship, resulting in a lower wall tension than would otherwise be present in a ventricle with a high systolic pressure and/or large intracavitary volume. However, these compensatory mechanisms may be outstripped by advancing severity of disease or may fail by adversely affecting diastolic function of the cardiac muscle or by excessively increasing demand on the coronary arterial supply.

CLINICAL EVALUATION OF VALVAR DISEASE

Valvar abnormalities often cause cardiac symptoms (dyspnea, fatigue, chest pain) and/or signs (abnormal heart sounds, murmurs, venous or arterial pulses, precordial impulses, etc.). It is often possible for a clinician with knowledge of the pathophysiology of valvar disease to establish an accurate bedside diagnosis of most valve abnormalities, singly or in combination, by assimilation of the historical and physical findings. Appropriate noninvasive laboratory techniques may be used to add precision to the bedside diagnosis, whereas invasive studies are usually reserved for the preoperative evaluation of patients who are deemed to be candidates for cardiac surgery.

HEART SOUNDS, MURMURS, AND PULSES IN VALVAR DISEASE

Almost without exception, valvar lesions produce abnormal heart sounds and murmurs that can be detected by cardiac auscultation. These abnormalities may be characterized by extra heart sounds (opening snaps, ejection sounds, clicks, or gallop sounds), alterations in intensity or timing of heart sounds, or heart murmurs. Heart sounds, also called transients, result from the abrupt deceleration of a moving column of blood as a result of impact on valve leaflet tissue or the ventricular walls. Murmurs result from disturbed or turbulent flow, often through malformed valves. The timing, quality, and precordial location of these auscultatory phenomena establish the valve abnormalities responsible for these events.

In addition to altering heart sounds, valvar lesions often result in abnormal pulses, which can be detected by inspection and/or palpation of the precordium, the carotid arteries, and the jugular veins.

In the following sections dealing with specific valvar disorders, the characteristic auscultatory abnormalities will be integrated with the pressure recordings and the functional anatomical alterations responsible for them. Intracardiac imaging techniques, principally x-ray motion pictures (cineangiography) and echo-Doppler ultrasonography, in concert with recording of heart sounds and murmurs have established the causation of most of these auscultatory events. A house officer who is able to comprehend the interrelationship of cardiac events and their external manifestations can readily translate bedside findings into an accurate hemodynamic assessment.

MITRAL STENOSIS

Stenosis of the mitral valve most commonly results from the inflammatory changes associated with acute rheumatic fever. Acute rheumatic fever is relatively rare among those born and raised in the United States but is almost endemic in third-world countries and among the populace inhabiting crowded living or working environments in which Group A β-hemolytic streptococcal pharyngitis can spread rapidly. Most newly discovered cases of mitral stenosis in the United States occur among immigrants from Latin America, the Caribbean, and Asia. For unknown reasons, mitral stenosis is more prevalent in females.

The mitral orifice is restricted by commissural fusion, scarring, and/or calcification of the leaflets and variable degrees of subvalvar pathology (thickening and shortening of the chordae and elongation of the papillary muscles). The stenosed valve may become tapered like a funnel or may be rendered into a "fish mouth" configuration. Stagnation in the atrium may result in thrombus formation in the auricular appendage. Mural thrombosis and systemic embolism are common in mitral stenosis, especially if the left atrium is greatly enlarged and particularly if atrial fibrillation is present. Atrial fibrillation results from dilation of the atrium from the elevated pressure and inflammation and scarring of the atrial walls from the rheumatic process.

Hemodynamic Basis of Symptoms

Elevation of left atrial, pulmonary venous, and pulmonary capillary pressure results from the pressure gradient. The magnitude of pressure elevation is related to the severity of stenosis (reduction in valve area) and the rate of flow across the valve. The formulae of Gorlin and Gorlin define the relationship between pressure and flow in mitral stenosis:

$$\text{Mitral valve flow (mL/sec)} = \frac{\text{Cadiac out (mL/min)}}{\text{Diastolic filling time (sec/min)}}$$

$$\text{Mitral valve area (cm}^2) = \frac{\text{Mitral valve flow (mL/sec)}}{K \text{ Mitral valve pressure gradient}}$$

K is a constant derived from the gravity acceleration factor for blood and validated by correlation with surgical findings and is equal to 31.

These formulae reveal that the rate of mitral valve flow increases if there is either an increase in cardiac output or a decrease in diastolic filling time (as a result of an increase in heart rate). In exercise, the heart rate and cardiac output increase and the diastolic filling time decreases, greatly augmenting the mitral valve flow. The pressure gradient increases to the second power with any increase in flow; doubling the flow quadruples the gradient. Left atrial pressures in excess of 25 mm Hg exceed the oncotic pressure in the pulmonary capillaries and result in pulmonary edema.

When left atrial pressure rises, there is an obligate increase in pulmonary arterial and right ventricular pressure, termed "passive pulmonary hypertension," which is needed to maintain forward flow.

In some patients with mitral stenosis there is pronounced pulmonary vasoconstriction, which further elevates the pressures in the right ventricle and pulmonary artery—this phenomenon has been called "protective" pulmonary hypertension because the flow rate is limited by the constrictors proximal to the pulmonary capillaries and shifts the burden to the right heart.

Chronic left atrial hypertension and the associated fibrosis and scarring of the left atrial walls lead to intermittent or sustained atrial fibrillation. This arrhythmia imposes an additional hemodynamic burden on the left atrium and pulmonary capillaries because the ventricular rate increases uncontrollably, which shortens the diastolic filling time and further augments left atrial pressure. A vicious circle is created in which the shortened diastolic filling time raises the left atrial pressure while depriving the left ventricle of an adequate filling volume, which in turn leads to an inadequate systemic cardiac output, which triggers sympathetic neurohumoral hyperactivity, further augmenting the heart rate.

Pregnancy often provokes the symptoms in previously asymptomatic subjects with mitral stenosis because of the added burden of increased blood volume, shunting to the placenta increasing cardiac output, and the increased heart rate associated with labor and delivery.

Hemodynamic Basis for Physical Findings

Left atrial hypertension and the diastolic transvalvar gradient (Figs. 11.8 and 11.9) result in a pressure burden on the right ventricle and a unique abnormality of left ventricular filling. The pressure overload on the right ventricle may be detected by palpation of a right ventricular lift in the left parasternal area (see Fig. 11.6) and/or elevation of the jugular venous *a* wave. The left ventricular apical impulse is usually not displaced and is not forceful. If the right ventricle is greatly enlarged, the left ventricular

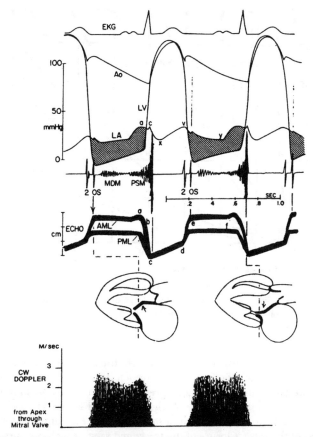

Figure 11.8.   Pressure, Sound, and Echo-Doppler Correlates in Mitral Stenosis. Stenosis of the valve results in an atrioventricular pressure gradient (shaded area) throughout diastole, elevated left atrial pressure, and a reduced rate of ventricular filling (no rapid filling wave or a wave are seen in the ventricular diastolic pressure). The M-mode echocardiogram demonstrates a thickened mitral valve with parallel anterior diastolic excursions of both leaflets as a result of commissural fusion that joins the two leaflets. The Doppler velocities average 2 M/sec across the mitral valve, indicative of a 16 mm Hg gradient. The sounds and murmurs will be described in the text.

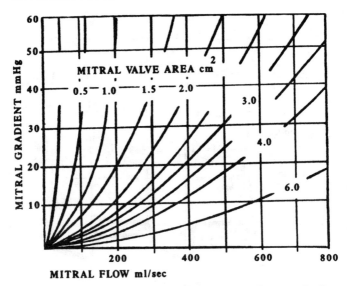

Figure 11.9. The Relationship of Mitral Flow to the Pressure Gradient Across the Mitral Valve with Different Valve Areas. A normal valve area is >3 cm^2; critical stenosis occurs when the valve area is <1 cm^2.

impulse may be displaced or obscured by the dominant chamber. The transvalvar gradient causes the left atrial pressure to rise above left ventricular diastolic pressure, which causes the mitral valve to close late and open early, as shown in Figure 11.10.

The heart sounds in mitral stenosis reflect the pathophysiology of the valve. Closure of the thickened valve at high pressure, when the rate of ventricular pressure rise is at its steepest, results in a loud first sound. The failure of the valve leaflets to open normally because of commissural fusion results in the early diastolic opening snap. Turbulent flow through the mitral valve results in a rumbling mid-diastolic murmur. Mid-diastole is defined as the period of time from mitral valve opening until either diastasis or atrial systole occur. Diastasis usually does not occur in mitral stenosis because the left atrial and ventricular pressures fail to equilibrate. If sinus rhythm is present, a crescendo presystolic murmur (PSM) is heard, merging with a very loud first heart sound.

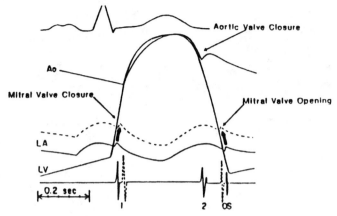

Figure 11.10. Mitral Stenosis—The Effect of Increased Atrial Pressure on the First Sound and Opening Snap. The interval between the second sound (2) and opening snap (OS) is shortened by further elevation of left atrial pressure, which could result from tachycardia, increased cardiac output, or increasing stenosis. The first sound (1) becomes increasingly delayed as diastole encroaches further on ventricular systole because of the longer time required for left ventricular contraction to develop a pressure greater than atrial pressure.

The interval between aortic closure and mitral valve opening, the second sound-to-OS interval, can be timed by listening with a stethoscope. If the two events have timing similar to the two syllables in the word butter, the interval is approximately 80 msec. Intervals less than 80 msec imply a significantly elevated left atrial pressure (Fig. 11.10).

There has been debate about the presence of a "presystolic murmur" in atrial fibrillation, because atrial systole is absent. However, as shown in Figure 11.12, it is often possible to detect a crescendo terminus to the mid-diastolic murmur during rapid heart rates.

Natural History

The natural history of mitral stenosis depends on the severity of obstruction, the rate of progression, the burdens placed on the heart (multiple pregnancies, manual labor), and the presence of

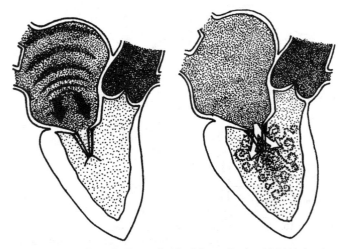

Figure 11.11. Diastolic Events in Mitral Stenosis. As atrial blood enters the mitral valve sleeve during isovolumic relaxation under high pressure, the funnel-like mitral valve fails to open fully (left) and the advancing column of blood is abruptly decelerated by impact against the fused mitral leaflets (black arrows), generating an opening snap. Turbulent flow through the restricted orifice results in a mid-diastolic murmur (right), often followed by a crescendo presystolic murmur.

complications such as atrial fibrillation, embolism, and endocarditis. Although the factors that determine the rate of progression are not fully known, the earlier the attack(s) of acute rheumatic fever, as well as the presence of recurrent reactivation by streptococcal infections, undoubtedly play a role (Figure 11.11).

It is not unusual to encounter children or young adults from third-world countries with severe mitral stenosis, disproportionate pulmonary hypertension, and a loud murmur of tricuspid regurgitation obscuring the physical findings of mitral stenosis. Among immigrants from Latin America, the condition is often discovered when severe left heart failure complicates a pregnancy or a respiratory infection. It should be emphasized that any cause of tachycardia, with or without an increase in cardiac output, will increase the mitral valve flow rate and magnify the left atrial pressure.

In the example depicted in Figure 11.13, the shortening of

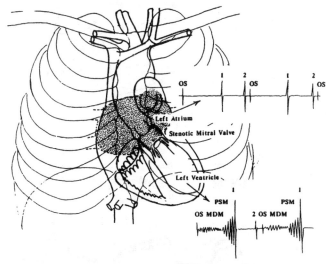

Figure 11.12. Mitral Stenosis with Atrial Fibrillation. The variable lengths of diastole will cause beat-to-beat changes in the timing and intensity of the opening snap, the intensity of the first heart sound, and the character of the diastolic murmur. During long diastolic cycles, the mid-diastolic murmur will fade out before the first heart sound, the first sound will be soft, and the ensuing opening snap relatively late because of decompression of the left atrium. During short cycles or tachycardia, there may be a "presystolic" accentuation of the mid-diastolic murmur, a loud first sound, and an early opening snap because the atrium has not had time to decompress.

the diastolic filling time in the face of an increased cardiac output augments the transmitral flow rate by 50%:

$$\text{from:} \ \frac{34{,}000 \ \text{mL/min}}{34 \ \text{sec/min}} = 100 \ \text{mL/sec}$$

$$\text{to:} \ \frac{3{,}900 \ \text{mL/min}}{26 \ \text{sec/min}} = 150 \ \text{mL/sec}$$

The most tragic complication of mitral stenosis is systemic embolism, particularly when the target is the cerebral vasculature with permanent neurological residua. Embolism may occur in sinus rhythm but is most often associated with atrial fibrillation or the interconversion from atrial fibrillation to sinus rhythm

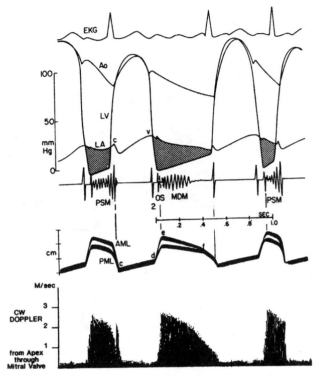

Figure 11.13. The Effect of Mild Exercise on Mitral Stenosis. Note that the left atrial pressure more that doubles with only a 15% increase in cardiac output.

when the atrial contraction purges the clot from the stagnant atrium. Chronic anticoagulation reduces the likelihood of embolism.

A potentially fatal complication of mitral stenosis is pulmonary hemorrhage resulting from rupture of high-pressure bronchial veins that drain into the left atrium, roughly analogous to esophageal varices in portal hypertension.

Laboratory Findings

Radiography

The radiographic manifestations of mitral stenosis may be subtle, because significant cardiac enlargement is uncommon. Left atrial

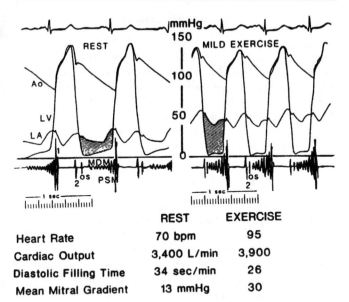

	REST	EXERCISE
Heart Rate	70 bpm	95
Cardiac Output	3,400 L/min	3,900
Diastolic Filling Time	34 sec/min	26
Mean Mitral Gradient	13 mmHg	30

Figure 11.14. Precordial Location of the Auscultatory Features of Mitral Stenosis. The opening snap is best heard at the base, over the region of the left atrium, because the shock wave is reflected back into the atrium (see Fig. 11.10). The opening snap can also be heard at the apex. The rumbling mid-diastolic murmur (MDM) and presystolic murmur (PSM) are often heard only at the apex, with the bell of the stethoscope applied lightly.

enlargement will cause straightening of the left superior cardiac border, will elevate the left main stem bronchus, and may produce a characteristic "double density" caused by superimposition of the ovoid density of the increased volume of blood in the chamber. Mitral valve calcification may be seen on radiographs or by fluoroscopy. The location of the left atrium and mitral valve can be seen in Figure 11.12.

If significant pulmonary hypertension is present, pulmonary artery dilation, an increase in upper lobe vascularity, and right heart enlargement may be seen. The elevated pulmonary venous pressure may produce an "antler" configuration of dilated upper lobe pulmonary veins. Kerley B lines, short horizontal markings at the lung bases extending to the lateral pleurae, are caused by interlobular edema and indicate chronic elevation of the left atrial and pulmonary venous pressures.

Electrocardiography

Left atrial enlargement may be manifest by broad and notched P waves in leads II and V1 or by large fibrillatory waves if atrial fibrillation is present. The left ventricle is characteristically normal or underdeveloped because of the diminished inflow, whereas the right ventricle bears a pressure burden. Therefore, there may be a vertical or right axis in the frontal plane. A rapid ventricular response to atrial fibrillation may cause ST-T changes suggestive of ischemic heart disease.

Echo-Doppler Ultrasonography

Diagnostic patterns of mitral stenosis are readily appreciated by echocardiography—in fact, mitral stenosis was the first lesion diagnosed by this procedure when it was documented in the 1950s. The mitral leaflets are thickened and fused, and both move ventrally in diastole (instead of the normal reciprocating motion) because the posterior leaflet is tethered to the anterior leaflet by commissural fusion. These changes can be seen on the M-mode and two-dimensional echocardiograms shown in Figures 11.8 and 11.13. The e-f slope of mitral M-mode echocardiogram has a reduced slope because the valve is held widely open through diastole by the pressure gradient.

The thickness and mobility of the fused leaflets and the presence or absence of subvalvar disease (chordal shortening and thickening) can provide important information regarding the feasibility of repair or balloon valvuloplasty. The mitral orifice can be viewed in cross section to estimate the orifice area.

The left atrial diameter is increased, whereas the left ventricular dimensions are normal. Left atrial thrombus may be seen by conventional echocardiography but is more readily detected by transesophageal echocardiography (TEE) because the probe is placed against the esophageal-atrial wall and can be rotated to scan the atrium and auricular appendage. The right ventricle may be enlarged and have thickened walls because of hypertrophy. In mixed lesions, for example mitral stenosis and regurgitation, the left ventricular dimensions will reflect the volume overload.

The continuous wave Doppler signal from transmitral flow (see Figs. 11.8 and 11.13) can provide accurate estimation of the diastolic gradient across the valve and, by the use of empiric formula (the pressure half-time), an accurate assessment of valve orifice area can be derived.

Therapy

The natural history of mitral stenosis can be significantly improved by medical therapy designed to maintain a slow heart rate (<70 beats per minute at rest and <100 with mild exertion) and thus maintain an adequate diastolic filling time. β-adrenergic blocking agents (propranolol, nadolol, metoprolol, or atenolol) are effective at controlling the ventricular rate in sinus rhythm or atrial fibrillation, whereas digoxin is only effective if chronic atrial fibrillation is present. Anticoagulation with Coumadin is mandated when intermittent or chronic atrial fibrillation is present.

The mid-diastolic and presystolic murmurs are very often confused with systolic murmurs but should be readily differentiated at the bedside by noting that they precede the carotid pulse and that the first heart sound is loud. A potentially tragic confusion of the presystolic murmur with a systolic murmur all too frequently occurs when a house officer evaluates a critically ill young female in the setting of infection or pregnancy, hears a murmur, believes that the murmur is systolic, and recommends "afterload reduction" or inotropic agents. Inotropic and vasodilator agents will cause tachycardia and worsen an already critical condition. The likelihood of mitral stenosis should always be considered when acute dyspnea complicates pregnancy or any cause of tachycardia, particularly in a patient who is a Latina. Diuretics should be used sparingly, because excessive volume depletion will reduce cardiac output and augment tachycardia.

Because mitral stenosis is a manifestation of rheumatic heart disease, rheumatic fever prophylaxis is indicated for patients who are exposed to crowded living or working conditions or who have children at home. Additional antibiotic prophylaxis for endocarditis is also indicated for dental procedures or potentially contaminated interventions (urethral catheterization, cytoscopy, colonoscopy, etc.).

When symptoms are present despite heart rate control, mitral valve repair (commissurotomy) or replacement can improve exercise capacity and relieve symptoms. The relief afforded by commissurotomy may last for more than a decade. The threat of

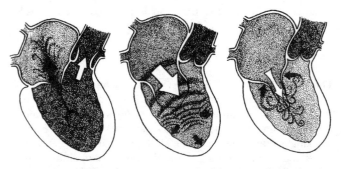

Figure 11.15. The Murmurs of Mitral Regurgitation. In systole, a high velocity jet (left black arrow) causes turbulent flow into the left atrium throughout systole. Torrential mitral inflow occurs in mid-diastole (white arrow; center), rapidly distending the ventricular chamber, causing a third heart sound. In the wake of the rapid filling wave, eddy currents around the mitral valve initiate closure, so that the remaining outflow through the narrowed valve produces a mid-diastolic murmur indicated by the turbulent flow pattern (right).

systemic embolism is not reduced by prosthetic mitral valve replacement, so a commissurotomy leaving a natural tissue valve should be attempted if feasible. Catheter balloon valvuloplasty has been successful in relieving mitral stenosis in flexible, noncalcified valves but is a technically demanding procedure that is not widely available.

MITRAL REGURGITATION

Incomplete systolic closure of the mitral orifice may result from pathological changes in the structural elements of the valve (leaflets, chordae, annulus, papillary muscles), left ventricular functional abnormalities, or interactions between structural and functional elements. Four types of mitral regurgitation will be discussed: chronic, acute, intermittent, and mitral prolapse. Mitral prolapse is the underlying etiology for a spectrum of mild, to chronic, to acute forms of mitral regurgitation but has many unique features that set it apart from other forms of mitral regurgitation.

Mitral regurgitation almost always produces a systolic murmur and frequently causes diastolic auscultatory events as well. The basis for these systolic and diastolic events in all forms of mitral regurgitation is illustrated in Figure 11.15.

Pathophysiology

Chronic Mitral Regurgitation

Hemodynamically significant mitral regurgitation produces a volume overload of the left heart, because both chambers must contain an increased amount of blood proportional to the volume of regurgitant flow: the left atrium in systole and the left ventricle in diastole. The volume overload affects the heart differently when it progresses slowly, as in chronic rheumatic heart disease, than when it develops suddenly, because of ruptured chordae tendineae, papillary muscle infarction, or infective endocarditis. In chronic regurgitation, a progressive increase in the compliance of the left heart chamber permits dilatation without a significant elevation of filling pressure, whereas in acute valvar incompetence, the left heart is subjected to markedly elevated filling pressures (Figures 11.16 and 11.17).

Chronic mitral regurgitation is usually well tolerated, because the heart can compensate for the volume overload with increased compliance and an increase in ventricular stroke volume. Therefore, there is minimal back pressure on the pulmonary veins and hence little or no dyspnea. Pregnancy is usually well tolerated because ventricular afterload is reduced by the virtual A-V fistula through the placental circulation. Symptoms of fatigue due to low cardiac output may occur late in the disease when the heart has become markedly enlarged after chronic exposure to the volume overload or when ventricular afterload increases because of hypertension or the peripheral vascular changes of aging.

Acute Mitral Regurgitation

Acute mitral regurgitation is poorly tolerated, despite the fact that the left heart chambers may be subjected to a lesser volume overload compared with chronic regurgitation. Left ventricular diastolic pressure and left atrial pressure during ventricular systole (the v wave) increase markedly because of the poorly tolerated volume load so there is considerable back pressure on the pulmonary veins and resultant severe dyspnea. Forward cardiac output may also be compromised by the inability of the left heart chambers to accommodate a sufficient volume to maintain normal forward stroke volume in the face of back leakage. The tall v waves and elevated left ventricular diastolic (filling) pressure are shown in Figure 11.17.

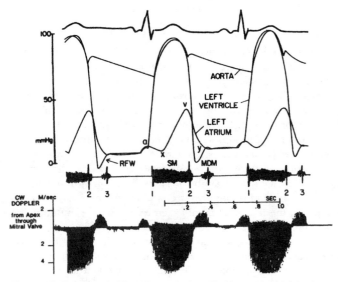

Figure 11.16. Chronic Mitral Regurgitation. The increasing atrial volume from regurgitant flow into the left atrium during ventricular systole results in a tall *v* wave, the increased forward flow in early diastole in a rapid *y* descent in the left atrium, and an exaggerated ventricular rapid filling wave (RFW) in the left ventricle. There is a holosystolic murmur (SM) and a mid-diastolic murmur (MDM) best heard at the apex. The mitral regurgitant Doppler velocity is nearly uniform throughout systole, reflecting the well-maintained ventricular-atrial gradient. The direction of the transmitral flow signal is away from the apical transducer.

The left heart chambers must be able to dilate and increase the stroke volume to compensate for mitral regurgitation. If the ability of the ventricle to "relax" is compromised by hypertrophy or ischemia or cannot increase its stroke volume because of ischemic ventricular dysfunction or infarction, a small amount of regurgitation may be poorly tolerated.

Acute mitral regurgitation as a result of the noncompliant left heart chambers does not significantly displace the apical impulse but produces an exaggerated left ventricular rapid filling wave palpable at the cardiac apex and audible as a third heart sound (*3* in Fig. 11.17). The minimally enlarged left atrium is able to contract forcefully and may produce an exaggerated *a*

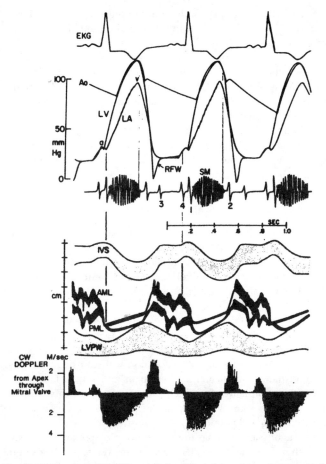

Figure 11.17. Acute Mitral Regurgitation. The tall v waves and elevated left ventricular diastolic (filling) pressure characterize acute mitral regurgitation. The murmur length is abbreviated because the left atrial pressure nearly equals left ventricular systolic pressure ("ventriculoid v waves"). The mitral valve echocardiogram demonstrates erratic motion because of flail leaflets. The Doppler signal representing the mitral regurgitant jet has a late systolic decline because of the declining ventricular-atrial systolic gradient.

wave, which causes a presystolic apical impulse and a fourth heart sound (*4* in Fig. 11.17). During systole, the limited compliance of the left atrium resists late systolic regurgitant flow from the left ventricle. Atrial pressure rises rapidly with a "ventriculoid" configuration with v waves that may reach 75–100 mm Hg. The resulting systolic murmur (SM), unlike the chronic regurgitant murmur, is not holosystolic but has a late systolic termination. The murmur may be harsh rather than blowing and may be confused with an "ejection murmur." The Doppler signal is directed away from the apical transducer, but unlike chronic mitral regurgitation, the late systolic velocity is attenuated because of the high v waves in the left atrium.

Mitral Prolapse

The valve in mitral prolapse is usually thickened and redundant, so that it is literally too big to guard the mitral orifice competently during systole. This disproportion becomes increasingly exaggerated as the ventricle loses volume through ventricular ejection. The functional anatomy of prolapse is demonstrated in Figure 11.18.

The volume of regurgitant flow in mitral prolapse is usually relatively small, although some patients may develop progressively severe regurgitation or rupture of chordae. However, symptoms are frequently out of proportion with the relatively mild hemodynamic impairment. Chest pain and severe fatigue are common complaints, for which there is no satisfactory explanation. Patients may also complain of palpitations, which can be attributed to arrhythmias.

The physical findings in mitral valve prolapse are so unusual that they remained unexplained for many years, until the condition was first clarified by x-ray motion pictures in the 1960s. These studies revealed that there is a disproportion between the enlarged and redundant mitral valve leaflets and normal-sized left heart chambers. Consequently, the valve cannot be maintained in a subanular position throughout systole, the billowing leaflet(s) prolapse into the left atrium, and the valve becomes incompetent. When prolapse occurs, portions of the valve leaflets referred to as "scallops" slip from their position of coaptation with the opposite leaflet and slide toward the atrium under the driving force of the systolic rise in ventricular pressure. Once the scallops lose the

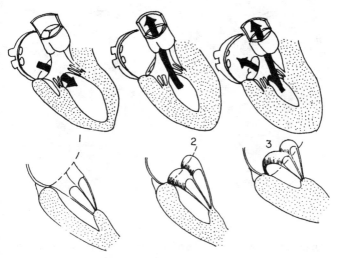

Figure 11.18. Functional Anatomy of Mitral Prolapse. Three phases of the cardiac cycle in the left heart are indicated: (1) diastole, (2) early systole, and (3) late systole. In early systole, the mitral valve is competent. By late systole, the left ventricular cavity is smaller and the distance between the mitral annulus and papillary muscle has shortened. The leaflet billows back into the atrium, rendering the valve incompetent. The prolapse produces a click, and the incompetent valve produces a late systolic murmur (Fig. 11.19).

structural support of their opposite member, only chordal restraints prevent their complete avulsion, as shown in Figures 11.18 and 11.19 (see also Fig. 11.20).

The timing of the click and murmur is quite variable and changes with activity or body position in a predictable manner. Interventions that decrease ventricular filling tend to exaggerate the disproportion and lead to earlier prolapse; therefore, standing causes an earlier click and a longer and often louder murmur. Squatting increases venous return and increases ventricular afterload, so the click and murmur occur later in systole. The effects of postural changes on heart (left ventricular) volume and these volumetric changes in the timing of the click and murmur are demonstrated in Figure 11.21.

Although the cause of the arrhythmias that are commonly present in mitral prolapse is unknown, it is believed that the

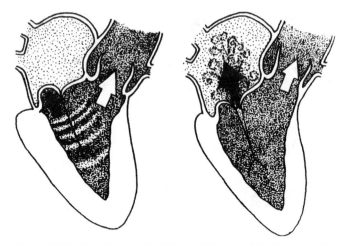

Figure 11.19. The Basis for the Click and Murmur of Mitral Prolapse. The abrupt checking of the billowing posterior leaflet in midsystole (left; black arrow) causes a sharp sound that propagates toward the apex. When the leaflets lose apposition (right), there is a high velocity, turbulent jet into the left atrium in late systole.

abnormal stresses imposed on the mitral leaflets and their support structures might be contributory.

Ischemic Mitral Regurgitation (Papillary Muscle Dysfunction)

A structurally normal mitral valve may become acutely incompetent in patients with ischemic heart disease, as a result of ischemia or infarction of the papillary muscle and/or the underlying ventricular myocardium. Several syndromes have been described in patients with ischemic heart disease. Infarction of a papillary muscle usually leads to severe acute mitral regurgitation that is poorly tolerated by the impaired ischemic ventricle. The hemodynamic effects and clinical findings resemble those presented in Figure 11.17 and require urgent operative intervention.

Another syndrome is acute, intermittent mitral regurgitation which may appear and resolve repeatedly. An example of this syndrome is illustrated in Figure 11.22.

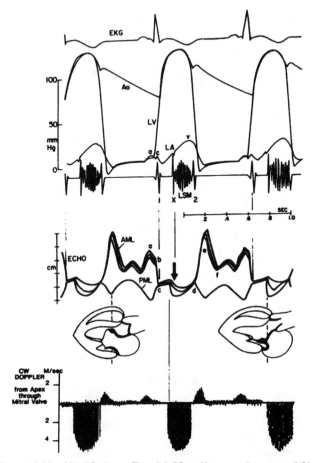

Figure 11.20.   Mitral Prolapse. The click (X) and late systolic murmur (LSM) of mitral prolapse are correlated with the leaflet excursions on the mitral valve echo. At the time of valve closure, immediately after the first heart sound (1), the valve is competent. Prolapse is seen as a dorsal dipping (vertical arrow) of the mitral leaflets between the *c* and *d* points on the echo and is correlated with the midsystolic click and the beginning of a high-velocity regurgitant Doppler jet. The velocities remain high because there is a large systolic ventriculoatrial gradient, indicative of mild mitral regurgitation.

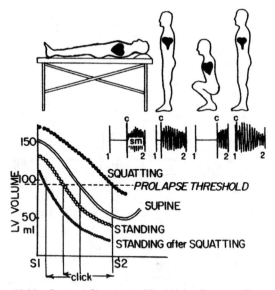

Figure 11.21. Postural Changes in Mitral Valve Prolapse. The prolapse threshold is the minimum LV volume required to prevent prolapse of the mitral valve. Any LV volume less than the threshold will result in prolapse and an ensuing systolic murmur (SM).

Natural History

Chronic Mitral Regurgitation

Chronic mitral regurgitation is often well tolerated despite its severity because of the compensatory increase in compliance of the left heart chambers, the lack of pulmonary venous hypertension, the infrequent incidence of systemic embolization, and the relatively minor energy expenditure of the volume workload imposed on the ventricle. However, mitral regurgitation is often self-perpetuating, in that ventricular, annular, and atrial dilation may progressively increase the severity of the valve incompetence. Easy fatigue is the principal symptom, and its insidiousness usually limits the ambition of the individual to engage in sufficient activity to recognize exercise intolerance. It is often difficult to justify mitral valve replacement in individuals with mitral regurgitation because of the mildness of their symptoms and the potential mor-

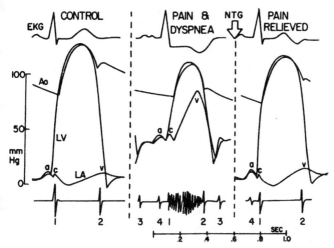

Figure 11.22. Mitral Regurgitation in Ischemic Heart Disease. Mitral regurgitation in ischemic heart disease may be intermittent in a Jekyll-Hyde fashion, producing severe disabling symptoms relieved by administration of nitroglycerin (TNG). The murmur of mitral regurgitation may be heard only during angina attacks.

bidity of prosthetic valves (thromboembolism, structural failure, etc.). However, if the decision to replace the valve is postponed until the left heart chambers are irreparably dilated, the operative mortality is high and the results are less optimal than with earlier surgery.

Acute Mitral Regurgitation

Acute mitral regurgitation is usually so poorly tolerated that emergency operative intervention is required. The sudden volume overload imposed on the noncompliant left heart chambers, combined with the loss of forward stroke volume, leads to marked back pressure on the pulmonary veins and poor systemic perfusion. Reflex vasoconstriction, triggered by low cardiac output, augments the regurgitant fraction. This vasoconstriction can be temporarily ameliorated by the use of vasodilators, which lower the resistance to forward ejection and thus increase the cardiac output and reduce the back pressure.

Mitral Valve Prolapse

Mitral valve prolapse is believed to have a benign prognosis for most patients with this condition, despite the not infrequent complex of symptoms (chest pain, palpitations, syncope, easy fatigue, etc.). In a small percentage of patients with mitral prolapse, progressive mitral regurgitation or severe valvar regurgitation from chordal rupture or infective endocarditis may develop. The redundancy of the leaflet material makes surgical repair of prolapsing mitral valves with severe regurgitation an attractive alternative to valve replacement.

Rarely, serious ventricular tachyarrhythmias may occur and lead to syncope or sudden death. Myocardial infarction in the absence of coronary artery disease and, presumably, embolic cerebral vascular accidents have also been reported.

It is not known whether the prolapsing valve apparatus is responsible for the symptoms or whether autonomic dysfunction, coronary artery spasm, and occult A-V bypass tracts, all of which have been suggested, are responsible.

Intermittent Mitral Regurgitation

Intermittent mitral regurgitation is usually a result of ischemic heart disease and may improve with medical measures directed at improving the coronary perfusion or by revascularization (angioplasty or bypass surgery).

Laboratory Findings

Radiography

The volume overload of the left heart chambers resulting from chronic mitral regurgitation enlarges both the left atrium and left ventricle, but the changes in the lung field are less striking than those of mitral stenosis, because the pulmonary venous pressure is not greatly elevated and the degree of pulmonary artery hypertension is less marked. In some instances, the heart may be massively enlarged in a nearly asymptomatic patient.

In acute mitral regurgitation, the chest radiograph may resemble mitral stenosis because there is marked pulmonary venous and pulmonary arterial hypertension without marked chamber enlargement. Acute pulmonary edema, with a butterfly distribution of perivascular haziness, may be seen in patients with acute or intermittent severe valvar regurgitation.

Electrocardiography

Because the left ventricle receives and ejects an increased volume of blood, there may be an increase in the left precordial R-wave voltage. As in mitral stenosis, left atrial enlargement may be manifest by broad, notched, or diphasic P waves or by coarse atrial fibrillatory waves. When ischemic heart disease underlies the mitral regurgitation, the ECG may reveal evidence of infarction or ischemic ST-T changes.

Echo-Doppler Ultrasonography

Although echocardiography is not as helpful in establishing the diagnosis of mitral regurgitation as it is in mitral stenosis, the technique will demonstrate the extent of increase in atrial and ventricular dimensions and may suggest the underlying etiology of the mitral regurgitation. Rheumatic mitral regurgitation may be detected by the echocardiography demonstration of thickened or fused leaflets (see Figs. 11.8 and 11.13), whereas prolapse will produce wide diastolic excursions and posterior systolic slippage (see Fig. 11.20). When chordal rupture results in acute mitral regurgitation, the "flail" leaflets will produce bizarre chaotic diastolic excursion, as shown in Figure 11.17, with an anterior diastolic excursion of the posterior leaflet. Vegetations from endocarditis produce thick, shaggy-appearing echoes, which move in the direction of the leaflet to which they are attached.

Continuous-Wave Doppler

Continuous-wave Doppler interrogation of the regurgitant mitral valves provides invaluable information regarding the severity of mitral regurgitation. A holosystolic high-velocity signal (see Fig. 11.16) indicates a left atrial pressure that is not greatly elevated, whereas late systolic attenuation indicates that tall v waves are present, as shown in Figure 11.17. The high velocity confined to late systole in mitral prolapse, shown in Figure 11.20, indicates well-tolerated mitral regurgitation confined to late systole.

Color Flow Doppler

Color flow Doppler (see Chapter 4) is also useful in assessing the location and extent of the regurgitant jet. If the blue jet (away from the transducer) extends into the pulmonary veins, severe regurgitation is present.

Therapy

Chronic Mitral Regurgitation

Medical. Digoxin is used for its inotropic effect and, if atrial fibrillation is present, to control ventricular response. However, patients with predominate mitral regurgitation tolerate relatively fast heart rates without difficulty. Therefore, aggressive digitalization aimed at decreasing the ventricular response below 70 is seldom necessary. Afterload reduction (hydralazine, prazosin, or angiotensin-converting enzyme inhibitors) is effective in decreasing the regurgitant fraction and increasing cardiac output. Warfarin is indicated in predominant mitral regurgitation in the setting of atrial fibrillation. Bacterial endocarditis prophylaxis is recommended. Rheumatic fever prophylaxis is indicated if the valve lesion is rheumatic.

Surgical. Mitral valve replacement is indicated for symptomatic patients with declining ventricular function or increasing heart size if cardiac catheterization demonstrates significant mitral regurgitation.

Acute Mitral Regurgitation

The accurate, early diagnosis of acute mitral regurgitation and immediate attempts at medical stabilization with afterload reduction (even if systolic pressure is normal) and diuretics are of paramount importance. Cardiac catheterization and mitral valve replacement should quickly follow, even for patients who are poor surgical candidates, because the mortality of this lesion without surgery is extremely high.

Mitral Valve Prolapse

β-blockers have been effective in controlling the "adrenergic" symptoms such as tachycardia, palpitations, and anxiety-provoked arrhythmias. It is believed that some of the arrhythmias may have their basis in the abnormal stresses put on the valve leaflets and papillary muscles by the prolapsing valve. By decreasing the ventriculovalvular disproportion, the amount of mitral prolapse may be reduced. This effect may explain the drug's utility in lessening arrhythmias.

Additional antiarrhythmic agents for ventricular extra systoles or atrial fibrillation may be required. Because of the tendency toward long QT intervals in mitral prolapse, quinidine or other type IA agents should not be used as a first-line drug to treat ventricular ectopy.

Chest pain and fatigue are more difficult symptoms to control. Often, reassuring the patient (when appropriate) that he or she does not have coronary artery disease, combined with treatment with β blockers, can improve otherwise incapacitating symptoms.

We believe that antibiotic prophylaxis for dental procedures and potentially "dirty" surgery is indicated for all patients with auscultatory evidence of mitral prolapse.

Some surgeons have claimed that mitral valve plication and/or annuloplasty may improve disabling symptoms, even for patients with hemodynamically insignificant mitral valve regurgitation. These observations suggest that the valve plays a primary role in the symptomatology.

MIXED MITRAL VALVE DISEASE

Rheumatic heart disease often produces a combination of commissural fusion and shrinkage of the leaflets, so the valve is both stenotic and regurgitant. A similar combination may occur after valve surgery, because mitral stenosis surgery inadvertently results in valvar incompetence. Combined mitral valve disease results in a double impact on the left heart chambers because they are subjected to a volume overload from the regurgitation, and the obligatory increase in diastolic mitral inflow magnifies the atrioventricular gradient and thus subjects the left atrium and pulmonary veins to a pressure overload as well.

The physical findings are a combination of stenosis and regurgitation, with a left parasternal heave from right ventricular pressure overload and an outward and downward displaced left ventricular lift. Auscultation may reveal the mid-diastolic and presystolic murmurs of mitral stenosis, along with the holosystolic murmur of mitral regurgitation. The dominant condition may be difficult to ascertain, but the presence of a third heart sound or an increased left ventricular impulse suggests dominant regurgitation, whereas the lack of ventricular displacement and a barely perceptible ventricular apex beat suggest dominant stenosis.

The symptoms and natural history also depend on the dominant lesion, with fatigue favoring dominant regurgitation and dyspnea favoring dominant stenosis. Mixed lesions tend to cause marked left atrial enlargement with attendant stagnation, thrombosis, and propensity to embolism.

Laboratory Findings

The laboratory assessment of mixed mitral valve disease reveals findings similar to those of the individual component lesions and will usually reflect the impact of the dominant lesion. For example, when mitral stenosis dominates, the addition of mitral regurgitation actually enhances the impact of the stenosis, because there is an obligatory increase in diastolic flow rate to compensate for the regurgitant venous pressure and a systolic pressure overload to the right heart.

When mitral regurgitation dominates, the left ventricle will be enlarged by radiography and echocardiography, and the ECG may demonstrate evidence of left ventricular hypertrophy.

TRICUSPID VALVE DISEASE

The tricuspid valve can be affected by congenital and acquired lesions of the leaflets as well as by functional impairment of the right ventricle.

Rheumatic fever may render the tricuspid valve stenotic or incompetent, but virtually always in conjunction with rheumatic mitral valve disease. Right ventricular pressure overload from pulmonary hypertension, particularly when the right ventricle is dilated, can produce functional tricuspid regurgitation. Tricuspid regurgitation can also result from destruction of the valve in infective endocarditis or from the carcinoid syndrome.

Pathophysiology

Tricuspid stenosis elevates the right atrial pressure in response to the rate of flow across the valve in a manner similar to, but to a lesser degree than, the left-sided events in mitral stenosis. Exercise capacity is usually limited by low cardiac output rather than by high venous pressure proximal to the stenosis (as in the case with mitral stenosis).

The hemodynamic impact of tricuspid regurgitation depends largely on the status of the right ventricle and the pulmonary vascular bed. If pulmonary hypertension or impaired right ventricular function is present, the lesion is poorly tolerated and atrial arrhythmias, hepatic congestion, ascites, and edema of the lower extremities complicate a low cardiac output state. If the right ventricle and pulmonary vascular resistance are normal, complete absence of tricuspid valve leaflets is remarkably well tolerated.

Hemodynamic Basis of Physical Signs

Right heart hemodynamics are greatly influenced by the negative intrathoracic pressure effects of inspiration, and this respiratory influence affects the bedside manifestations of tricuspid valvar lesions. The augmented venous return during inspiration increases flow across the tricuspid valve, the magnitude of the jugular venous pulse waves, and the intensity of tricuspid murmurs as shown in Figures 11.23 and 11.24.

When tricuspid stenosis is present, the jugular venous *a* waves are greatly augmented (Fig. 11.23). As in mitral stenosis, the auscultatory complex of tricuspid stenosis consists of an early diastolic opening snap, a diastolic rumble with presystolic augmentation, and a loud first sound, but these events are markedly augmented by inspiration or the Muller maneuver (inspiration with a closed glottis) and best heard along the left sternal border. Because mitral valve disease often coexists with tricuspid stenosis, the presence of prominent *a* waves and the inspiratory augmentation of an additional parasternal murmur provides evidence of the tricuspid pathology.

Tricuspid regurgitation presents a volume load to the right heart chambers, which is manifested by systolic jugular venous and hepatic pulsations, and a left parasternal diastolic impulse (which results from the large volume of to-and-fro flow across the valve). On auscultation, a third heart sound, representing augmented early diastolic inflow, and a holosystolic murmur (SM) are both heard along the left sternal border and are aug-

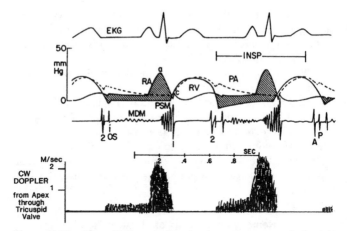

Figure 11.23. Tricuspid Stenosis. Prominent *a* waves are seen in the right atrium (and jugular veins), and there is a diastolic gradient between the atrium and ventricle (shaded area). The gradient, presystolic murmur, and Doppler velocity signal increase with inspiration because of the augmented venous return.

mented by inspiration, as shown in Figure 11.24, or with the Muller's maneuver.

Natural History

The impact of tricuspid valve disease on life expectancy is heavily dependent on the presence or absence of associated left heart lesions and/or the status of the pulmonary vascular resistance. Isolated tricuspid regurgitation has been well tolerated in a large number of patients who were subjected to surgical removal of the tricuspid valve because of the presence of valve infection. On the other hand, elevated pulmonary pressure in association with tricuspid regurgitation can diminish right heart output and lead to profound right heart failure and passive congestion of the liver and abdominal viscera.

Laboratory Findings

Clues to the presence of rheumatic tricuspid valve disease by laboratory studies may be subtle, because the invariably associated

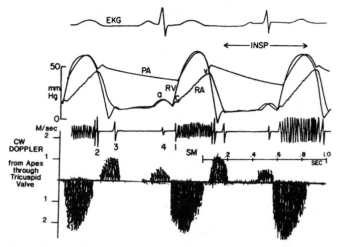

Figure 11.24. Tricuspid Regurgitation. Pulmonary hypertension is present and causes the tricuspid regurgitation to be more severe than when right ventricular afterload is normal. The holosystolic murmur (SM) and tall *v* waves result from systolic regurgitation, and the third sound and rapid filling wave from increased diastolic inflow. The fourth sound is due to atrial contraction into the hypertrophied and poorly compliant right ventricle. Inspiration increases right heart flow and murmur intensity.

left-sided valvular disease usually dominates the radiological, electrocardiographic, and echocardiographic findings. A prominent bulging of the right heart border indicates right atrial enlargement, but this finding is not diagnostic of intrinsic disease of the tricuspid valve.

Echocardiography can define tricuspid valve abnormalities, especially the presence of vegetations, and continuous wave Doppler interrogation of a tricuspid regurgitant jet can lead to an accurate estimation of right ventricular pressure as discussed in Chapter 4.

Therapy

The impact of tricuspid regurgitation is greater when there is pulmonary hypertension, often present due to concomitant mitral valve disease. If the mitral valve must be replaced and there is organic tricuspid regurgitation, the residual stenosis inherent in the prosthetic valve maintains a high pulmonary arterial pressure, especially with exercise. Therefore, tricuspid valve annuloplasty or replacement is often required in combined mitral and tricuspid disease. Severely symptomatic tricuspid stenosis usually requires valve replacement because commissurotomy is rarely successful. Concomitant mitral stenosis is almost invariably present, but its signs and symptoms may be masked by the low output through the right heart.

AORTIC STENOSIS

Pathophysiology

Stenosis of a semilunar valve or ventricular outflow tract results in a pressure overload—an elevation of ventricular pressure to overcome the obstruction. The ventricular pressure contour assumes a pointed top or steep triangular ("isometric") contour in place of the normal rounded or plateau ("isotonic") shape. The arterial pressure pulse downstream from the obstruction rises slowly (low dp/dt), the arterial pulse pressure is diminished, and the duration of ventricular ejection lengthens as shown in Figure 11.25.

The pressure difference or gradient between the ventricle and the artery is proportional to the square of the flow rate across the orifice and, therefore, quadruples as the flow doubles.

The anatomical site of the pressure drop (gradient) can be determined by catheter withdrawal tracings across the outflow tract. In addition to valvar stenosis, two other sites of discrete (fixed) stenosis can be localized: subvalvar and supravalvar. Coarctation of the aorta is a fourth site of discrete stenosis, but it will not be discussed further here.

Figure 11.26 illustrates catheter withdrawal tracings from three types of left ventricular outflow tract stenosis, and the site of the pressure drop determines the site of the lesion. A high-peaked pressure in the left ventricular body and slow-rising pressure in the aorta are common to all three examples.

Subvalvar and supravalvar stenotic lesions are congenital. Valvar aortic stenosis can be congenital or acquired or a combination of congenital nonstenotic deformity and acquired deposition of calcium due to the wear and tear of resulting turbulence. Another

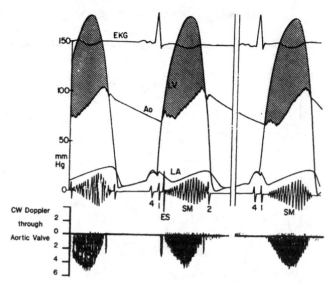

Figure 11.25. Aortic Stenosis—Flexible Versus Calcified Valve. The hemo-dynamic and auscultatory effects of aortic stenosis are depicted in a patient with a flexible valve (left) and a calcified valve (right). Both examples demonstrate a pressure gradient (shaded area) and pressure contours typical of aortic stenosis. The patient with a flexible valve exhibits an ejection sound (ES), because the valve is still mobile. Both patients have late-peaking crescendo-decrescendo systolic murmurs (SM) and fourth sounds (4) because of the increased strength of atrial contraction.

form of aortic stenosis may be the result of senile degenerative processes that progressively sclerose the leaflets in elderly patients. Typically, the congenitally stenotic aortic valve is bicuspid or unicuspid, with initially flexible leaflets that dome upward in systole and that may close competently during diastole. The valve in acquired aortic stenosis has thickened, rigid, fibrotic, or calcified leaflets, with the addition of fusion of the commissures in rheumatic heart disease. With the passage of two to three decades, deformed valves acquire calcium and these depositions may be sufficiently dense and extensive to obscure the etiology of the underlying valve disease.

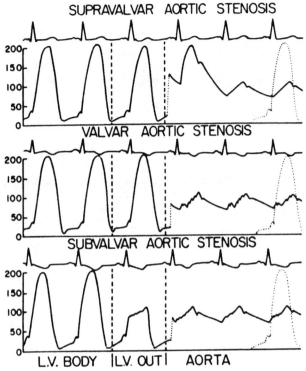

Figure 11.26. Aortic Stenosis—Three Types of Discrete Stenosis. Catheter withdrawal tracings are recorded in three types of discrete (fixed) outflow obstruction. The high-peaked pressures in the LV body (left) and slow-rising pressures in the aorta (right) are similar in all three examples. As the catheter is withdrawn to the subvalvar area (LV out) in the bottom strip, the low systolic pressure indicates a subvalvar obstruction. In valvar stenosis (middle strip), the fall in systolic pressure occurs as the catheter is pulled across the valve. In supravalvar stenosis (upper strip), the proximal aortic pressure is high, and the pressure drop occurs as the catheter is withdrawn farther up the ascending aorta.

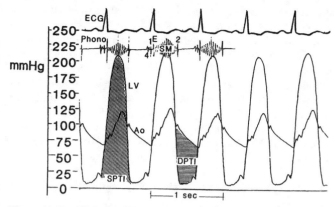

Figure 11.27. Supply/Demand Imbalance of Aortic Stenosis. SPTI represents the systolic pressure time index, proportional to the work expended by left ventricular systole, and DPTI is the diastolic pressure time index, the time available for coronary perfusion and the pressure delivering it. Aortic stenosis results in an abnormally high left ventricular pressure and a low aortic pressure, which increases SPTI and decreases DPTI. The shaded areas demonstrate that the magnitude of the SPTI greatly exceeds the DPTI.

Hemodynamic Basis of Symptoms

To generate the high left ventricular pressures required to overcome the resistance imposed by the stenotic outflow tract lesion, concentric hypertrophy develops and leads to a thick-walled, nondilated chamber with reduced compliance.

The left ventricle is threatened with a supply/demand imbalance as a result of performing excessive pressure work and receiving inadequate coronary perfusion. Figure 11.27 illustrates this dilemma.

This increased oxygen consumption of the hypertrophied, hypertensive ventricle, combined with the relatively low aortic and coronary perfusion pressure, leads to a myocardial supply/demand imbalance, which is augmented by exercise when increased flow requirements necessitate even greater left ventricular hypertension, and peripheral vasodilation may produce a lower coronary perfusion pressure. An increase in flow across a stenotic valve requires an increase in pressure gradient to the second power; therefore, doubling the flow rate would quadruple the pressure gradient. Consequently, a left ventricle that is ischemic or in borderline compensation at rest is rendered increasingly ischemic with and after exercise. Exertional dyspnea (due to increased filling pressure of the ischemic and hypertrophic ventricle), angina, syncope, and sudden death are frequent manifestations. The actual mechanism of syncope and sudden death is unknown, but it is possible that activation of left ventricular baroreceptors by the hypertensive left ventricle may be responsible for an abrupt fall in output through a negative-feedback mechanism. The low coronary perfusion pressure may induce acute left ventricular dysfunction or arrhythmias.

Hemodynamic Basis of Physical Signs

All types of discrete aortic stenosis (congenital or acquired; valvar, subvalvar, or supravalvar) have a sustained left ventricular impulse and a reduced rate of rise of the arterial upstroke. The outflow tract obstruction retards ejection, and the hypertrophied left ventricle "squeezes" blood out by a sustained thickening rather than the normal rapid shortening of the contractile elements. The aortic pressure pulse is blunted by the obstruction, and the turbulence generated by flow through the stenotic orifice leads to the slow-rising, shuddering, saw-toothed arterial impulse as shown in Figures 11.25, 11.26, and 11.27 (see also Fig. 11.28).

The systolic murmur of valvar aortic stenosis is usually well transmitted to the carotid arteries and may be transmitted in an altered form by "filtering out" the harsh components to the apex, where it may resemble the murmur of mitral regurgitation. A palpable murmur, or "thrill," is often present at the site of maximum murmur intensity on the chest wall.

In discrete subaortic stenosis, the murmur is best heard along the left sternal border, whereas in supravalvar aortic stenosis, the murmur is loudest at the upper right sternal border. A click is not generated in either condition, because there are no moving parts.

Natural History

Because a "good ventricle" can compensate for outflow obstruction with hypertrophy, aortic stenosis may be well tolerated for many years. However, the obstruction is progressive and the increasing demands of hypertrophy become more costly; cardiac

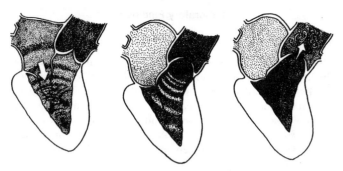

Figure 11.28. The Murmur and Heart Sounds of Aortic Stenosis. The stiff left ventricle receives less than a normal amount of passive filling and requires a vigorous "atrial kick" to achieve an adequate end-diastolic volume. This presystolic outward thrust may be felt at the apex and is accompanied by a fourth heart sound (left). If the aortic valve is mobile, as in congenital valvar aortic stenosis, a loud ejection sound or "click" is heard approximately 0.1 second after the first sound at the apex, and this click initiates the murmur. This sound is caused by the abrupt cessation of upward movement of the fused domelike valve when the valve fails to open (center). The turbulence generated by the high flow across the stenotic orifice produces a harsh crescendo-decrescendo midsystolic murmur and thrill best appreciated immediately downstream from the lesion, e.g., over the ascending aorta (second right parasternal interspace) in valvar aortic stenosis (right). The duration of the murmur and lateness of its peak intensity are directly related to the gradient and inversely related to the stenotic orifice size.

decompensation or sudden death may insidiously or abruptly terminate this previously asymptomatic interlude. Congenital aortic stenosis has a bimodal distribution with early symptomatology in those born with severe obstruction and a later symptom onset in the fourth decade in those with initially minimal obstruction who acquire increasing stenosis.

Rheumatic aortic stenosis usually becomes symptomatic in the fifth decade, or approximately 30 years after the attack of rheumatic fever. Because rheumatic aortic stenosis rarely occurs without other valvar involvement, principally mitral, the symptoms may reflect the multivalvar affliction. Degenerative aortic stenosis rarely becomes symptomatic before 65 years of age and is the most common form of aortic stenosis seen in patients 70 years of age and older.

Laboratory Findings

Radiography

The overall cardiac size in aortic stenosis may be normal, because the hemodynamic impairment often results in concentric hypertrophy of the left ventricle with a small diastolic chamber size. Late in the course of the disease, the left ventricle may dilate. In congenital aortic stenosis, the ascending aorta is usually dilated ("poststenotic dilation"). In adults older than 50 years of age, valvar calcification may be seen on radiographs, but fluoroscopy permits detection of milder degrees of calcification and permits evaluation of the leaflet excursions.

Electrocardiography

Although the ECG may be surprisingly normal (particularly in females) in patients with significant stenosis, tall R waves over the left precordium are usually present. The presence of ST-T changes ("left ventricular strain") often indicates a severe degree of obstruction and an enhanced probability of sudden death. Left atrial enlargement—broad P waves—are often present.

Echo-Doppler Ultrasonography

The characteristic echocardiographic appearance in aortic stenosis is an increased echo density of the aortic valve with reduced systolic excursions of the leaflets. The left ventricle is often normal in size, with increased wall thickness. In young patients with aortic stenosis, the aortic leaflet excursions may appear normal as the "domed" valve projects into the aortic root and the bases of the leaflets seem to separate widely. An asymmetrically placed diastolic closure line may indicate a bicuspid valve. Discrete subvalvar or supravalvar stenosis can be seen on two-dimensional echocardiograms.

Continuous wave Doppler interrogation of the aortic valve (see Fig. 11.25) can accurately estimate the transaortic pressure gradient. This technique provides an ideal means of following patients with mild or asymptomatic lesions. The accuracy of the Doppler gradient measurement is predicated on the ability to interrogate the jet within 20° of its vector. It should also be recognized that a relatively small gradient (<30 mm Hg) can result from low flow across a severely stenotic valve in a patient with left ventricular dysfunction.

A pressure gradient can also be recorded in the left ventricular outflow tract in a condition unrelated to the conditions described above—hypertrophic cardiomyopathy. Unlike the discrete obstructive lesions previously discussed, the aortic upstroke (dp/dt) is more rapid than normal as are the rate and degree of ventricular emptying. In all of the discrete forms of aortic outflow obstruction noted earlier, the rate of ventricular emptying is retarded. In hypertrophic cardiomyopathy, the pressure gradient varies paradoxically with interventions that decrease ventricular filling; unlike discrete forms of stenosis, the gradient increases with decreases in filling. These paradoxical findings have generated considerable debate and controversy about the significance of these pressure gradients.

Therapy

A most useful diagnostic test in the elderly patient (>60 years of age) with suspected aortic stenosis is cardiac fluoroscopy. Significant aortic stenosis will almost invariably demonstrate a calcified and immobile aortic valve. Because mitral annular calcification may simulate the murmur of aortic stenosis, this condition can be ruled in or out. If the coronary arteries are heavily calcified and there is little or no valve calcification, coronary artery disease with papillary muscle dysfunction simulating the murmur of aortic stenosis should be suspected. Echocardiography and Doppler imaging will help confirm the diagnosis.

Critical aortic stenosis (aortic valve area less than 1.0 cm^2) usually presents with one or more of the classical symptom triad: angina, syncope, and dyspnea. The occurrence of these symptoms implies a poor prognosis with a 5-year mortality greater than 50%, even under optimal medical therapy. Therefore, confirmation of the aortic stenosis by cardiac catheterization and subsequent aortic valve replacement is indicated for these patients, even if there is decreased left ventricular function.

AORTIC REGURGITATION

Backflow of blood into the left ventricle results from the failure of coaptation of the aortic valve leaflets, either because of valvar or aortic root disease. Congenital bicuspid aortic valves or rheumatic scarring of the leaflets may cause stenosis, regurgitation, or a combination of obstruction and incompetence. Aortic root pathology, as seen in tertiary syphilis, Marfan's syndrome, Erdheim's medial necrosis, ankylosing spondylitis, dissecting aneurysm, etc., can also lead to regurgitation with minimal valvar pathology.

Chronic aortic regurgitation can be well compensated for by left ventricular dilatation or an increase in compliance so that the stroke volume of the left ventricle can increase to accommodate the obligatory backflow. The increased "volume work" of the heart is less energy consuming than the pressure work of aortic stenosis. Unlike aortic stenosis, exercise may be well tolerated because peripheral arteriolar dilation and tachycardia promote forward flow and diminish backflow.

Hemodynamic Basis of Symptoms

The compensatory adaptations to chronic aortic regurgitation become self-defeating in that the ventricle cannot dilate indefinitely and the low aortic diastolic pressure cannot provide adequate perfusion pressure for the coronary arteries. The left ventricle may have to pump 10–20 L/min to maintain a net output of 5 L/min, and the resulting dilation and hypertrophy leads to a massive increase in heart size, or "corbovinum."

The earliest symptoms may result from the increased pounding sensation from the wide pulse pressure in the systemic arteries with systolic hypertension from the increased stroke volume and a low diastolic pressure resulting from an increased rate of aortic runoff. The increased excursions of the volume-overloaded left ventricle may also produce discomfort. The supine increase in venous return, combined with resting bradycardia, may greatly overload the left ventricle at rest and lead to orthopnea and paroxysmal nocturnal dyspnea. Chest pain may result from inadequate coronary perfusion when the aortic diastolic pressure falls and the left ventricular diastolic pressure rises in severe or poorly tolerated aortic regurgitation. Chronic aortic regurgitation is depicted in Figure 11.29.

Acute aortic regurgitation, resulting from infective endocarditis, traumatic valve rupture, disruption of a prosthetic valve suture line, or dissecting aneurysm leads to a unique and often misdiagnosed condition. The left ventricle is faced with a sudden

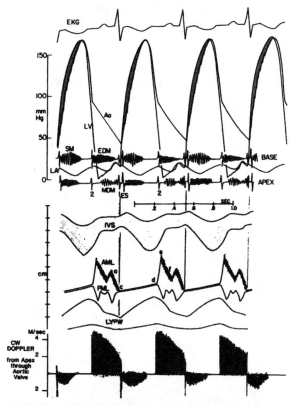

Figure 11.29. Chronic Aortic Regurgitation. The increased stroke volume and increased diastolic runoff lead to a wide aortic pulse pressure. The regurgitant blood causes a decrescendo early aortic diastolic murmur (EDM), and vibratory fluttering and functional stenosis of the mitral valve, and a left ventricular volume overload. The two phases (MDM and PSM) of the apical diastolic Austin Flint murmur correspond to the two closing movements (*e-f* and *a-c*) of the mitral echogram. Vigorous systolic ejection generates an ejection sound (ES), systolic murmur (SM), and increased excursions of the ventricular walls on the echo.

increase in volume that it cannot tolerate, and the ventricular diastolic pressure abruptly rises, often to 50–60 mm Hg, as shown in Figure 11.30.

This rapid rise in left ventricular diastolic pressure "precloses" the mitral valve, thus protecting the pulmonary vascular bed from the intolerably high pressure. Patients with acute aortic regurgitation often suffer an acute decrease in cardiac output and have dyspnea from the elevated left atrial pressure.

Hemodynamic Basis of Physical Signs

The diagnostic bedside manifestations of chronic aortic regurgitation result from the increased left ventricular stroke volume and aortic pulse pressure. The bed may oscillate with each systole, and the dramatic carotid pulsations may lead to bobbing of the head (Musset's sign). Other eponyms abound: Quincke's capillary pulsations, Corrigan's water hammer arterial pulses, Traube's pistol shot, Duroziez's to-and-fro murmurs over the femoral artery, and Hill's marked augmentation of the femoral artery systolic pressure (see Fig. 11.31).

Sustained isometric hand grip markedly increases the peripheral resistance and, in turn, the quantity of aortic regurgitation and the intensity of the diastolic murmurs.

Acute aortic regurgitation presents strikingly different clinical findings. Unlike chronic aortic regurgitation, the pulse pressure is not increased, because the quantity of aortic diastolic backflow is reduced by the overfilled left ventricle, the diastolic pressure of which "holds up" the diastolic pressure as shown in Figure 11.30. The aortic diastolic regurgitant murmur may be shortened. The limited compliance of the ventricle also reduces the ability of the ventricle to increase its stroke volume, and the systolic "flow" murmur may be soft or absent.

Another consequence of the left ventricle's inability to accept a sudden increase in volume loading is the mitral preclosure, which leads to a unique, loud, mid-diastolic crescendo-decrescendo murmur (MDM) and is probably a distorted Austin Flint murmur caused by abrupt narrowing of the mitral orifice during preclosure. The first heart sound is not heard at the onset of systole because of the mitral valve preclosure, and mitral valve closure may be represented by a mid-diastolic sound in the midst of the Austin Flint murmur.

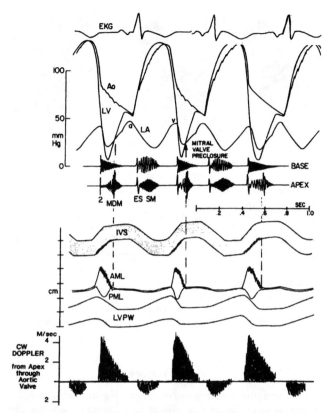

Figure 11.30. Acute Aortic Regurgitation. The relatively noncompliant, non-dilated LV is overfilled by regurgitant blood, and the rapidly rising LV diastolic pressure "precloses" the fluttering mitral valve in mid-diastole and inhibits late diastolic aortic regurgitation. Preclosure is caused by LV/LA pressure crossover and generates a loud crescendo-decrescendo mid-diastolic murmur (MDM). The "squared off" diastolic excursions of the LV walls on the echocardiogram represent the inhibition of further volume increases in the acutely overloaded ventricle.

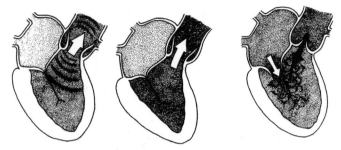

Figure 11.31. The Murmurs of Aortic Regurgitation. Aortic regurgitation causes an increased left ventricular stroke volume and diastolic runoff of blood to the left ventricle, which accounts for the physical signs (left). The precordium is active, with an outward and downward displacement of the apex beat, demonstrating a rapid diastolic filling wave and increased systolic early peaking midsystolic crescendo-decrescendo "ejection" or "flow" murmur at the base (center). The aortic backflow leads to a decrescendo diastolic blow best heard along the course of the regurgitant stream at the left sternal border. The aortic valve backflow interacts with the mitral valve inflow to produce a mitral stenosislike apical diastolic rumbling murmur with presystolic accentuation (right). This murmur was first described more than 100 years ago by Flint and is believed to result from dynamic decreases in mitral orifice size in mid- or late diastole caused by the aortic regurgitant jet and left ventricular distention.

Natural History

The compensatory mechanisms in chronic regurgitation may permit two to three decades of absent or minimal symptoms, but because of the inherent limitations of these compensations, rapid deterioration occurs after decompensation sets in. This rapid decline often results from irreversible left ventricular dilatation and dysfunction, and considerable efforts have been expended to try to prevent these manifestations by proper timing of valve replacement. At present, concerns about the relative morbidity and mortality associated with valve replacement compared with that of the natural history do not warrant valve replacement in asymptomatic individuals.

The natural history of unoperated acute aortic regurgitation is sufficiently poor to warrant urgent valve replacement after the diagnosis has been established, even in the face of active valvar infection.

Laboratory Findings

Radiography

In chronic aortic regurgitation, the left ventricular portion of the cardiac silhouette is enlarged because of dilation and hypertrophy. Because the left ventricular compliance increases in compensation for the volume overload, the left atrial and pulmonary venous pressures are not increased, and the left atrium is, therefore, not enlarged and the pulmonary vascularity seems normal. The aorta may be dilated in congenital bicuspid aortic valve, dissecting aneurysm, and diseases of the aortic root.

In contrast, acute aortic regurgitation may present with severe hemodynamic embarrassment without significant cardiac enlargement. Although the left atrium and pulmonary veins are "protected" by mitral valve preclosure, pulmonary congestion may be seen in severe, decompensated acute aortic regurgitation.

Electrocardiography

The ECG in chronic aortic regurgitation usually demonstrates tall left precordial R waves and may have associated peaked T waves with S-T elevation, the "diastolic overload pattern," or the "strain" pattern seen in aortic stenosis, with T inversion.

Acute aortic regurgitation invariably demonstrates tachycardia on the ECG, but there are no other consistent ECG findings.

Echo-Doppler Ultrasonography

Chronic aortic regurgitation presents a characteristic and diagnostic echo pattern of increased left ventricular dimensions and excursions combined with fine fluttering of the anterior mitral leaflet echo (see Fig. 11.28). The aortic root may be dilated, and the aortic valve closure line may be asymmetrically placed in bicuspid aortic valve disease. A double aortic wall may be seen in dissecting aneurysm.

Acute aortic regurgitation presents a diagnostic echo appearance with tachycardia, minimally increased left ventricular size with exaggerated wall motion, and preclosure of the fluttering mitral valve echo (see Fig. 11.30). Occasionally, shaggy vegetations may be seen in the aorta during systole and the left ventricle during diastole.

Continuous wave Doppler interrogation of aortic regurgitation provides useful hemodynamic information. The velocity of the regurgitant jet provides an estimate of the relationship of aortic diastolic pressure to left ventricular diastolic pressure; the aortic diastolic pressure can be approximated by a sphygmomanometer recording of the blood pressure (see Chapter 4). The contrast between the holodiastolic signal from chronic aortic regurgitation and the attenuated signal from acute aortic regurgitation is apparent on inspection of Figures 11.29 and 11.30.

Color flow Doppler imaging provides a qualitative evaluation of the magnitude of aortic regurgitation from the breadth of the regurgitant jet and the distance that it travels toward the apex.

Therapy

Chronic Aortic Regurgitation

Medical. Digitalis and subacute bacterial endocarditis (SBE) prophylaxis are indicated. Afterload reduction is indicated if hypertension is present. Noninvasive evaluation may be performed at regular intervals to assess the severity of the aortic regurgitation and the left ventricular function. Clues to the increasing severity of the aortic regurgitation (AR) and decline in left ventricular (LV) function include a history of paroxysmal nocturnal dyspnea, the presence of increasing pulse pressure (>100 mm Hg) or diminishing aortic diastolic pressure (<50 mm Hg), a loud solitary mid-diastolic Austin Flint murmur, an S3, an increasing cardiomegaly, an increasing internal left ventricular dimension (systolic internal diameter of >5.5 cm on echocardiogram), and a declining ejection fraction at rest or with exercise.

Surgical. Optimal timing of aortic valve replacement is important to prevent irreversible myocardial damage. If consideration of the above parameters indicates severe AR and/or LV dysfunction, confirmed at cardiac catheterization, aortic valve replacement is recommended. Postoperative studies have shown a decrease in heart size with improved LV function.

Acute Aortic Regurgitation

Acute aortic regurgitation is a potentially reversible illness that carries a poor prognosis if treated by medical means alone. Prompt clinical diagnosis (physical examination and echocardiograms are most helpful), medical stabilization (bedrest, diuretics, afterload reduction), and early surgical intervention usually lead to a favorable outcome. Even in the setting of active bacterial endocarditis, aortic valve replacement must not be postponed if decompensation is present.

MIXED AORTIC VALVE DISEASE

The addition of aortic regurgitation to aortic stenosis leads to the necessity for a larger stroke volume (to compensate for the backflow) and a resulting marked increase in transvalvar gradient. Because the ventricle must dilate to accommodate the regurgitant flow, the systolic wall tension generated and oxygen consumed by the left ventricle are higher in mixed aortic lesions than in pure aortic stenosis with the same left ventricular pressure. Patients with mixed lesions are often symptomatic at an earlier age than those with pure lesions.

The dominance of stenosis or regurgitation can often be detected by the arterial pressure—a wide arterial pulse pressure and rapid upstroke would favor dominant aortic regurgitation and a narrow, slow-rising pulse would favor aortic stenosis.

Laboratory Findings

Radiography

The left ventricle will be enlarged, and the aortic root is often dilated in mixed aortic valve lesions.

Electrocardiography

Because the coexistence of stenosis and regurgitation increases the systolic outflow and the magnitude of the systolic left ventricular pressure, marked left ventricular hypertrophy may be seen on the ECG.

Echo-Doppler Ultrasonography

Mixed aortic valve lesions present a composite echocardiographic appearance with the left ventricular dimensions, reflecting the impact of the dominant lesion. The aortic root echocardiogram may demonstrate an asymmetric closure line or increased echo-density, suggesting calcification of the valve. Doppler interrogation will reveal an outflow tract gradient as well as an aortic regurgitant jet.

PULMONARY STENOSIS

Outflow obstruction of the right ventricle may be at valvar, sub-valvar, or supravalvar level and is usually congenital in etiology. Rarely, rheumatic disease, carcinoid heart disease, pericardial constriction, and intracardiac tumors can obstruct outflow from the right ventricle. This section will deal only with isolated pulmonary stenosis and not the many complex forms of congenital heart disease in which pulmonary stenosis may be present.

Congenital valvar pulmonary stenosis results from fusion of the cusps into a thickened, fibrous dome and is almost always associated with hypertrophy of the subvalvar infundibulum, which may increase in severity in response to the hypertrophy stimulus.

Supravalvar or peripheral pulmonary artery stenosis may be in a single area in the main pulmonary artery or scattered throughout the pulmonary branches; it most often results from intrauterine rubella infection.

Isolated subvalvar pulmonary stenosis is usually caused by hypertrophied anomalous muscle bundle(s) within the right ventricle and not infundibular hypertrophy.

Hemodynamic Basis of Symptoms

The severity of right ventricular outflow obstruction increases with time as a result of disproportionate physical growth, increasing hypertrophy, or progressive scarring of the valve. The right ventricle compensates with a progressive concentric hypertrophy, leading to a small, stiff, thick-walled chamber. Some patients with severe obstruction (gradients higher than 100 mm Hg) tolerate the lesions remarkably well, but exercise limitations or syncope, fatigue, and chest pain are the most common symptoms.

Hemodynamic Basis of Physical Signs

In right ventricular outflow obstruction, the hypertrophic right ventricle has reduced compliance and requires an augmented right atrial contraction *a* wave for filling (Fig. 11.32). This power-ful *a* wave may actually open the pulmonary valve and initiate flow to the pulmonary artery, and it can be detected as a presys-tolic wave in the jugular veins. The powerful and sustained right ventricular contraction can be felt along the left parasternal area,

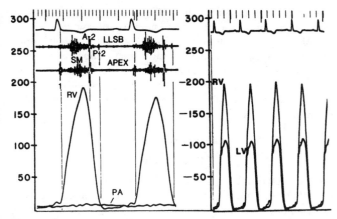

Figure 11.32. Pulmonary Valvar Stenosis. The obstructed pulmonary valve results in a peaked elevated RV pressure and a low pulmonary artery (PA) pressure. The powerful RA and RV a waves often exceed PA diastolic pressure and open the pulmonic valve. There is a crescendo-decrescendo systolic murmur (SM). The components of the second heart sound are split (aortic, A-2; pulmonic, P-2) with P-2 being delayed (left). RV pressure is elevated and exceeds LV pressure (right).

and the turbulent flow may produce a thrill in the second left parasternal interspace in valvar stenosis and the third or fourth parasternal interspace in subvalvar disease. The turbulence leads to poststenotic dilatation of the pulmonary artery, and the systolic bulge of this artery may be felt in the second left parasternal interspace. On auscultation, a loud left parasternal fourth heart sound, an early click (in valvar stenosis only), and a late-peaking crescendo-decrescendo parasternal systolic murmur indicate significant outflow obstruction. The pulmonic closure sound is soft and delayed and may not be appreciated. The hemodynamic and auscultatory findings in valvar pulmonic stenosis are shown in Figure 11.32.

Natural History

Severe pulmonary stenosis may require operative intervention in infancy or childhood. Because obstruction usually progresses, patients that survive childhood may be detected while they are asymptomatic by physical examination or progressive fatigue and exercise intolerance. Right heart failure is not common.

After operative intervention or balloon valvuloplasty in pulmonary stenosis, a malignant outflow tract stenosis or "suicide ventricle" will develop in some patients; this is believed to be caused by the relief of the valvar stenosis that previously distended the subvalvar region. Subvalvar muscle resection is therefore indicated in these cases.

Laboratory Findings

Radiography

The characteristic radiographic appearance of pulmonic stenosis consists of dilatation of the main and left pulmonary arteries (poststenotic dilatation), combined with a slight upward tipping of the apex (right ventricular hypertrophy) and normal peripheral lung fields. Occasionally, the right atrium will be enlarged.

Electrocardiography

Right ventricular hypertrophy (tall R waves in the right precordial leads and vertical or right axis deviation) will be almost invariably present in significant pulmonary stenosis. Tall, peaked P waves may indicate right atrial enlargement.

Echo-Doppler Ultrasonography

Because the pulmonic valve is difficult to demonstrate by echocardiography, the echocardiogram is rarely diagnostic in pulmonary stenosis. However, the presence of right ventricular hypertrophy and hypertension, the latter by Doppler interrogation of the tricuspid regurgitant jet, can be diagnostic of pulmonary stenosis. Rarely, the pulmonary outflow jet can be measured by Doppler, allowing an estimate of the pressure gradient across the pulmonic valve. It should be noted that the pulmonary artery pressure in pulmonic stenosis is always less than 20 mm Hg, so that the magnitude of the gradient can be calculated by subtracting 10–20 mm Hg from the tricuspid regurgitation-derived right ventricular pressure.

PULMONARY REGURGITATION

Pulmonary valvar regurgitation can result from congenital deformity or absence of the valve cusps or may be functional in response to an increase in pulmonary vascular resistance (pulmonary hypertension). Valvar pulmonary regurgitation with normal pulmonary artery resistance is rare enough to be a medical curiosity; it is most often benign. Pulmonary hypertension, on the other hand, is a serious and life-limiting condition, and the presence or absence of associated pulmonary regurgitation is of no significant consequence. Pulmonary hypertension, secondary to mitral stenosis, represents a reversible form of pulmonary hypertension, and the pulmonary regurgitant murmur (Graham Steell's murmur) may disappear after mitral surgery.

Suggested Reading

Carabello BA, Crawford FA. Valvular heart disease. N Engl J Med 1997; 337:32.

Criley JM, Criley D, Zalace C. The physiologic origins of heart sounds and murmurs: the unique interactive guide to cardiac diagnosis. Boston: Little, Brown and Co, 1997 (CD-ROM program).

Criley JM, Siegel RJ. New techniques should enhance, not replace, bedside diagnostic skills in cardiology, Part 1. Bull Mod Concepts Cardiovasc Dis 1990;59:19.

Criley JM, Siegel RJ. New techniques should enhance, not replace, bedside diagnostic skills in cardiology, Part 2. Bull Mod Concepts Cardiovasc Dis 1990;59:25.

Dajani AS, Taubert KA, Wilson W, et al. Prevention of bacterial endocarditis: recommendations by the American Heart Association. JAMA 1997;277:1794.

Chapter 12

Congenital Heart Disease

INTRODUCTION

Because many patients who survive to adulthood with congenital heart disease are potentially operable and because the natural history of many congenital heart disease lesions, particularly those with either high pulmonary blood flow or cyanosis, is associated with progressive disability and premature death, it is important for the house officer to recognize the need to establish a presumptive diagnosis and initiate steps leading to a definitive diagnosis.

Congenital heart disease (CHD) may permit survival into adult life because of certain favorable factors:

1. The lesion is mild.
2. Multiple lesions counterbalance one another.
3. Compensatory mechanisms have taken place.
4. The lesions have been surgically corrected or palliated.

At the same time, certain complications may take place that render the clinical presentation less clear in the adult with CHD than in the child:

1. Acquired valvular, vascular, or myocardial disease.
2. Infective endocarditis.
3. Embolic phenomena.
4. Pulmonary hypertension.
5. Congestive failure.
6. Arrhythmias.
7. Surgical misadventures.

A well-focused noninvasive workup with the availability of the imaging capability of contemporary echographic, Doppler, scintigraphic, and magnetic resonance imaging technology is capable of establishing a definitive diagnosis in most cases. In many instances, the anatomical information established by noninvasive means is sufficiently accurate to render invasive procedures redundant. It is important to emphasize the necessity for a presumptive diagnosis not only in choosing the appropriate diagnostic modalities but in guiding their application. An unfocused diagnostic effort may yield ambiguous or misleading results.

The diagnostic value of the history, cardiac physical examination, and the "routine" laboratory tests will be emphasized in this chapter. The choice of appropriate secondary (specialized noninvasive) and tertiary (invasive) studies should take into consideration the differential diagnostic possibilities afforded by the clinical evaluation.

The secondary diagnostic studies permit detection and quantitation and, to a lesser extent, localization of shunts. For example, radionuclide scintigraphy can rule in right-to-left shunts by detection of intravenously injected radiolabeled microspheres in the renal parenchyma but cannot localize the site of shunting. Similarly, intravenous injection of a radionuclide that can be tracked by placement of scintigraphic cursors over the lung fields will detect early recirculation curves compatible with left-to-right shunting but cannot distinguish the site of shunting. These radionuclide studies may falsely diagnose shunts when there is delayed transit through the right heart due to tricuspid regurgitation or when certain high-flow states are present.

Two-dimensional (2D) echocardiography can define atrial and ventricular septal defects but can be falsely positive in suggesting atrial defects because of echo "dropout" and can miss ventricular septal defects and right ventricular outflow obstruction.

Color flow Doppler imaging, a technique in which two-dimensional echocardiography is combined with color-coded signals that designate flow toward and away from the transducer, as well as high velocity or turbulent flow, may almost eliminate the need for angiography for critically ill infants and some adults. Once again, a strong presumption of congenital heart disease and a specific differential diagnosis should be present to use this technique appropriately.

Magnetic resonance imaging (MRI) can render superb images of the heart, particularly when the image acquisition is gated to the electrocardiogram (ECG) and appropriate image planes ("slices") are used.

This chapter will alert the physician to the more common forms of CHD that may be encountered in the adult. Because surgical techniques have evolved, rendering more and more patients with CHD amenable to palliative or corrective surgery, a high index of suspicion of CHD is warranted when patients' cardiac findings cannot be explained on the basis of acquired heart disease.

RECOGNITION

A significant CHD lesion will usually present with two or more of the following findings.

1. A precordial murmur. (If the murmur is continuous, a diagnosis of CHD is virtually ensured.)
2. Chamber enlargement or hypertrophy.
3. Abnormal pulmonary vascularity on chest roentgenogram.
4. Abnormal cardiac silhouette on chest roentgenogram.
5. Cyanosis with or without clubbing or polycythemia.
6. Abnormal ECG.

CLASSIFICATION OF CONGENITAL HEART DISEASE

Anatomical

There are three basic anatomical or structural abnormalities that may be present singly or in combination in an adult patient with CHD.

1. **Obstruction** to transvalvar or great artery flow. (If obstruction is complete, it is termed "atresia.")
2. **Communication** between chambers or great vessels.
3. **Transposition** of great arteries and/or veins. (This category also includes anomalous connection of systemic veins to the left heart or pulmonary veins to the right heart.)

Functional

The anatomical abnormalities in turn lead to four types of functional abnormalities that may also occur alone or in combination.

1. Ventricular or atrial enlargement or hypertrophy.
2. Systemic or pulmonary hypertension.

3. Left-to-right shunting: pulmonary blood flow (PBF) >systemic blood flow (SBF).
4. Right-to-left shunting: arterial O_2 desaturation with SBF > PBF.

Because it is the functional sequelae that usually permit clinical recognition of CHD, it is important to understand the interrelationships between the anatomical defects and the functional results.

OBSTRUCTIONS

Obstructions to ventricular outflow or great vessel flow produce a pressure drop (gradient) across the obstruction with a higher-than-normal pressure and hypertrophy of the upstream ventricle. Obstruction to ventricular inflow leads to dilatation and hypertrophy of the upstream atrium.

The pressure gradient across a stenotic outflow tract is associated with increased velocity (gradient = $4 \times$ velocity^2), and murmur intensity is proportional to velocity to the fourth power (Fig. 12.1). Therefore, a long, late-peaking murmur suggests severe stenosis because it implies a long, late-peaking gradient.

An **exception to this rule** occurs when the ventricle with outflow obstruction has an alternate outlet as in the tetralogy of

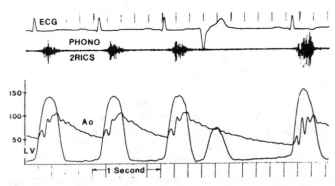

Figure 12.1. Aortic Stenosis. The relationship of the pressure gradient to the murmur is demonstrated in the postextrasystolic beat in a patient with aortic stenosis. The increase in the left ventricular-aortic pressure gradient is matched by an increase in murmur intensity and duration.

Fallot, in which case a short (or absent) systolic murmur is associated with severe obstruction (or atresia) of the pulmonary outflow tract.

Significant pulmonary stenosis is almost invariably associated with ECG manifestations of right ventricular hypertrophy (RVH). Therefore, the absence of RVH virtually rules out pulmonary stenosis. The absence of left ventricular hypertrophy (LVH) on ECG is less reliable in ruling out aortic stenosis.

The flow disturbance caused by **valvar stenosis** or coarctation usually leads to enlargement, or poststenotic dilatation, of the portion of the great artery downstream from the stenotic lesion. An **exception to this rule** occurs in the tetralogy of Fallot because the alternate outflow pathway (aorta) diminishes pulmonary blood flow and therefore turbulence; low pulmonary blood flow ensues, and the pulmonary artery is small.

Subvalvar and supravalvar stenoses are usually not associated with poststenotic dilatation. One exception is the tetralogy of Fallot with infundibular stenosis and absence, not atresia, of the pulmonary valve leaflets; the main pulmonary artery may have aneurysmal dilatation.

COMMUNICATIONS

Communications between chambers, great vessels, or great vessels and chambers behave predictably. If the communication is sufficiently large (**nonrestrictive**), it will equalize the pressure in the communicating chambers or great vessels. For example, a ventricular septal defect (VSD) as large as the aortic orifice will equalize the pressures in the right and left ventricles. On the other hand, a small (**restrictive**) VSD will obstruct flow across the defect and will maintain a significant pressure difference between the ventricles.

Flow across a restrictive ventricular septal defect has high velocity because of the pressure drop across the defect (systemic pressure minus normal right ventricular pressure, approximately an 80 mm Hg pressure gradient) and results in velocities comparable to those in severe aortic or pulmonic stenosis. Therefore, there will be a holosystolic murmur in patients with restrictive ventricular septal defects.

When there is a restrictive communication between the aorta (Ao) and the pulmonary artery (PA) (e.g., a small patent ductus arteriosus), there is a large pressure gradient and resulting increase in flow velocity, which phasically increases in systole and decreases in diastole, leading to a **continuous murmur** that reaches a peak in late systole. Similarly, a continuous murmur results from a restrictive communication between the aorta and a right heart chamber (e.g., ruptured sinus of Valsalva aneurysm).

Conversely, a nonrestrictive ventricular septal defect has no pressure drop across the septum and consequently has flow velocities comparable to that of aortic or pulmonary outflow, so that flow through these large defects usually produces little or no murmur.

Flow through an atrial septal defect (ASD) occurs throughout the cardiac cycle and is not associated with a pressure drop across the septum. The most common murmur of atrial septal defect is systolic, and results from the two- to fivefold increase in right ventricular outflow that is associated with high velocity and a pressure gradient. A rumbling mid-diastolic murmur that results from the high volume of right ventricular inflow may be heard in the tricuspid area.

As a general rule, the presence of a systolic or continuous murmur in a patient with congenital heart disease is a favorable sign, because it suggests high-flow velocities and a potentially remediable defect. This maxim is particularly helpful for a cyanotic patient, because it implies pulmonary stenosis or atresia and a low pulmonary artery pressure. Alternatively, the absence of a significant systolic murmur or the presence of only a diastolic murmur is usually an ominous sign, suggesting the lack of either a significant left-to-right shunt or pulmonary stenosis, or the presence of pulmonary hypertension. When pulmonary vascular obliterative changes are present, most forms of definitive or palliative surgery are contraindicated.

The direction of flow is dictated by the resistance to flow downstream from the chambers communicating through the defect. The resistance to flow downstream can be increased by a stenotic valve, a noncompliant ventricle, or an increase in pulmonary vascular resistance (PVR) or systemic vascular resistance (SVR). The relationship of PVR to SVR determines the direction of flow through a VSD or patent ductus arteriosus (PDA) and the relationship of right ventricular (RV) versus left ventricular (LV)

Table 12.1
Shunt Determination in Congenital Heart Disease

Site of communication	Predominant shunt L → R if	Predominant shunt R → L if
Atrial septal defect (ASD)	Tricuspid valve (TV) normal and RV compliance normal	TV abnormal* or RV compliance abnormal**
Ventricular septal defect (VSD)	VSD restrictive or VSD nonrestrictive with normal RV outflow tract and PVR <SVR	VSD nonrestrictive with RV outflow obstruction (tetralogy of Fallot) or PVR >SVR (Eisenmenger's)
Patent ductus arteriosus (PDA)	PDA restrictive or PVR <SVR	PDA nonrestrictive and PVR >SVR

PVR = peripheral vascular resistance; SVR = systemic vascular resistance.
* Stenosis, atresia, severe Ebstein's anomaly.
** Pulmonary hypertension, stenosis, or chronic volume overload.

compliance determines the direction of flow through an ASD (Table 12.1).

TRANSPOSITION

Transposition (and obligatory shunts due to anomalous connections) defects rarely exist in isolation, because most of them are associated with communications or other abnormalities that tend to compensate for the anomaly and contribute to adult survival.

Transposition of the great arteries (TGA), in which the aorta arises from the right ventricle and the pulmonary artery from the left ventricle, is incompatible with survival unless compensated for by associated communications or **ventricular inversion.** Additional **obstruction** of the right ventricular outflow tract also aids in permitting adult survival because it prevents development of pulmonary hypertension. The following diagrams show combinations that permit adult survival with TGA.

1. **TGA with VSD and obstruction of RV outflow.** Without a VSD, only O_2 desaturated blood would circulate through systemic arteries. Excessive pulmonary blood flow and pulmonary hypertension are moderated by RV outflow obstruction.

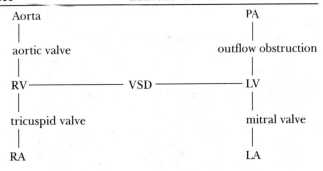

2. **Corrected TGA** (ventricular inflow inversion). Ventricular inflow inversion permits the anatomic RV to receive saturated blood from the left atrium (LA) and the LV to receive right atrial (RA) blood. The systemic arterial blood is therefore fully O_2 saturated.

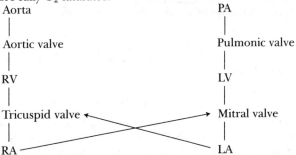

Anomalous pulmonary venous connection allows O_2-saturated blood to enter the right atrium (RA) or systemic veins, resulting in an obligatory left-to-right shunt and an increase in pulmonary blood flow.

1. Total anomalous pulmonary venous connection results in all of the pulmonary veins draining into the RA or a systemic vein and must be associated with an ASD to permit survival. There is a right-to-left shunt at the atrial level and massive pulmonary blood flow.

2. Partial anomalous pulmonary venous connection (APVC) results in an obligatory venous return from one lobe or the entire right lung into the right heart and an increase in pulmonary blood flow. Partial APVC is often associated with an

ASD (usually of the sinus venosus type), but survival does not depend on it.

Summary of Functional Considerations

In the absence of transposition, left-to-right shunts increase pulmonary blood flow (PBF) and right-to-left shunts reduce PBF. Most communications result in left-to-right shunts unless there is a downstream obstruction (e.g., outflow stenosis) or resistance to flow (e.g., hypertrophied RV). Transposition of the great arteries always requires compensatory defects for survival.

COMMON ACYANOTIC FORMS OF CONGENITAL HEART DISEASE PERMITTING ADULT SURVIVAL

Lesion   Clinical/Laboratory Findings

A. OUTFLOW TRACT LESIONS
1. **Bicuspid Aortic Valve**
   a. Without hemodynamic impairment

1. Early systolic click, short mid-systolic murmur at second right intercostal space.
2. Eccentric closure line of aortic valve on echocardiogram.
3. **Significance:** may develop increasingly severe aortic stenosis and/or aortic regurgitation in later life. Prone to infective endocarditis.

   b. With aortic stenosis (Fig. 12.2)

1. Males/females = 4/1.
2. Delayed carotid upstroke.
3. Sustained LV lift.
4. Early systolic click, midsystolic murmur at R base, transmitted to carotids and apex.

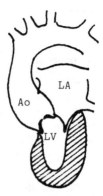

Figure 12.2.

5. LVH on ECG.
6. **Significance:** see no. 3 above. If symptomatic or associated with significant ECG changes, should be evaluated by Doppler study and/or cardiac catheterization. Surgery increases survival.

c. With aortic regurgitation

Note: All forms of discrete LV outflow obstruction share common clinical features: slow pulse upstroke, midsystolic murmur, LVH on ECG, etc. The differentiating features will be outlined under each lesion.

1. Bounding pulses, bisferiens carotid pulse.
2. Click, systolic murmur as in AS.
3. Diastolic blow along left sternal border (LSB).
4. LVH on ECG.
5. **Significance:** may be well

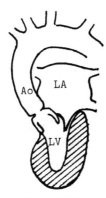

Figure 12.3.

tolerated for years. Indications for operative intervention outlined in Chapter 11.

2. **Supravalvar Aortic Stenosis**
   (Fig. 12.3)

   1. Abnormal facies and dentition with mental retardation ("What, me worry?" —Alfred E. Neumann) common.
   2. Different blood pressure (BP) in arms (R >L).
   3. No click. Midsystolic murmur at R base, loud A2.
   4. Echo may demonstrate narrow aorta above valve.
   5. **Significance:** may be familial.
   Cardiac catheterization indicated if lesion suspected.

3. **Discrete Subvalvar Aortic Stenosis**
   (Fig. 12.4)

   1. Slow carotid upstroke.

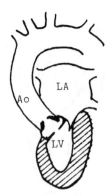

Figure 12.4.

2. No click. Midsystolic murmur along LSB.
3. Soft murmur of AR common.
4. Echo may demonstrate constriction of LV outflow tract and early closure of aortic valve.
5. **Significance:** may develop secondary hypertrophy and resemble hypertrophic cardiomyopathy. Cardiac catheterization indicated if lesion suspected. Turbulence in outflow tract results in trauma to aortic valve leaflets.

4. **Coarctation of Aorta** (Fig. 12.5)

1. Hypertension in upper extremities, slow-rising pulses and low BP in legs.
2. Visible collateral arteries on back.
3. Rib notching on chest radiograph.

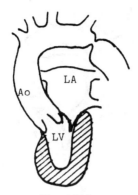

Figure 12.5.

4. Echo from suprasternal notch may demonstrate co-arctation.
5. **Significance:** often overlooked as cause of hypertension. Operation best in young patients. May be managed with antihypertensive therapy in older individuals.

Note: This lesion is often associated with a bicuspid aortic valve.

5. **Hypertrophic Cardiomyopathy (HCM)**
   (See Chapter 13)
   (Fig. 12.6)

1. Often familial history of heart disease or sudden death; patient may be asymptomatic or have dyspnea, syncope, or chest pain.
2. Brisk carotid upstroke, sustained apical impulse.
3. S4 and loud mid- to late

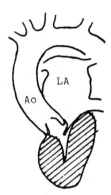

Figure 12.6.

systolic murmur that increases with Valsalva.
4. LVH on ECG — often striking.
5. Echo can be diagnostic (see Chapter 4).
6. **Significance:** appropriate therapy (SBE prophylaxis, β blockers, antiarrhythmics, avoidance of exercise) may lower mortality even for asymptomatic patients. Operation does not lower mortality.

6. **Subvalvar Pulmonic Stenosis**
   a. Rare as isolated lesion.
   b. May coexist with HCM or VSD.
7. **Valvar Pulmonic Stenosis** (Fig. 12.7)

1. May have round facies.
2. Prominent jugular venous *a* wave.
3. RV lift, with systolic thrill and murmur at upper

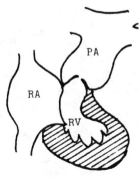

Figure 12.7.

LSB. P2 soft and late, click may be heard.
4. LVH, RAE on ECG.
5. Poststenotic dilatation of PA on radiograph.
6. **Significance:** if no RVH, pulmonary stenosis is unlikely. If present, cardiac catheterization is indicated. Surgery is low risk; good results can be anticipated.

8. **Supravalvar Pulmonic Stenosis**
   a. Usually a result of maternal rubella infection during pregnancy
   b. Usually bilateral and multiple
B. **LEFT-TO-RIGHT SHUNTS**
1. **Atrial Septal Defect**
   (Fig. 12.8)
   a. Ostium secundum

1. Most common ASD, females/males = 2/1.
2. Mitral prolapse present in 1/3.
3. Often not symptomatic

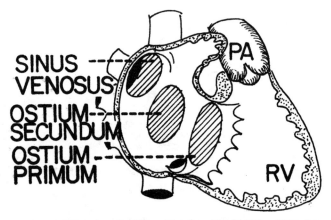

Figure 12.8. Right Anterior Oblique Diagram of the Right Heart Chambers. Diagram demonstrates the location of the three common types of atrial septal defects. Sinus venosus defects are in the superior dorsal atrial septum and are almost invariably associated with partial anomalous pulmonary venous drainage into the right atrium. Ostium secundum defects result from excessive resorption of the embryologic septum primum; these defects are usually large and may be fenestrated. Ostium primum defects result from failure of fusion of the embryologic endocardial cushion and septum primum, resulting in an inferior defect associated with mitral and tricuspid valve deformities (cleft septal leaflets with or without regurgitation).

until fourth to sixth decade.
4. RV and PA lift; fixed, split S2, with midsystolic murmur. Ejection click common.
5. Enlarged right heart and pulmonary plethora on chest radiograph; "hilar dance" on fluoroscopy.
6. Shunt can be confirmed and quantitated by radionuclide angiography.
7. RSR' or RSR'S' in V1 common, with normal or right

axis. P-R may be pro-
longed.
Atrial fibrillation in older
patients.

8. Significance: because lesion has low-risk repair
   and may become inoper-
   able in later life (as RV
   fails and pulmonary hypertension develops, R-L
   shunt occurs) cardiac catheterization is indicated
   when lesion is suspected.
   Operation is indicated if
   heart enlarged and PBF:
   SBF is > 2:1. SBE prophylaxis usually not required
   (unless mitral prolapse
   murmur present).

(Fig. 12.9)
Note: All types of ASD share common features as outlined
under ostium secundum. Differentiating features will be
noted under other defects.
b. Sinus venosus

1. Often associated with partial anomalous pulmonary
   venous connection.
2. **Significance:** low-risk surgery can close defect and
   reroute anomalous pulmonary veins.

c. Ostium primum

1. Left and superior axis deviation of ECG plus RSR′S′
   highly suggestive of diagnosis.
2. Mitral regurgitant murmur
   may be present.
3. Surgery carries slight risk
   of acquired heart block.

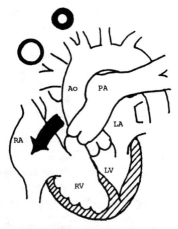

Figure 12.9. Atrial Septal Defect. In this depiction of a young patient with an ASD, there is a left-to-right shunt because the RV compliance (distensibility) is greater than that of the LV. With a large (nonrestrictive) ASD, the pressures in the atria are equal and the flow follows the line of least resistance. The pulmonary vascular resistance (thin circle adjacent to the right pulmonary artery) is low, permitting high flow without elevation of the pulmonary artery pressure. The right heart chambers and PA are dilated to accommodate the high flow (volume overload).

d. Miscellaneous

Mitral valve may require repair, rarely replacement.

1. Defects may be multiple (ostium primum + secundum) or entire septum may be absent (''single atrium'').
2. Various eponyms are associated with ASD complexes:
    a. Holt-Oram syndrome: hypoplastic thumb + ostium secundum ASD.
    b. Ellis-van Creveld syndrome: polydactyly + single atrium.

c. Lutembacher's syndrome: mitral stenosis (probably rheumatic) + ASD.

2. **Ventricular Septal Defects**
   a. Maladie de Roger

   1. Small VSD.
   2. Left parasternal thrill with loud holosystolic murmur at fourth left intercostal space.
   3. Chest radiograph and ECG may be normal.
   4. Cardiac catheterization unnecessary. Lesion can be confirmed by Doppler study.
   5. **Significance:** clinical course usually benign. SBE prophylaxis is indicated.

   (Fig. 12.10)
   b. Large VSD with L-R shunt

   1. Relatively rare in adults (most large VSDs develop pulmonary hypertension in childhood).
   2. Heart enlarged with active RV and LV. Holosystolic murmur at lower left sternal border. S2 split, not fixed.
   3. Lesion can be confirmed by Doppler study.
   4. Radionuclide shunt study will confirm and quantitate shunt.
   5. **Significance:** may be associated with aortic regurgitation due to loss of support of valve. Cardiac catheteri-

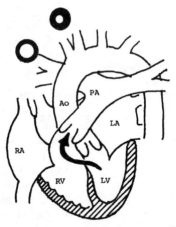

Figure 12.10. Maladie de Roger. A small (restrictive) ventricular septal defect that serves to limit the magnitude of the left-to-right shunt and does not increase the right heart pressure significantly. The pulmonary vascular resistance (indicated by the thin circle opposite the right pulmonary artery) is normal.

zation is indicated, and surgery indicated if large L-R shunt confirmed and PVR not greatly increased.

Note: Septal defects can be supracristal or infracristal relative to the crista supraventricularis.

3. **Patent Ductus Arteriosus**

1. Females/males = 2/1.
2. Continuous murmur peaking at S2, best heard in left infraclavicular area.
3. If shunt large, heart will be enlarged and pulmonary vascularity will be increased.
4. **Significance:** complete restoration to normal is

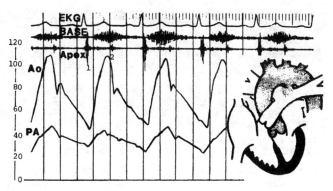

Figure 12.11. Patent Ductus Arteriosus. The Ao pressure is higher than the PA pressure throughout the cardiac cycle, which results in pulsatile continuous flow and a murmur at the base, which spills through and obscures the second heart sound. The PA pressure is elevated to 50/25 because of the high flow state (PBF/SBF = 5/1), but the pulmonary vascular resistance is normal.

possible with low-risk surgery in young patients. In older patients, risk increases due to friability of ductus and aortic isthmus. Rarely, ductus may recur if ligated and not divided.

(Fig. 12.11)

4. Other Causes of "Continuous Murmurs" That May Simulate PDA in Acyanotic Patients
   a. Anomalous origin of left coronary artery from pulmonary artery
   b. Coronary—cameral fistulae (coronary artery to cardiac chamber)
   c. Pulmonary arteriovenous (AV) fistulae
   d. Congenital or acquired AV fistulae

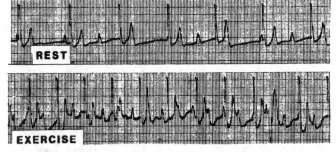

Figure 12.12. Congenital Complete Heart Block. An electrocardiographic rhythm strip at rest demonstrates dissociated atrial and ventricular complexes with a ventricular rate of 43. With exercise, the ventricular rate is 80.

    e. VSD with aortic regurgitation

    f. Ruptured sinus of Valsalva aneurysms (aorta to right heart chamber)

    g. Venous hum

    h. Coarctation of aorta

    i. Pulmonary artery branch stenoses

C. **CONGENITAL COMPLETE HEART BLOCK** (Fig. 12.12)

    1. May be familial.

    2. Heart rate of <50, pulse bounding, jugular venous cannon *a* waves, variable S1.

    3. Systolic (flow) murmur along LSB, often mistaken for VSD.

    4. High mortality in first year of life, usually stable course in first three to four decades.

D. **CORRECTED TRANSPOSITION OF GREAT ARTERIES** (Fig. 12.14)

    1. May have no associated lesions, but following are commonly found:

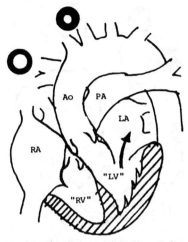

Figure 12.13.   Corrected Transposition of the Great Arteries. The congenital "correction" consists of inversion of the inflow tracts of the two ventricles, so that the trabecular RV, with its tricuspid valve, links with the LA and its pulmonary venous (oxygenated) blood, and the LV, with its bicuspid (mitral) valve, receives RA blood. Thus, the "RV" that pumps blood to the PA is morphologically an LV, and the Ao receives blood from an "LV" that has the architecture of an RV. Left AV valve incompetence is common (arrow). Corrected transposition may be associated with ventricular septal defect and subpulmonic stenosis (not shown), and if the subpulmonic stenosis is sufficiently severe, cyanosis may result.

    a. Heart block.
    b. Abnormal left AV valve (Ebstein's deformity, with left AV valve regurgitation).
    c. VSD with or without subpulmonic stenosis.
    d. Dextrocardia.

(Fig. 12.13)
Corrected transposition is almost invariably a levo transposition, in which the aorta is to the left of the pulmonary artery as a result of the embryonic bulboventricular loop bending to

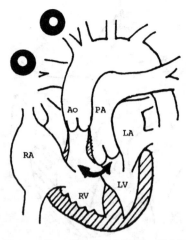

Figure 12.14. Transposition of the Great Arteries. This invariably cyanotic condition is illustrated here for comparison with corrected transposition. There is an obligatory desaturation of the Ao blood, because the RV receives systemic venous blood and is in continuity with the Ao. Survival depends on admixture, in this example, at ventricular level. Because the pulmonary vascular bed is not protected by outflow tract stenosis in this example, the pulmonary vascular resistance is elevated (thickened circle). The aorta is to the right of the pulmonary artery.

the left, instead of the normal rightward anterior loop. A leftward loop would be concordant with the rest of the body in situs inverses, in which dextrocardia would be "normal," but when it occurs in situs solitus (normal body position), there is often a discordant dextrocardia or dextroposition. Therefore, a levo transposition can be anticipated when the heart is in the right thorax, and corrected transposition can be suspected when there is dextrocardia with minimal disability.

COMMON CYANOTIC FORMS OF CONGENITAL HEART DISEASE PERMITTING ADULT SURVIVAL

Lesion   Clinical/Laboratory Findings

A. SEPTAL DEFECTS WITH DOWNSTREAM RESISTANCE
1. Tetralogy of Fallot
   (Fig. 12.15)

a. Nonrestrictive VSD
b. RV outflow obstruction
c. RV hypertrophy
d. "Overriding aorta"

1. Severity of outflow stenosis will determine degree of cyanosis.
2. History of cyanosis at birth, cyanotic spells, and squatting in childhood.
3. Exercise increases degree of cyanosis.
4. Cyanosis (rest or with exercise), clubbing, single S2, outflow stenosis murmur.
5. ECG: RVH or biventricular hypertrophy.
6. Radiograph: boot-shaped heart (small pulmonary artery, apex tipped up).
7. Hematocrit will reflect mean daily level of arterial desaturation unless patient is iron depleted.
8. Many adults with Tetralogy of Fallot have had palliative systemic pulmonary shunts created. If patent, a continuous murmur will be heard.
9. **Significance:** potentially correctable in most cases. Cardiac catheterization and consideration of surgery indicated in all suspected cases.

(Fig. 12.15)
2. Eisenmenger's Complex (Large VSD with Pulmonary Hypertension)

1. Development of pulmonary hypertension in childhood

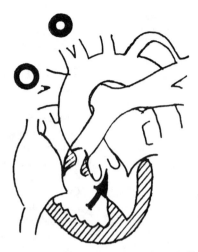

Figure 12.15. Tetralogy of Fallot (with Blalock-Taussig Shunt). There is a large nonrestrictive ventricular septal defect and obstruction to outflow of the RV at two levels: infundibular and valvar. The PA is underdeveloped and the RV is hypertrophic because it generates systemic pressure. There is a right-to-left shunt (arrow) directly from the RV into the Ao because the resistance to aortic outflow is less than through the stenotic RV outflow tract. A palliative left Blalock-Taussig shunt (subclavian-PA anastomoses), which increases the quantity of oxygenated blood entering the LV and therefore raises the Ao blood oxygenation, is shown. The normal pulmonary vascular resistance is indicated by the thin circle adjacent to the right pulmonary artery.

Note: If the right ventricular outflow tract or the main pulmonary artery is atretic (absent or completely interrupted), the pulmonary arteries derive their blood from bronchial collaterals. This severe form of tetralogy is often called a "type IV truncus arteriosus." In this situation, the only murmurs heard are the continuous murmurs from the systemic-pulmonary collaterals. Although the entire right ventricular outflow traverses the VSD into the aorta, this flow produces no murmur because it is a nonrestrictive defect.

diminishes L-R shunt, cyanosis increases as shunt reverses (R-L).

2. Dyspnea on exertion but no LV failure.
3. Hemoptysis.
4. Heart size small because of balanced shunt. Main PA dilated but peripheral vessels constricted.
5. On examination, RV and PA impulse, single or narrowly split S2, murmur of pulmonary regurgitation (no VSD murmur).
6. **Significance:** "fixed " high pulmonary vascular resistance precludes cardiac surgical correction, but with careful medical management (treatment of arrhythmias, phlebotomy for hematocrit higher than 60%, etc.) reasonable longevity is possible.

(Fig. 12.16)
3. Eisenmenger Reaction (ASD or PDA with Pulmonary Hypertension)
   a. ASD with reversed shunt

1. A late complication of large ASD, usually after fifth decade. The shunt reverses when RV fails and/or pulmonary vascular resistance increases.
2. Right heart and pulmonary arteries enlarged because f large intracardiac shunt three to four decades.

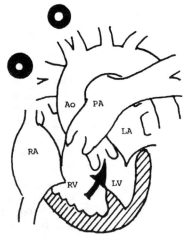

Figure 12.16. Eisenmenger's Complex. There is a large nonrestrictive VSD, and the pulmonary vascular bed is unprotected from the resulting systemic RV pressure. The shunt (arrow) is right to left because the pulmonary arteriolar resistance (thick circle) exceeds systemic vascular resistance. The pulmonary hypertension is irreversible and closure of the VSD would be fatal.

3. RV lift, widely split S2, murmur of tricuspid, and/or pulmonic regurgitation.
4. ECG: right bundle branch block (RBBB) or rsR′, atrial fibrillation common.
5. **Significance:** cardiac catheterization indicated to assess pulmonary vascular resistance. Surgical closure of ASD is possible if resistance is less than 5 units or decreases markedly with oxygen breathing.

(Fig. 12.17)
b. Patent ductus

1. Size of PDA is large and

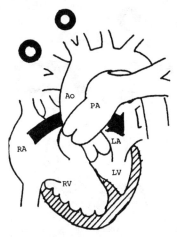

Figure 12.17. Atrial Septal Defect with Reversed Shunt. The Eisenmenger's reaction results from many years of exposure to high pulmonary blood flow that leads to dilated, hypertrophic, failing RV, which becomes less receptive to atrial inflow than the LV. The pulmonary vascular resistance (thickened circle) rarely exceeds systemic vascular resistance with ASD, and its effect on the shunt is indirect; the elevated pressure leads to RV hypertrophy and eventually a decreased ejection fraction. The resulting thickened RV with a large end-systolic volume resists diastolic filling.

pulmonary hypertension is usually established early in life.

2. Reversed flow through PDA is extracardiac, so heart is not enlarged.

3. On examination, feet are cyanotic and clubbed, fingers acyanotic. No murmur, or murmur of pulmonary regurgitation.

4. **Significance:** inoperable, but patients may do quite well with conservative management.

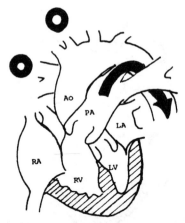

Figure 12.18. Patent Ductus with Shunt Reversal. There is a large nonrestrictive ductus, which results in equalization of pressures in the Ao and PA. When the pulmonary vascular resistance exceeds systemic resistance, there is shunt reversal, with desaturated blood entering the descending thoracic aorta (arrow) and causing cyanosis of the lower extremities (differential cyanosis).

(Fig. 12.18)

"Reversed differential cyanosis," or blue fingers and pink toes, can be seen when there is transposition of the great arteries (TGA) with a PDA and pulmonary hypertension.

A common misconception is that differential cyanosis and reversed differential cyanosis can result from a PDA in combination with a coarctation of the aorta. It should be noted that the aortic pressure downstream from a coarctation is at systemic level (mean pressure 70–90 mm Hg) so that it would be necessary to have pulmonary hypertension for right-to-left shunting through a PDA, with or without a coarctation.

4. Ebstein's Anomaly of the Tricuspid Valve

1. Abnormally placed and deformed tricuspid valve.
2. Hypoplastic right ventricle.
3. Frequently associated

with patent foramen ovale.

4. Degree of cyanosis dependent on degree of inadequacy of tricuspid valve (obstruction and/or regurgitation) and abnormal RV function.

5. Auscultation often reveals multiple heart sounds: split S1 ("sail sound" of late tricuspid closure), split S2 (RBBB), S3, and S4. Murmurs may be present in systole (tricuspid regurgitation), diastole, or presystole.

6. ECG: wide, bizarre RSR' complex in V1. Right atrial enlargement. Atrial fibrillation common.

7. Associated with Wolff-Parkinson-White syndrome.

8. Radiograph: enlarged heart, especially right atrium, with decreased pulmonary vascularity.

9. Echocardiography: diagnostic enlargement of anterior tricuspid leaflet, displaced septal leaflet, and delayed closure of anterior leaflet.

10. **Significance:** may present with arrhythmias in middle age.

(Fig. 12.19)

OPERATIVE INTERVENTIONS IN CONGENITAL HEART DISEASE

Operations for congenital heart defects can be divided into **palliative or definitive** categories. Although terms such as "total correc-

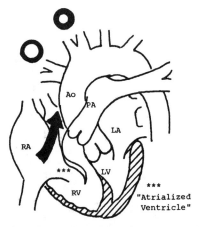

Figure 12.19. Ebstein's Anomaly. The tricuspid valve is deformed and the RV walls are hypoplastic. A patent foramen ovale permits right-to-left shunting (arrow) and causes variable cyanosis. The pulmonary arteriolar resistance is normal. The displaced tricuspid valve creates an "atrialized ventricular chamber" (***) that is upstream of the tricuspid valve but within the RV walls. The tricuspid valve is often incompetent.

tion'' and ''curative'' are used as synonyms for definitive procedures, these terms (with rare exceptions) reflect unwarranted optimism. Two procedures that can be truly curative (in that the heart can be completely normal afterward) are ligation with division of a small patent ductus and suture closure of an ASD in childhood. All other procedures entail certain compromises such as ventriculotomy construction of conduits or may leave residual functional abnormalities such as chamber enlargement, impaired contractility, conduction defect, outflow obstruction, valvar regurgitation, or persistent or new murmurs.

Palliative operations are usually associated with lower risk than definitive procedures and thus can be used as temporizing measures that permit survival of critically ill patients until a more definitive intervention can be undertaken. Most palliative procedures actually add new defects and therefore may increase the complexity of the later definitive repair. However, this theoretical disadvantage is counterbalanced by the improved functional status and maturity of the patient.

Tables 12.2 and 12.3 define palliative and definitive procedures and the clinical indications for their use.

Table 12.2
Palliative Procedures in Congenital Heart Disease

CHD type	Procedure	Purpose
Nonrestrictive VSD with normal great vessel orientation or transposition of the great vessels	Pulmonary artery banding	↓ excessive pulmonary blood to prevent pulmonary hypertension

Transposition of the great arteries	1. Creation of atrial septal
	  a. catheter balloon or blade septostomy (Rashkind)
	  b. Surgical excision of posterior interatrial septum (Blalock-Hanlon)
	2. Venous return inversion
	  a. right pulmonary vein-right atrial anastomosis (Baffes)
	Complete "atrial switch"
		Brings oxygenated blood in right atrium, right ventricle, and aorta
		↑ oxygenation of RA and aortic blood, improves mixing

TGA with VSD and pulmonary	Excision of atrial septum, baffle inserted to route pulmonary venous blood through tricuspid valve to RV, caval blood through mitral valve to LV (VSD not repaired) (palliative Mustard-Senning)	Brings oxygenated blood to RA and RV to improve aortic oxygen saturation
Tetralogy of Fallot Pulmonary atresia Tricuspid atresia	Subclavian-pulmonary artery anastomosis (end-to-side) (Blalock-Taussig)	↑ pulmonary blood flow and oxygenation of aortic blood
Tricuspid atresia	Right ventricular bypass a. superior vena cava to right pulmonary artery end-to-end anastomosis (Glenn) b. descending aorta-left pulmonary artery anastomosis (side-to-side) (Potts) c. Ascending aorta to right pulmonary artery (side-to-side) (Waterston-Cooley)	↑ pulmonary blood flow and oxygenation of aortic blood

The Potts and Waterston-Cooley procedures have theoretical advantages over the Blalock-Taussig shunt: greater flow, better systemic oxygenation, and avoidance of sacrificing the subclavian artery. In addition, the Blalock-Taussig anastomosis may become progressively restrictive as the patient grows, leading to decreasing flow, declining systemic oxygenation, and a rising hematocrit. However, the ease of ablating the subclavian-pulmonary anastomosis at the time of definitive repair compared to the technical complexicity of closing a Potts or Waterston-Cooley shunt has lead to a greater use of the original "blue baby operation."

Table 12.3
Definitive Operative Treatment of Complex Congenital Heart Disease

CHD type	Procedures
Tetralogy of Fallot Double outlet right ventricle (DORV) Transposition (when combined with Rastelli procedure—see below) Pulmonary atresia with ASD or VSD DORV or TGA (when combined with internal tunnel patch from left ventricle to aorta)	Intracardial repair: Closure of VSD by patch, enlargement of outflow tract by resection, or resection plus patch; with DORV or transposition, septal defect patch is fashioned to connect LV and aorta Extracardiac conduit from right ventricle to pulmonary artery, with or without valve (Rastelli)
TGA without pulmonary hypertension	"Atrial switch"—excision of atrial septum with creation of a baffle-septum that routes all of pulmonary venous return through the tricuspid valve to RV and caval blood through the mitral valve to LV. Clsoure of VSD and/or repair of pulmonic stenosis if present (Mustard/Senning) "Atrial switch"—aorta and pulmonary arteries are separated from their semilunar valves and translocated to alignment with appropriate ventricle, coronary arteries are anastomosed (usually via grafts) to the translocated aorta
Tricuspid atresia, single ventricle with pulmonic stenosis or atresia	Right atrium to pulmonary artery oversewing of tricuspid and/or pulmonic valve (Fontan)

Suggested Reading

Foster E. Congenital heart disease in adults. West J Med 1995;163:492.

Higgins CB, Silverman NH, Kesting-Sommerhoff BA, Schmidt KG. Congenital heart disease: echocardiography and magnetic resonance imaging. New York: Raven Press, 1990.

Kaplan S. Congenital heart disease after childhood: an expanding patient population-natural adult survival patterns. J Am Coll Cardiol 1991; 18:319.

McNamara DG. The adult with congenital heart disease. Curr Probl Cardiol 1989;14:63.

Perloff JK, Child JS. Congenital heart disease in adults. Philadelphia: WB Saunders, 1991.

Chapter 13

The Cardiomyopathies

DEFINITION AND CLASSIFICATION

The cardiomyopathies are defined as diseases of the myocardium associated with cardiac dysfunction. They have recently been classified into four groups: 1) dilated cardiomyopathy, 2) hypertrophic cardiomyopathy, 3) restrictive cardiomyopathy, and 4) arrhythmogenic right ventricular cardiomyopathy (1). Previously, the cardiomyopathies were defined as "heart muscle disease of unknown cause" and were differentiated from heart muscle disease of known cause. They are now classified by the dominant pathophysiology or, if possible, by etiological or pathogenetic factors.

DILATED CARDIOMYOPATHY

This group is characterized by poor myocardial systolic function. Left ventricular, and often right ventricular, contractility is diminished, leading to a decrease in cardiac output and increased end-systolic and end-diastolic ventricular volumes and pressures (2). Cardiomegaly, resulting more from dilatation than hypertrophy, is invariably present. There is evidence to suggest that reduced ability of the sarcoplasmic reticulum to accumulate calcium plays a major role in the altered excitation-contraction coupling in patients with dilated cardiomyopathy (3). The reported annual incidence of the idiopathic form in the United States is between 5 and 8 cases per 100,000 persons (2,4) and is the cause of congestive heart failure (CHF) in approximately 25% of all cases of CHF (5).

Etiologies include the following:

- idiopathic
- familial/genetic
- viral and/or immune

- alcoholic/toxic
- associated with a recognized cardiovascular disease (e.g., hypertension, ischemic heart disease)

Clinical Profile

Patients most commonly present with signs and symptoms of congestive heart failure, with symptoms of left-sided failure predominating (see Chapter 10). In addition, it is not uncommon for the patient to present with signs of a myocardial, cerebral, renal, or mesenteric infarction or a pulseless, blue extremity due to an embolus from a mural thrombus. Sudden death is frequent in patients with a dilated cardiomyopathy and is most commonly the result of ventricular arrhythmias or conduction system disease (2).

Murmurs are frequently heard during cardiac auscultation and are not themselves indicative of primary valvular disease. A holosystolic mitral or tricuspid regurgitation murmur is very common and is due to ventricular dilatation and resultant lateral displacement of the papillary muscles, which inhibits leaflet coaptation. Annular dilatation may also occur and serve as the major mechanism for functional mitral regurgitation. Occasionally, an apical "diastolic rumble" may also be heard and is due either to increased early diastolic atrioventricular flow, the result of mitral regurgitation, or a loud summation gallop.

The chest radiograph most commonly shows cardiomegaly and evidence of pulmonary venous and arterial hypertension.

The electrocardiogram is almost always abnormal. In addition to evidence of ventricular and atrial enlargement, Q or QS waves and poor R wave progression across the anterior precordial leads are frequently seen. Atrioventricular (AV) nodal and intraventricular conduction defects, particularly left bundle branch block, and arrhythmias, particularly atrial fibrillation and premature ventricular depolarizations, are common associated findings.

The characteristic echocardiographic findings (see Chapter 4) in a patient with a congestive cardiomyopathy reflect poor contractile function: decreased ejection fraction, decreased velocity of circumferential fiber shortening, increased end-systolic and end-diastolic volumes, chamber enlargement, and regurgitant murmurs.

Management

The goal of therapy is to alleviate the symptomatic manifestations of congestive heart failure (see Chapter 10). Additional interventions in the case of cardiomyopathy with known etiology will be dictated by the underlying disease, such as complete abstinence in the case of alcoholic cardiomyopathy. The true natural history of the disease is difficult to determine, because asymptomatic cardiomegaly may precede clinical manifestations for months to years. Recent data suggest that the 5-year mortality is approximately 20% (2). Death may result from progressive heart failure or from ventricular arrhythmias, which accompany left ventricular dysfunction (see Chapter 15, Sudden Cardiac Death). Dilated cardiomyopathy is currently the most common reason for cardiac transplantation. Novel therapies have been described and are currently under investigation (6).

HYPERTROPHIC CARDIOMYOPATHY

Hypertrophic cardiomyopathy (HCM) is characterized by an increased ventricular muscle mass without associated increase in cavity size and asymmetric hypertrophy of the septum (7). The disorder is most commonly familial (the majority have autosomal dominant transmission) and mutations in sarcomere contractile proteins have been demonstrated (8). This disorder has also been called hypertrophic obstructive cardiomyopathy (HOCM), idiopathic hypertrophic subaortic stenosis (IHSS), and muscular subaortic stenosis (MSS), to name a few.

Hemodynamically, hypertrophic cardiomyopathy is characterized by poor diastolic function of the left ventricle due to reduced compliance. The decrease in compliance is reflected in an increased left ventricular (LV) end-diastolic pressure and impedance to diastolic filling. Systolic function is maintained (normal cardiac output, ejection fraction and end-diastolic volume). A systolic pressure gradient between the body of the left ventricle and the outflow tract may be recorded in some patients at rest or after provocation (i.e., exercise, Valsalva maneuver, or isoproterenol infusion) (Fig. 13.1). Proposed explanations for this gradient include: (*a*) dynamic outflow obstruction by the hypertrophied septum, (*b*) outflow obstruction by the anterior leaflet of the mitral valve during systole, and (*c*) forceful, exaggerated LV contraction with late systolic isometric contraction. The

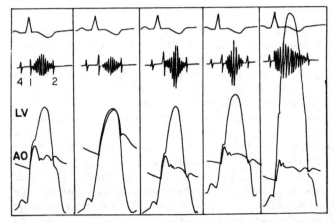

Figure 13.1. Pressure Gradients in HCM. Variable pressure gradients between the left ventricular cavity (LV) and the aorta (AO) may be recorded during cardiac catheterization of a patient with HCM. AO and LV pressure recordings and a phonocardiogram demonstrate characteristic hemodynamic and auscultatory findings in HCM. The LV-AO pressure gradient may be present at rest (control) as shown here, may appear spontaneously during the course of the hemodynamic study, or may manifest itself only after provocation. Interventions that decrease ventricular filling (Valsalva maneuver), lower arterial resistance (vasodilators such as amyl nitrate), or increase the force of ventricular contraction (isoproterenol or postectopic beat) may provoke the appearance of a gradient and systolic murmur not present at rest or enhance an existing LV-AO gradient and systolic murmur as shown here. Increasing the impedance to LV ejection using a vasopressor agent will decrease the magnitude of the gradient. Provocation of a pressure gradient in a patient without other evidence of HCM should not be considered diagnostic of HCM because such a gradient can be produced in normal hearts and in patients with other cardiac conditions.

variability of the gradient and the fact that the left ventricle ejects nearly its entire volume during the first half of systole suggests that true obstruction or impediment to outflow does not occur. The presence of symptoms and the higher apparent death rate in symptomatic patients without pressure gradients renders the significance of the pressure gradient unclear (9).

Clinical Profile

Dyspnea on exertion, chest pain that may be anginal in character, palpitations, and/or syncope are the major symptoms in patients with hypertrophic cardiomyopathy. A family history of sudden death or "heart failure" is not uncommon. This disease may present as sudden death, particularly in younger patients during or after exercise (8).

Physical examination reveals large dominant *a* waves in the jugular venous pulse and a jerky carotid pulse or "pulsus bisferiens." A sustained late systolic left ventricular impulse preceded by a presystolic thrust is noted on palpation of the precordium. A variable mid- to late-systolic murmur and a fourth heart sound may be heard at the apex and left sternal border. The intensity of the systolic murmur is increased by standing and during the strain phase of the Valsalva maneuver.

The chest radiograph is usually normal. Left ventricular and left atrial hypertrophy are frequently but not always noted on the electrocardiogram. Small Q waves in leads V4 through V6 and an R/S ratio in V1 greater than 0.2 are suggestive of hypertrophic cardiomyopathy. Less frequently, prominent Q waves in II, III, and aVF are seen and are presumed to result from hypertrophy of the upper septum.

On the echocardiogram, an increase in the thickness of the interventricular septum with a lesser increase in the thickness of the LV posterior basal wall is seen (septum to posterior wall thickness ratio of greater than 1.3—a reflection of asymmetric septal hypertrophy [ASH]). Additional echocardiographic features include decreased systolic thickening of the septum, systolic anterior motion (SAM) of the anterior leaflet of the mitral valve, decreased E-to-F slope of the mitral valve, a normal or reduced LV end-diastolic dimension, and midsystolic closure of the aortic valve (see Chapter 4). It should be noted that asymmetric septal hypertrophy on the echocardiogram is not pathognomonic of hypertrophic cardiomyopathy and has been observed in a number of other conditions: systemic arterial hypertension with valvular aortic stenosis, in healthy athletes, after insertion of prosthetic aortic valves, after inferior myocardial infarction, and in hypothyroid heart disease.

Management

The clinical course of patients with hypertrophic cardiomyopathy is variable and not clearly related to the measured systolic pressure gradient. Recent data indicate 1- and 5-year survival rates of 95% and 92%, respectively (10). β-adrenergic blockade remains the mainstay of therapy and is most useful in alleviating the chest pain associated with this disease. The primary rationale for β-blockade therapy is based on the premise that prevention of exercise tachycardia aids in ventricular filling and reduces the oxygen demands of the ventricle. Additional benefits are the antiarrhythmic effects of β blockers and the possible blocking of the "hypertrophying" influence of circulating catecholamines. Calcium-blocking agents (i.e., verapamil) have also been used in selected patients and have been found to alleviate symptoms. The rationale for their use is based on their demonstrated effects on myocardial contractility (a decrease in contractility improves the O_2 supply:demand ratio). However, verapamil may cause serious hemodynamic complications and should be used cautiously. Myectomy for symptomatic patients' nonresponse to medical therapy has been performed for more than three decades and may provide symptomatic benefit. However, there are limited data available to suggest that either medical or surgical therapy alters the course of the disease or the incidence of sudden death (8). Dual-chamber pacing has also been shown to be beneficial in symptomatic patients who have not responded to medical therapy (11). The mechanism by which pacing alleviates symptoms is unknown.

RESTRICTIVE CARDIOMYOPATHY

This group is characterized by restricted filling and reduced diastolic volume of either or both ventricles with normal or nearly normal systolic function and wall thickness. Interstitial fibrosis may be present. There is usually only a modest increase in ventricular cavity size (12). The major hemodynamic fault is a decrease in ventricular compliance, which produces a distinctive early diastolic "dip and plateau" configuration of right and left ventricular pressures. However, the left ventricular end-diastolic pressure characteristically is higher than right ventricular end-diastolic pressure and serves to distinguish a restrictive cardiomyopathy from constrictive pericarditis, which may mimic it (see Chapter 14). Ventricular end-diastolic volume is usually normal or decreased. Cardiac output may be normal or decreased, depending on the extent of replacement of contractile myocardium and the limitation to ventricular filling.

A restrictive cardiomyopathy may be present in the absence of demonstrable systemic disease or cause (idiopathic) or it may occur in association with other diseases, e.g., amyloidosis, endomyocardial disease with or without eosinophilia.

Clinical Profile

Patients may present with signs and symptoms of congestive heart failure, which is of diastolic origin (see Chapter 10).

Physical findings may mimic those of constrictive pericarditis in that a rapid "y" descent of the jugular venous pulse, Kussmaul's sign, and pulsus paradoxus can be noted in patients with restrictive cardiomyopathies. Cardiac auscultation usually reveals a third and fourth heart sound and murmurs of mitral and tricuspid regurgitation may be heard. Chest radiograph usually shows a normal or slightly enlarged cardiac silhouette. The electrocardiogram may be normal. Intraventricular conduction delay and arrhythmias (ventricular and supraventricular) are not uncommon. Echocardiography may demonstrate symmetric wall thickening with variable degrees of chamber enlargement. Diffuse hypokinesis may also be noted.

Management

The natural history of the idiopathic form is variable (12). Initial management should be undertaken to alleviate the symptoms of congestive heart failure.

ARRHYTHMOGENIC RIGHT VENTRICULAR CARDIOMYOPATHY

This cardiomyopathy is characterized by progressive fibro-fatty replacement of the right ventricular myocardium. The disease begins as a focal regional process followed by global right ventricular involvement. The septum and left heart are typically spared. It is most commonly of familial origin with autosomal dominant inheritance and incomplete penetrance (13,14). The typical presentation is sudden death in a young individual (15).

SPECIFIC CARDIOMYOPATHIES

This term is now used to describe heart muscle disease that is associated with specific cardiac or systemic disorders. They may present with the characteristic features of a dilated or restrictive cardiomyopathy or have features of both. Included within this group are the following:

- ischemic cardiomyopathy (16)
- valvular cardiomyopathy
- hypertensive cardiomyopathy
- inflammatory cardiomyopathy: usually defined as myocarditis associated with cardiac dysfunction. Myocarditis is diagnosed histologically by established methods. Idiopathic, autoimmune, and infectious forms have been described. An infectious etiology is common and pathogens include human immunodeficiency virus (HIV), enterovirus, adenovirus, cytomegalovirus (CMV) (17)
- metabolic cardiomyopathy: included in this group are the cardiomyopathies associated with hyperthyroidism and acromegaly, familial storage diseases and infiltrations (e.g., hemochromatosis, glycogen storage disease, Hurler's syndrome), nutritional disorders (e.g., beriberi), and amyloidosis (primary, secondary, senile, or hereditary) (18,19)
- general systemic disease: includes primarily those disorders broadly classified as connective tissue or collagen-vascular disorders, e.g., systemic lupus erythematosus (SLE), scleroderma, polyarteritis nodosa. Infiltrative and granulomatous disease would also fall into this category (e.g., sarcoidosis, leukemia, lymphoma) (20,21)
- muscular dystrophies and neuromuscular disorders
- sensitivity and toxic reactions: alcohol, anthracyclines, cocaine (22,23)
- peripartum cardiomyopathy

References

1. Report of the 1995 World Health Organization/International Society and Federation of Cardiology Task Force on the Definition and Classification of Cardiomyopathies. Circulation 1996;93:841.
2. Dec GW, Fuster V. Idiopathic dilated cardiomyopathy. N Engl J Med 1994;331:1564.
3. Meyer M, Schillinger W, Pieske B, et al. Alterations of sarcoplasmic reticulum proteins in failing human dilated cardiomyopathy. Circulation 1995;92:778.
4. Manolio TA, Baughman KL, Rodeheffer R, et al. Prevalence and etiology of idiopathic dilated cardiomyopathy (Summary of a National Heart, Lung, and Blood Institute Workshop). Am J Cardiol 1992;69:1458.

5. Brown CA, O'Connell JB. Myocarditis and idiopathic dilated cardiomyopathy. Am J Med 1995;99:309.

6. Fazio S, Sabatini D, Capaldo B, et al. A preliminary study of growth hormone in the treatment of dilated cardiomyopathy. N Engl J Med 1996;334:809.

7. Wigle ED, Rakowski H, Kimball BP, et al. Hypertrophic cardiomyopathy. Clinical spectrum and treatment. Circulation 1995;92:1680.

8. Seidman CE, McKenna WJ, Watkins HC, et al. Molecular genetic approaches to diagnosis and management of hypertrophic cardiomyopathy. In: Braunwald E, ed. Heart disease. A textbook of cardiovascular medicine. New York: WB Saunders, 1992:77–83.

9. Criley JM, Siegel RJ. Subaortic stenosis revisited: the importance of the dynamic pressure gradient. Medicine 1993;72:412.

10. Cannan CR, Reeder GS, Bailey KR, et al. Natural history of hypertrophic cardiomyopathy. A population-based study, 1976 through 1990. Circulation 1995;92:2488.

11. Nishimura RA, Symanski JD, Hurrell DG, et al. Dual-chamber pacing for cardiomyopathies: a 1996 clinical perspective. Mayo Clin Proc 1996;71:1077.

12. Kushwaha SS, Fallon JT, Fuster V. Restrictive cardiomyopathy. N Engl J Med 1997;336:267.

13. McKenna WJ, Thiene G, Nava A, et al. Diagnosis of arrhythmogenic right ventricular dysplasia/cardiomyopathy. Br Heart J 1994;71:215.

14. Marcus FI, Fontaine G. Arrhythmogenic right ventricular dysplasia/cardiomyopathy. A review. PACE 1995;18:1298.

15. Thiene G, Nava A, Corrado D, et al. Right ventricular cardiomyopathy and sudden death in young people. N Engl J Med 1988;318:129.

16. Cheng TO. Congestive heart failure in coronary artery disease. Am J Med 1991;91:409.

17. Pisani B, Taylor DO, Mason JW. Inflammatory myocardial diseases and cardiomyopathies. Am J Med 1997;102:459.

18. Adams PC, Kertesz AE, Valberg LS. Clinical presentation of hemochromatosis: a changing scene. Am J Med 1991;90:445.

19. Cohen AS. Amyloidosis. In: Isselbacher KJ, Braunwald E, Wilson JD, et al., eds. Harrison's Principles of Internal Medicine. 13th ed. San Francisco: McGraw-Hill, 1994:1625–1630.

20. Sturfelt G, Eskilsson J, Nived O, et al. Cardiovascular disease in systemic lupus erythematosus. A study of 75 patients from a defined population. Medicine 1992;71:216.

21. Newman LS, Rose CS, Maier LA. Sarcoidosis. N Engl J Med 1997;336:1224.

22. McCall D. Alcohol and the cardiovascular system. Curr Probl Cardiol 1987;12:353.

23. Mouhaffel AH, Madu EC, Satmary WA, et al. Cardiovascular complications of cocaine. Chest 1995;107:1426.

Chapter 14

Pericardial Heart Disease

The pericardium consists of a serous or loose fibrous membrane (visceral pericardium), beneath which lies the myocardium, and a dense collagenous sac (parietal pericardium), which surrounds the heart. Under normal conditions, up to 50 mL of fluid may be present in the space between the visceral and parietal pericardium. The pericardium supports the heart and limits its movement within the mediastinum, serves as a barrier to the spread of infection from the lungs and pleural, (should sudden cardiac dilatation occur), and may modify the ventricular pressure–volume (compliance) relationship as preload is increased (1,2).

Because its layers are serosal surfaces (lined with mesothelial cells) and because of its proximity and attachments to other structures (pleura, diaphragm, sternum, and myocardium), the pericardium may be involved in a number of systemic or localized disease processes. The clinical presentations of pericardial disease are variable and are dependent not only on the response of the pericardium to an injury (exudation of fluid, fibrin, or inflammatory cells, granuloma formation, fibrous proliferation, or calcification) but also on how the response affects cardiac function.

The following discussion highlights the clinical presentation and evaluation of acute pericarditis, cardiac tamponade, and constrictive pericarditis.

ACUTE PERICARDITIS

Symptoms and Signs

Most patients with acute pericarditis will complain of retrosternal or precordial chest pain. The pain is most often, but not always, "pleuritic" in character (worsened with deep inspiration, movement, or lying down) and relieved by sitting up, leaning forward, and by taking shallow inspirations. Because the pain may be aggravated by inspiration, the patient may complain of shortness of breath. Additional symptoms most often will be determined by the underlying etiology.

A pericardial friction rub is the most common and important physical finding in pericarditis. It is most often triphasic in character, consisting of a systolic component during ventricular systole, an early diastolic component occurring during the early phase of ventricular filling, and a presystolic component synchronous with atrial systole. The friction rub is less commonly biphasic—a systolic component with either an early diastolic or presystolic component.

A single component or monophasic rub is rare (<20% of cases) and is usually systolic. The friction rub is best heard at the cardiac apex with the patient sitting up or in the hands-and-knees position. It may be transient and its presence does not preclude the presence of a large pericardial effusion.

Chest Radiograph

A routine chest radiograph may be of value in acute pericarditis but not necessarily in diagnosis, because heart size may be normal with a small pericardial effusion. The presence of a pericardial friction rub in association with pleuropulmonary or mediastinal abnormalities may assist in establishing an etiology, e.g., neoplastic or infectious.

Electrocardiogram

The electrocardiogram may be diagnostic, especially if followed over time (3). In the acute phase (stage 1), the ST segment vector is directed anteriorly, inferiorly and leftward, causing ST segment elevation (reflecting subepicardial injury) in the precordial leads, especially in V5 and V6 and in leads I and II (see Fig. 1.4). ST segment elevation in V6 is usually greater than 25% of the T-wave amplitude (4). An isoelectric or depressed ST segment is commonly seen in V1. PR segment depression may be noted in leads II, aVF, and V4–V6. In stage 2, the ST segment begins, returning to the isoelectric line, and T-wave amplitude decreases. T-wave inversion in those leads previously showing ST segment elevation is noted during stage 3. At this time, the ST segment is isoelectric. Stage 4 is characterized by resolution of the electrocardiographic abnormalities. Additional electrocardiogram (ECG) abnormalities may be noted during pericarditis and include atrial arrhythmias (usually insignificant) and, if a large effusion is present, low-voltage QRS complexes and electrical alternans. The latter phenomena are due to the "insulating" effect of the pericardial fluid and the pendulum motion of the heart within the pericardium at a frequency one-half of the heart rate.

Etiology

Common causes of pericarditis/pericardial effusion include the following:

- **Idiopathic.** Commonly preceded by a febrile illness or "viral syndrome." In most cases, the etiology is not established.
- **Infections.**

  Viral—Coxsackie virus (especially group B), echovirus, adenovirus, mumps virus, influenza virus, and Ebstein-Barr virus. Human immunodeficiency virus (HIV) is becoming an increasingly recognized cause of pericarditis (5). Viral pericarditis is frequently associated with a myocarditis and cardiac enzyme elevation; in this instance, the term "myopericarditis" is used.

  Bacterial—usually the result of spread from a contiguous myocardial abscess or pleuropulmonary focus (pneumonia or empyema) or after thoracic surgery or trauma. *Staphylococcus aureus* and *Streptococcus pneumoniae* are the most common organisms (6,7). Infection is often polymicrobial and anaerobic organisms more common if the focus of origin is a mediastinitis secondary to an orofacial or dental infection. Mycobacteria should be considered in populations at risk. Pericarditis may occur during acute rheumatic fever.

  Other infectious agents—mycoplasma, histoplasma, coccidioidomycosis, nocardia, actinomycosis, Q fever, Lyme disease.
- **Connective tissue disease.** Scleroderma, systemic lupus, mixed connective tissue disease, rheumatoid arthritis, polymyositis/dermatomyositis (8).
- **Malignancy.** Most commonly metastatic from breast or lung. However, lymphoma, leukemia, and melanoma have a high incidence of metastasis to the pericardium. Adenocarcinoma

of unknown origin may also present as pericarditis or cardiac tamponade (9).

- **Uremia.** Usually treatable by dialysis or more frequent dialysis in those already on dialysis.
- **Drug-induced.** "Lupus syndrome" due to procainamide, hydralazine, isoniazid, or diphenylhydantoin. The anthracycline antineoplastic agents, such as doxorubicin, may cause pericarditis in addition to the more common myocardial toxicity.
- **Postmyocardial (Q wave) infarction (Dressler's syndrome)** (10).
- **Postpericardiotomy.** Incidence as high as 30% within 2–4 weeks after open heart surgery, often associated with pulmonary infiltrate and/or pleural effusion. Probably of immunologic origin and different than the acute pericarditis that may occur within the first week after a transmural (Q wave) myocardial infarction.
- **Mediastinal radiation therapy.**
- **Myxedema.**
- **Sarcoidosis.**

LABORATORY ASSESSMENT

In addition to careful history and physical examination, the following laboratory studies may be of value in establishing an etiologic diagnosis (11).

- Complete blood count (CBC) and differential: May suggest infection or leukemia.
- Erythrocyte sedimentation rate (ESR): usually elevated but not specific for pericarditis or its etiology. May be useful in following course and assessing response to therapy if pericarditis is due to an inflammatory process (infection, autoimmune disorder).
- Blood urea nitrogen (BUN) and creatinine.
- Blood cultures
- Serology: acute and convalescent phase viral titers, antinuclear antibody (ANA), double-stranded (DNA), RA latex, HIV, toxoplasma and mycoplasma titers.
- Tuberculosis (TB) skin test and sputum for acid-fast staining and TB culture
- Electrocardiogram.
- Chest radiograph.
- Echocardiography: to confirm the presence of pericardial fluid,

to rule out a contiguous cardiac process (endocarditis, myocardial abscess), and to assess for cardiac compromise (12).
- Pericardiocentesis: indicated in suspected cardiac tamponade and occasionally indicated as a diagnostic procedure, especially if infection or malignancy is suspected.

Noninvasive evaluation of patients with pericarditis will yield a specific etiology in only approximately 15% of cases (11,13). Pericardiocentesis findings increase the likelihood of a specific diagnosis by approximately another 10%. If pericarditis and pericardial effusion are recurrent and life-threatening, pericardioscopy and pericardial biopsy may be useful (14).

Therapy

Therapy is most appropriately directed at the underlying etiology if a treatable cause can be defined. Chest pain may be alleviated with the use of salicylates or nonsteroidal anti-inflammatory drugs. Corticosteroid therapy for several days may be necessary to treat severe pain. Patients with viral myopericarditis should be placed on bed rest and frequently assessed for signs and symptoms of declining left ventricular function. Echocardiography may be helpful in differentiating depressed myocardial contractility from cardiac tamponade or constriction. Corticosteroids have been instilled directly into the pericardial space to treat uremic pericarditis. Instillation of antineoplastic agents or sclerosing agents into the pericardial space has been used in malignant causes of pericarditis.

It is not unusual for the patient to have one or more relapses of acute symptoms weeks or months after apparent resolution. If these episodes continue to recur, a trial of corticosteroid therapy may be more effective than other anti-inflammatory drugs. Colchicine has been shown to be an effective agent in small, uncontrolled clinical trials (15). Rarely, pericardiectomy is indicated to relieve recurrent symptoms or as prophylaxis against constrictive pericarditis.

CARDIAC TAMPONADE

Intrapericardial pressure is normally subatmospheric. An increase in the quantity of intrapericardial fluid, whatever the cause, results in a rise in the intrapericardial pressure. The initial portion of the pericardial pressure–volume curve is relatively flat, i.e., relatively large increases in intrapericardial volume produce small changes in intrapericardial pressure. The curve becomes steeper as the fibrous and relatively inelastic parietal pericardium is "stretched." Eventually, continued fluid accumulation will raise the intrapericardial pressure to a level that exceeds the normal filling pressure of the ventricles (16). When this occurs, ventricular filling is restricted and cardiac tamponade is present. The slope of the pressure-volume curve of the pericardial sac and the point at which cardiac tamponade occurs is dependent on the following:

- **The rate of fluid accumulation.** With slow accumulation, large volumes of fluid can be more readily accommodated due to gradual stretching of the pericardium.
- **Pericardial compliance.** A previously diseased and thickened pericardium is likely to be less distensible.
- **Intravascular volume.** Tamponade will inhibit cardiac output to a greater extent during hypovolemia.

The pathophysiology of cardiac tamponade is complex but explains a number of physical and hemodynamic findings. Pulsus paradoxus is one of the most consistent and important clinical features of cardiac tamponade. An understanding of its genesis may be of help in understanding the physiology of tamponade.

Pulsus Paradoxus

As originally described in constrictive pericarditis, a paradoxical arterial pulse is said to be present when the cardiac rhythm is regular and there are apparent "dropped beats" in the peripheral pulse during inspiration. Manometrically, pulsus paradoxus is present when there is a greater than 10 mm Hg decrease in systolic blood pressure during inspiration in the supine position. A few mm Hg of inspiratory decrease in arterial pressure is normal.

Pulsus paradoxus results from the inspiratory decrease in left ventricular filling, caused by the dominance of augmented right heart filling (during inspiration) in the confined intrapericardial space. Inspiration creates a negative intrathoracic pressure that causes the left heart filling pressure to fall. As the pulmonary vasculature becomes more compliant and the left atrium and its

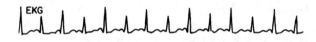

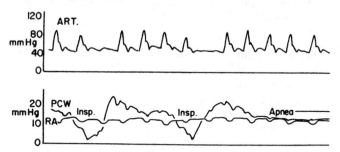

Figure 14.1. Pulsus Paradoxus. From the description of the mechanism of pulsus paradoxus, it should be apparent that ventricular filling in tamponade (and constrictive pericarditis) is dependent upon systemic venous pressure (18).

tributaries are subjected to a negative pressure, the overfilled extrathoracic systemic venous reservoir provides a more constant pressure head for right heart filling. Therefore, the right heart dominates the limited intrapericardial cardiovascular space during inspiration and this augmented filling is translated into increased right heart output, which in turn causes a rise in left heart filling pressure as inspiration ends and expiration begins (16).

Figure 14.1 demonstrates the phasic swings in left heart filling pressure (pulmonary capillary wedge [PCW]) and the relatively constant right atrial pressure (RA), resulting in inspiratory inhibition of left heart filling and marked decrease in arterial pulse amplitude—the paradoxical pulse. During apnea, there is an equilibration of atrial pressures, with "equal sharing" of the limited intrapericardial space and a steady arterial pressure.

Pulsus paradoxus is not diagnostic of cardiac tamponade and it may be noted in the following:

- constrictive pericarditis
- restrictive cardiomyopathy

- shock
- pulmonary embolism
- asthma or severe obstructive airway disease
- tension pneumothorax.

Pulsus paradoxus may be absent in tamponade in the following settings (16):

- hypovolemia
- chronic left ventricular dysfunction manifest by elevated left ventricular diastolic pressure
- atrial septal defect
- pulmonary arterial obstruction
- severe aortic regurgitation

Etiology

The most common causes of nontraumatic cardiac tamponade and their approximate frequency are as follows (2):

- malignant disease—55%
- idiopathic pericarditis—15%
- uremia—15%
- bacterial or mycobacterial infection—5%
- anticoagulant therapy—5%
- connective tissue disease—5%

Signs and Symptoms

The symptoms associated with cardiac tamponade are nonspecific. The patient will most commonly complain of intolerance to minimal activity and dyspnea. Congestive failure might well be diagnosed and inappropriate and potentially dangerous therapy (diuresis) instituted if a careful history and attention to salient physical findings are ignored (17).

Physical Examination

Physical examination commonly reveals a decreased systolic blood pressure with a narrow pulse pressure and pulsus paradoxus. The absence of pulsus paradoxus >15 mm Hg suggests that a pericardial effusion is not hemodynamically significant. A value >25 mm Hg usually separates true tamponade from lesser degrees of cardiac filling impairment (18,19). Exceptions when an abnormal pulsus may not be present in the setting of tamponade are noted above. The neck veins are distended, and examination of jugular venous pulsations reveals a rapid "x" descent and attenuated or absent "y" descent. Tachycardia, a compensatory mechanism to maintain cardiac output, is usually present. The apical impulse is indistinct and the lateral border of cardiac dullness is displaced laterally. Cardiac auscultation commonly demonstrates "distant" heart sounds. Pulmonary rales are uncommon, but a pleural effusion may be present. There may be right upper quadrant tenderness caused by hepatic engorgement.

Chest Radiograph

Chest radiograph may or may not demonstrate enlargement of the cardiac shadow, depending on the volume of intrapericardial fluid. The rapid accumulation of a relatively small amount of pericardial fluid may produce tamponade with minimal enlargement of the cardiac silhouette. On the lateral chest radiograph, an epicardial fat pad line may be seen within the cardiac silhouette. The pulmonary vasculature usually appears normal. Additional chest x-ray findings will depend on the etiology, such as mediastinal adenopathy, a lung mass, infiltrate, etc.

Electrocardiogram

The electrocardiogram may demonstrate low voltage QRS complexes, ST segment elevation, and PR segment depression characteristic of pericarditis or electrical alternans (beat-to-beat variation in P-, R-, and T-wave amplitudes). Alternans is seen in only 10–20% of cases of tamponade, and 50–60% of these cases are neoplastic in origin.

Echocardiography

In addition to pericardial fluid, the following echocardiographic and Doppler echo findings have been described in cardiac tamponade (11,20):

- right atrial compression
- right ventricular diastolic collapse
- abnormal variations in ventricular dimension during respiration

- abnormal variation in atrioventricular (AV) valve flow velocities with respiration
- distended inferior vena cava without inspiratory collapse
- "swinging" heart

Cardiac Catheterization

If cardiac catheterization is performed, equalization of right atrial, right ventricular, pulmonary artery diastolic, pulmonary capillary wedge or left atrial, and left ventricular end-diastolic pressures will be recorded during suspended respiration (Fig. 14.1). The intracardiac diastolic pressure will approximate intrapericardial pressure. A "dip and plateau" configuration of ventricular pressure, characteristic of constrictive pericarditis and restrictive cardiomyopathy, is not seen.

Treatment

Volume expansion with normal saline will usually increase cardiac output and blood pressure but is, at best, only a temporary measure. Pericardiocentesis may dramatically improve the hemodynamic status of the compromised patient.

Pericardiocentesis is a lifesaving procedure for patients with tamponade, but the procedure is potentially hazardous and should be performed with considerable care and under optimal circumstances. The potential hazards of cardiac perforation and coronary artery laceration can be minimized, and the therapeutic and diagnostic yield can be enhanced by appropriate planning and attention to detail (21).

Whenever possible, pressure from a pulmonary artery or right atrial catheter should be monitored before, during, and after pericardiocentesis. The presence of tamponade may be confirmed by a prompt decrease in central venous pressure attendant with pericardial fluid aspiration and the recurrence of tamponade can be detected by an elevation of right heart pressures toward pre-pericardiocentesis levels.

Pericardiocentesis should be performed in the cardiac catheterization laboratory whenever circumstances permit. The availability of fluoroscopy, a defibrillator, adequate laboratory facilities (e.g., hematocrit centrifuge), and the ease of ECG and pressure monitoring and recording in such a setting enhance the safety and diagnostic yield. Pericardiocentesis is best performed with the aid of two-dimensional echocardiography to help guide the needle away from vital structures but can be done without imaging if echocardiography is not readily available and severe hemodynamic compromise is present.

The subxiphoid approach with the patient sitting at a 45° angle is the preferred technique. A 16- to 18-gauge spinal needle is inserted between the xiphoid process and the left costal margin at a 30–45° angle to the skin. Alternatively, a cathether over a needle (Seldinger technique) can be used and a pigtail catheter can be inserted and left in place for repeated aspiration if reaccumulation of fluid is expected. The needle is directed toward the left shoulder. The V-lead of an ECG monitor electrode can be attached to the needle to detect epicardial contact (ST segment elevation on the V lead recording) and prevent ventricular puncture. As much fluid as possible should be aspirated with samples sent for appropriate studies.

As noted above, if there is tamponade, monitoring of right heart pressures will confirm the diagnosis since withdrawal of fluid will cause a prompt falling filling pressure. If there is no fall in venous pressure despite fluid removal, the diagnosis of tamponade is in doubt.

CONSTRICTIVE PERICARDITIS

Constrictive pericarditis is clinically and pathologically distinct from acute pericarditis. After pericardial injury, a chronic reparative process characterized by fibrous thickening of the layers of the pericardium may occur. When this process advances to the point at which diastolic filling of the normally distensible cardiac chambers is prevented by a nondistensible, thickened pericardium, "constriction" is said to be present.

Etiology

By its nature, constrictive pericarditis is most commonly a chronic process and the result of a remote and/or occult episode of acute pericarditis or pericardial injury. Common causes include the following:

- previous open heart surgery
- idiopathic
- mediastinal radiation

- bacterial or tuberculous pericarditis
- renal failure

In nearly 50% of cases, a specific etiology is never determined and such cases are usually ascribed to a previous, clinically inapparent viral pericarditis (22,23).

Signs and Symptoms

The patient with constrictive pericarditis most commonly presents with symptoms that mimic congestive heart failure; edema and ascites are often more pronounced than orthopnea and dyspnea. Careful physical examination may provide the initial clues to the presence of constrictive pericarditis. Pulsus paradoxus may or may not be present. Although the neck veins are distended, the lungs are clear, the heart is not enlarged, and the precordium is not overactive. Examination of the jugular venous pulsations reveals a rapid "y" descent. **Kussmaul's sign,** inspiratory increase in venous pressure, may be noted. On cardiac auscultation, an early diastolic sound, a pericardial knock 60 to 120 msec after the second heart sound may be heard. A pericardial knock occurs later than an opening snap and slightly earlier than an S3 that it may mimic. Hepatosplenomegaly may be present along with ascites.

Chest Radiograph

The chest radiograph most commonly shows a normal or slightly enlarged cardiac silhouette and clear lung fields with normal pulmonary vasculature. Pericardial calcification may be seen in approximately 50% of patients with constrictive pericarditis and is best seen on a lateral chest radiograph.

Electrocardiogram

The electrocardiogram shows no diagnostic features.

Echocardiography

Echocardiography and chest computed tomography occasionally demonstrate pericardial thickening. Echocardiographic septal motion may be abnormal and the left ventricular wall shows

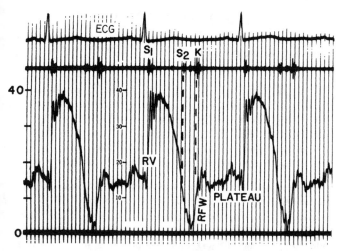

Figure 14.2. Constrictive Pericarditis. The characteristic diastole "dip and plateau" or "square wave" configuration of right ventricular (RV) pressure in constrictive pericarditis is demonstrated. A similar configuration was noted in the left ventricle. At the onset of diastole, inflow into the ventricles from the distended atria is rapid, producing an abrupt increase in intraventricular pressure corresponding to the rapid filling wave (RFW) shown in the figure. Later diastolic inflow is inhibited as the expanding ventricles encounter non-compliant pericardium. Early equalization of atrial and ventricular pressures and the near cessation of diastolic inflow result in a high-pressure plateau of equal magnitude in all cardiac chambers. A simultaneous phonocardiogram demonstrates the presence of a diastolic knock (K) occurring approximately 0.12 sec after the second heart sound (S2). This sound is heard during the rapid-filling phase of diastole as ventricular filling is suddenly inhibited by the constricting pericardium (time lines = 0.04 sec).

abrupt cessation of outward motion during early diastole. the pattern of transmitral flow variation observed with Doppler echo is comparable to that observed in cardiac tamponade. However, a prominent Y descent is often observed on hepatic vein or superior vena cava Doppler study (20,24).

CT and MRI

Both computed tomography (CT) imaging and magnetic resonance imaging (MRI) of the heart have been shown to be of diagnostic value in suspected constrictive pericarditis (25).

Cardiac Catheterization

Cardiac catheterization and hemodynamic assessment is the most important diagnostic study. Typical hemodynamic features include the following:

1. Rapid "x" and "y" descent in the right atrial pressure trace.
2. Early diastolic pressure "dip and plateau" configuration in the right ventricle (Fig. 14.2).
3. Equalization of increased diastolic pressures in the right atrium, right ventricle, LV, and pulmonary artery.
4. Elevated right ventricular and pulmonary arterial pressures.

These hemodynamic findings are by no means diagnostic of constrictive pericarditis. Similar pressures may be noted in patients with restrictive cardiomyopathy. Left heart catheterization may serve to differentiate between the two (see Chapter 13). In addition, characteristic Doppler echocardiographic abnormalities may serve to differentiate between the two (20,26).

Therapy

Surgical pericardial stripping is generally effective in symptomatic individuals.

References

1. Spodick DH. The normal and diseased pericardium: current concepts of pericardial physiology, diagnosis, and treatment. J Am Coll Cardiol 1983;1:240.
2. Lorell BH, Braunwald E. Pericardial disease. In: Braunwald E, ed. Heart disease. A textbook of cardiovascular medicine. 4th ed. Philadelphia: WB Saunders, 1992:45.
3. Spodick DH. Electrocardiogram in acute pericarditis. Distributions of morphologic and axial changes by stages. Am J Cardiol 1974;33: 470.
4. Ginzton LE, Laks MM. The differential diagnosis of acute pericarditis from the normal variant: New electrocardiographic criteria. Circulation 1982;65:1004.
5. Michaels AD, Lederman RJ, MacGregor JS, et al. Cardiovascular involvement in AIDS. Curr Probl Cardiol 1997;22:109.
6. Sagrista-Sauleda J, Barrabes JA, Permanyer-Miralda G, et al. Purulent pericarditis: review of a 20-year experience in a general hospital. J Am Coll Cardiol 1993;22:1661.
7. Brook I, Frazier EH. Microbiology of acute purulent pericarditis. A

12-year experience in a military hospital. Arch Intern Med 1996;156: 1857.

8. Langley RL, Treadwell EL. Cardiac tamponade and pericardial disorders in connective tissue diseases: case report and literature review. J Natl Med Assoc 1994;86:149.

9. Wilkes JD, Fidias P, Vaickus L, et al. Malignancy-related pericardial effusion. 127 cases from the Roswell Park Cancer Institute. Cancer 1995;76:1377.

10. Oliva PB, Hammill SC, Talano JV. Effect of definition on incidence of postinfarction pericarditis. Is it time to redefine postinfarction pericarditis? Circulation 1994;90:1537.

11. Permanyer-Miralda G, Sagrista-Sauleda J, Soler-Soler J. Primary acute pericardial disease: a prospective series of 231 consecutive patients. Am J Cardiol 1985;56:623.

12. Chandraratna PA. Echocardiography and Doppler ultrasound in the evaluation of pericardial disease. Circulation 1991;84(Suppl I):I–303.

13. Zayas R, Anguita M, Torres F, et al. Incidence of specific etiology and role of methods for specific etiologic diagnosis of primary acute pericarditis. Am J Cardiol 1995;75:378.

14. Nugue O, Millaire A, Porte H, et al. Pericardioscopy in the etiologic diagnosis of pericardial effusion in 141 consecutive patients. Circulation 1996;94:1645.

15. Adler Y, Zandman-Goddard G, Ravid M, et al. Usefulness of colchicine in preventing recurrences of pericarditis. Am J Cardiol 1994;73: 916.

16. Folwer NO. Cardiac tamponade. A clinical or an echocardiographic diagnosis? Circulation 1993;87:1738.

17. Hancock EW. Cardiac tamponade. Med Clin North Am 1979;63:223.

18. Cogwell TL, Bernath GA, et al. Effects of intravascular volume state on the value of pulsus paradoxus and right ventricular diastolic collapse in predicting cardiac tamponade. Circulation 1985;72:1076.

19. Curtiss EI, Reddy PS, Uretsky BF, et al. Pulsus paradoxus: definition and relation to the severity of cardiac tamponade. Am Heart J 1988; 115:391.

20. Zhang S, Kerins DM, Byrd BF 3rd. Doppler echocardiography in cardiac tamponade and constrictive pericarditis. Echocardiography 1994;11:507.

21. Spodick DH. The technique of pericardiocentesis. When to perform it and how to minimize complications. J Crit Illness 1995;10:807.

22. Cameron J, Oesterle SN, Baldwin JC, et al. The etiologic spectrum of constrictive pericarditis. Am Heart J 1987;113:354.

23. Fowler NO. Constrictive pericarditis: its history and current status. Clin Cardiol 1995;18:341.

24. Kronzon I, Tunick PA, Freedberg RS. Transesophageal echocardiog-

raphy in pericardial disease and tamponade. Echocardiography 1994; 11:493.

25. Masui T, Finck S, Higgins CB. Constrictive pericarditis and restrictive cardiomyopathy: evaluation with MR imaging. Radiology 1992;182: 369.

26. Hatle LK, Appleton CP, Popp RL. Differentiation of constrictive pericarditis and restrictive cardiomyopathy by Doppler echocardiography. Circulation 1989;79:357.

Chapter 15

Sudden Cardiac Death

DEFINITION AND INCIDENCE

Sudden cardiac death (SCD) is best defined as "natural death due to cardiac causes, heralded by abrupt loss of consciousness within 1 hour of the onset of acute symptoms, in a person with or without known preexisting heart disease, but in whom the time and mode of death are unexpected" (1). SCD is the leading cause of death in the United States, claiming approximately 350,000 individuals annually. Approximately 30% of victims have no prior symptoms of heart disease and SCD is often the first indication of clinical heart disease (2). Although the absolute number of cases of SCD has decreased in parallel with the reduction of overall cardiovascular mortality in the United States, the proportion of all cardiovascular deaths caused by SCD has remained relatively constant at 50%. SCD most commonly occurs in the out-of-hospital setting and is associated with a 80–90% mortality rate. There is still considerable debate regarding a universally acceptable definition of SCD (3). Definitions often vary between clinical investigations and this affects the reported incidence of various diseases as causes for SCD.

ETIOLOGY

The most common causes of SCD and their relative frequencies (4) include the following:

- coronary artery disease—70%
- cardiomyopathy—11%
- valvular and hypertensive heart disease—6%
- mitral valve prolapse with mitral regurgitation—4%
- long QT syndrome and Wolff-Parkinson-White syndrome (WPW)—8%
- other—1%

PATHOPHYSIOLOGY

Severe atherosclerotic coronary artery disease (CAD), i.e., >70% occlusion of one or more of the three major epicardial vessels, is found in most victims of SCD. The extent and degree of involvement is typically greater than that encountered in patients presenting with acute myocardial infarction (MI) or angina pectoris. Despite the severity of CAD, only approximately 30% of victims will have pathologic evidence of an acute thrombotic coronary occlusion or enzymatic evidence of acute myocardial infarction (in those victims who are successfully resuscitated). However, 70–80% will have evidence of prior infarction, myocardial fibrosis (scar), and depressed left ventricular function (1,5,6).

This myocardial substrate of obstructive coronary artery disease, chronic ischemia, and myocardial fibrosis is a predisposition to arrhythmias. Ambulatory monitoring has demonstrated that ventricular tachyarrhythmias most commonly precede or cause SCD (7). Ventricular fibrillation is typically preceded by frequent premature ventricular contractions (PVCs) or monomorphic or polymorphic ventricular tachycardia (VT). Bradyarrhythmias are less common (10–20% of monitored cases). Various "triggers" acting on the myocardial substrate have been described and include acute ischemia, electrolytic abnormalities (hypokalemia and hypomagnesemia), autonomic influences, circulating catecholamines, and cardioactive drugs that have proarrhythmia effects (8).

The very common occurrence of SCD in patients with chronic ventricular ectopy resulted in what has been called the "PVC hypothesis" of SCD. According to this theory, PVCs are an indicator of myocardial electrical instability and a harbinger of unstable and life-threatening arrhythmias. By inference, the more frequent or complex the ventricular ectopic activity, the greater the risk of SCD. The therapeutic implication of this hypothesis is that suppression of ventricular ectopic activity would decrease the risk of SCD. However, this hypothesis has been placed in question by several lines of evidence:

- There is a highly variable relationship between ventricular ectopy and the risk of SCD.
- Ventricular arrhythmias are related to the degree of myocardial contractile dysfunction, which is a risk factor for SCD.

- some patients with high-grade or complex ventricular ectopy have a benign prognosis.
- PVC suppression in asymptomatic patients has not been shown to prevent SCD.
- it is uncertain to what extent ventricular ectopy must be suppressed to protect against SCD.

RISK OF SCD

It has been estimated that the risk of SCD in the unselected adult population is 2 per 1000 persons per year. Therefore, screening of unselected patients is impractical. Based on the pathophysiology of SCD, it has been more practical to focus on patient groups with known heart disease and attempt risk stratification. Risk is best represented in relative terms and can be estimated as follows in terms of average annual risk (4):

- sudden death survivors (SCD not associated with acute MI)—10–30% average annual risk
- dilated cardiomyopathy—10%
- first year post-MI—5%
- hypertrophic cardiomyopathy—1–3%
- long QT syndrome—1–3%
- U.S. adult population—0.22%
- mitral prolapse without regurgitation—0.019%

APPROACHES TO THE PROBLEM OF SUDDEN CARDIAC DEATH

The Patient Who has Survived SCD

If SCD occurs during the course of an acute MI and the patient survives, the risk of SCD recurrence after discharge is no greater than that in the general post-MI population whose course is not complicated by primary ventricular tachycardia or fibrillation (9). In the absence of an acute infarction, the SCD recurrence rate approximates 50% at 2 years.

For patients who have been resuscitated from SCD, an aggressive assessment and management program should be pursued (10). However, the extent of evaluation and interventions should logically be guided by the likelihood of a meaningful functional recovery.

Transient abnormalities that may have facilitated or "triggered" the development of a sustained and hemodynamically unstable rhythm should be investigated. Such abnormalities would include, but are not limited to, serum electrolyte abnormalities, drug toxicity (particularly digoxin and the class Ia antiarrhythmics), or pacemaker malfunction in patients with permanent pacemakers.

Echocardiography should be performed to assess the presence of other cardiac causes of SCD other than coronary artery disease, particularly valvular heart disease and hypertrophic cardiomyopathy. Echocardiography will also allow a determination of wall motion and ejection fraction. **Radionuclide angiography** can also be performed to evaluate the ventricular function.

Cardiac catheterization should be performed to evaluate coronary anatomy and the extent of disease. Significant stenosis of the left main coronary artery, severe multivessel coronary artery disease, or a ventricular aneurysm detected at catheterization may dictate early surgical intervention.

The next logical step in the diagnostic and management program is to quantitate the frequency and complexity of ventricular ectopic electrical activity. **Ambulatory electrocardiographic monitoring (Holter monitoring)** for 24–48 hours is usually the first diagnostic modality used. However, electrocardiogram (ECG) monitoring has important limitations with respect to quantifying or defining the complexity of ventricular ectopic activity as well as allow assessment of drug effects on arrhythmia suppression and outcome. It has been estimated that 30–50% of patients with documented sustained ventricular tachycardia or cardiac arrest due to ventricular fibrillation will not demonstrate a significant number of PVCs during the monitoring period. Clinical studies also indicate that there is considerable spontaneous variation in the frequency and complexity of PVCs during ECG monitoring on a day-to-day basis. This spontaneous variation may complicate the evaluation of antiarrhythmic drug response and assessment of efficacy (11).

Intracardiac electrophysiologic study (EPS) is recommended for patients surviving a cardiac arrest without evidence of an acute Q-wave MI and for patients surviving cardiac arrest occurring more than 48 hours after the acute phase of MI in the absence of a recurrent ischemic event (12). EPS may be particularly useful in patients who do not have frequent high-grade ventricular ectopy during monitoring. Protocols for EPS generally vary from institution to institution but usually include the following:

- recording of spontaneous intervals
- assessment of sinus and atrioventricular (AV) node function
- assessment of ventriculoatrial conduction
- tachycardia induction with extra stimuli at different endocardial sites

During EPS, clinically relevant arrhythmias include sustained (>30 sec) monomorphic VT, the induction of polymorphic or monomorphic VT with hemodynamic collapse, or induction of VF. The optimal EPS protocol to evaluate SCD survivors remains controversial in that different extrastimuli techniques often yield different results with respect to arrhythmia inducibility. In the absence of antiarrhythmic drug therapy, ventricular tachyarrhythmias can be initiated during EPS in 70–80% of patients resuscitated from SCD. Sustained monomorphic VT is the most commonly induced rhythm (35–50%) in this group (12).

EPS is also used to determine drug efficacy in preventing arrhythmia induction. The ability to prevent induction of previously inducible sustained ventricular tachyarrhythmia is associated with a more favorable outcome during follow-up than is failure to identify a successful antiarrhythmic. Drug therapy can suppress arrhythmia induction in 25–80% of SCD survivors. This wide range of efficacy is most probably caused by extrastimuli methods. SCD survivors whose arrhythmias remain inducible are at more than twice the risk of recurrent cardiac arrest compared with patients who are noninducible. The prognostic significance of failure to induce arrhythmias at EPS seems to be dependent on or related to left ventricular (LV) function. Patients with depressed LV function and no obvious reversible cause of arrhythmias remain at risk for recurrent cardiac arrest. Patients with a documented ischemic mechanism for SCD who have normal LV function and noninducible arrhythmias at EPS are at low risk after treatment of the underlying ischemia (12).

EPS and Holter monitoring have both been used to assess the short and long-term efficacy of antiarrhythmic drugs in SCD survivors and other patients at high risk for SCD. The two approaches have been compared in a large, multicenter, controlled clinical trial and indicate that Holter monitoring leads to prediction of drug efficacy more often than EPS (77% versus 45%) (13). However, there was no difference between groups during the 6-year follow-up period in the number of deaths due to arrhythmic causes. Therefore, there was no significant difference in the success of drug therapy as selected by the two methods. Costs were significantly higher in the EPS group (14).

Optimal antiarrhythmic **drug therapy** in this patient group has yet to be defined (15). The ESVEM trial indicated that **sotalol,** a β blocker with class III properties, was more efficacious in preventing SCD and recurrences of arrhythmias when compared to imipramine, mexiletine, Pirmentol, procainamide, propafenone, or quinidine (16). Therapy with empiric **amiodarone,** when compared to therapy with other conventional antiarrhythmics guided by EPS and/or Holter monitoring, has been shown to decrease SCD recurrence but is associated with thyroid dysfunction and pulmonary toxicity, even at low doses (17). An ongoing trial comparing **metoprolol, amiodarone, propafenone, and implanted cardioverter-defibrillator (ICD)** therapy has shown increased mortality in the propafenone group and no difference in survival in the other treatment groups (18).

The AVID (Antiarrhythmics versus Implantable Defibrillators) trial, initiated in 1993, was halted in April 1997. Interim data analysis at that time indicated a 38% greater reduction in deaths in patients treated with ICDs when compared to the group treated with amiodarone or sotalol (19). The results of this trial are likely to simplify the management of patients at risk for sudden cardiac death.

The Patient with Dilated Cardiomyopathy

Dilated cardiomyopathy is the primary diagnosis in 7–23% of patients undergoing EPS after SCD not associated with acute MI (4). Approximately 50% of patients with dilated cardiomyopathy die from progressive congestive heart failure, and the remaining 50% of patients experience SCD most commonly as the result of ventricular tachyarrhythmias. There is a correlation between the degree of LV dysfunction and the risk of SCD (20). Asymptomatic, nonsustained ventricular tachycardia is common in patients with dilated cardiomyopathy who undergo Holter monitoring but suppression of PVCs does not improve survival in the asymptomatic patient. Routine EPS is not recommended in this patient group (12). The general approach to the patient with dilated cardiomyopathy and symptomatic ventricular arrhythmias is similar to that of the SCD survivor. Patients with marked LV dysfunction and complex ventricular ectopy on Holter monitoring commonly undergo EPS to assess arrhythmia inducibility. This patient group presents a number of problems when antiarrhythmic therapy is considered. Patients are at increased risk of toxicity due to altered drug pharmacokinetics (liver metabolism and renal excretion), some antiarrhythmics have negative inotropic effects, and virtually all antiarrhythmics exhibit proarrhythmia properties (21). Several studies suggest that low-dose **amiodarone** may be of value in this group. However, there are conflicting data that may be due to differences in outcomes between patients with ischemic cardiomyopathy and those with nonischemic causes of dilated cardiomyopathy (22,23). The role of ICDs remains to be determined. Patients may be spared death due to an arrhythmia, only to succumb to irreversible and progressive heart failure. This will limit the utility of ICDs when overall long-term mortality is selected as an end point.

The Patient who has Sustained an Acute MI

The incidence of SCD in patients with known coronary artery disease and prior myocardial infarction is 10–100 times that of the general population. Of those patients with SCD caused by coronary disease, approximately 50% will have a prior history of coronary disease.

Several clinical studies have identified "risk factors" associated with an increased prevalence of post-MI SCD. Such risk factors include *(a)* left ventricular dysfunction, *(b)* frequent ventricular arrhythmia, *(c)* late potentials detected by signal averaged electrocardiography, and *(d)* the ability to initiate sustained ventricular tachyarrhythmias during EPS (24,25). The indications for EPS in the post-MI patients are not well defined, but general recommendations include *(a)* patients surviving cardiac arrest occurring >48 hours after the acute phase of MI in the absence of a recurrent ischemic event, *(b)* patients surviving a cardiac arrest that occurred during the acute phase (<48 hours) of MI, *(c)* patients with cardiac arrest resulting from reversible ischemia, and *(d)* patients who are post-MI with other risk factors for future arrhythmic events such as low ejection fraction, positive signal average ECG, and frequent ventricular ectopy on Holter monitoring (12).

In the absence of contraindications, all patients who are post-

MI should be receiving **β blockers.** These drugs have both antiar-rhythmic and anti-ischemic properties and have been shown in numerous large scale studies to improve long-term survival (3 or more years) after acute myocardial infarction (26). These studies were reviewed in Chapter 9 (Myocardial Infarction). In practice, this group of drugs is frequently underused (27). Additional ben-eficial interventions in this group include lifestyle modification, serum cholesterol lowering, and daily aspirin therapy.

In contrast to β-blocker trials, a number of studies evaluating the routine use of **other conventional antiarrhythmic drugs** for post-MI patients have yielded negative results. These trials have been subjected to meta-analysis methods, which demonstrate a worse outcome or no difference in outcome for treatment groups, with the exception of amiodarone, when compared to groups who did not receive treatment or who received placebo (28,29). The study that received the most attention is the CAST (Cardiac Arrhythmia Suppression Trial) investigation (30,31). At the present time, there are no data to support the routine use of conventional antiarrhythmic drug therapy for PVC suppression in asymptomatic patients after myocardial infarction. The lack of a beneficial effect is most probably the result of proarrhythmic effects of the treatment drugs.

Amiodarone has been shown in several studies to be effica-cious in preventing SCD in post-MI patients (32,33). These stud-ies differ with respect to comparative study groups and the inclu-sion of patients at high or moderate risk of SCD or those who are asymptomatic. In the BASIS investigation, post-MI patients with frequent and complex but asymptomatic ventricular ectopy during Holter monitoring were randomized to individualized conventional antiarrhythmic therapy, empiric amiodarone (200 mg/day), or no antiarrhythmic therapy. At 1 year, the probability of survival was significantly greater in the amiodarone group when compared to the control group. A significant reduction in arrhythmic events was also observed in the amiodarone group. Significant benefits were not observed in the conventional treat-ment group (34). Patients treated with amiodarone who had pre-served left ventricular function (ejection fraction >40%) derived greater mortality benefit than those with ejection fraction <40% (35). Similar differences between amiodarone-treated patients and placebo-treated post-MI patients with asymptomatic high-grade ventricular ectopy was observed in the CAMIAT investigation (10% all-cause mortality at 2 years in the amiodarone group versus 21% in the placebo group) (36). Comparatively low doses of amiodarone have been used in amiodarone postinfarction trials, but noncardiac toxicity remains a problem. Presently, amiodarone seems to offer the greatest benefit to post-MI patients who require antiarrhythmic drug therapy but who cannot be given β blockers.

Data from the Coronary Artery Surgery Study (CASS) indicate that **revascularization** is beneficial in preventing SCD. Patients in high-risk subgroups with three-vessel disease and depressed LV function seem to derive the greatest benefit (37).

ICDs in selected patients may also decrease the risk of SCD. In patients who are post-MI with an ejection fraction <35% and complex ventricular ectopy, prophylactic ICD therapy has been shown to decrease mortality over more than 2 years of follow-up when compared to antiarrhythmic drugs, including amiodarone and β blockers, given empirically (38). Several ongoing studies are evaluating long-term efficacy as well as cost benefit (39,40).

References

1. Myerburg RJ, Castellanos A. Cardiac arrest and sudden cardiac death. In: Braunwald E, ed. Heart disease: a textbook of cardiovascular medicine. 4th ed. Philadelphia: WB Saunders, 1992:756.
2. Myerburg RJ, Kessler KM, Castellanos A. Sudden cardiac death: epidemiology, transient risk, and intervention assessment. Ann Intern Med 1993;119:1187.
3. Pratt CM, Greenway PS, Schoenfeld MH, et al. Exploration of the precision of classifying sudden cardiac death. Implications for the interpretation of clinical trials. Circulation 1996;93:519.
4. Gilman JK, Naccarelli GV. Sudden cardiac death. Curr Probl Cardiol 1992;17:695.
5. Farb A, Tang AL, Burke AP, et al. Sudden coronary death. Frequency of active coronary lesions, inactive coronary lesions, and myocardial infarction. Circulation 1995;92:1701.
6. Farb A, Burke AP, Tang AL, et al. Coronary plaque erosion without rupture into a lipid core. A frequent cause of coronary thrombosis in sudden coronary death. Circulation 1996;93:1354.
7. De Luna AB, Coumel P, Leclercq JF. Ambulatory sudden cardiac death: mechanisms of production of fatal arrhythmia on the basis of data from 157 cases. Am Heart J 1989;117:151.
8. Myerburg RJ, Kessler KM, Castellanos A. Sudden cardiac death. Structure, function, and time-dependence of risk. Circulation 1992; 85(Suppl I):I–2.

9. Tofler GH, Stone PH, Muller JE, et al. Prognosis after cardiac arrest due to ventricular tachycardia or ventricular fibrillation associated with acute myocardial infarction (the MILIS Study). Am J Cardiol 1987;60:755.

10. Waldo AL, Biblo LE, Carlson MD. General evaluation of out-of-hospital sudden cardiac death survivors. Circulation 1992;85(Suppl I): I–103.

11. DiMarco JP, Philbrick JT. Use of ambulatory electrocardiographic (Holter) monitoring. Ann Intern Med 1990;113:53.

12. Guidelines for Clinical Intracardiac Electrophysiological and Catheter Ablation Procedures. A report of the American College of Cardiology/American Heart Association Task Force on Practice Guidelines (Committee on Clinical Intracardiac Electrophysiologic and Catheter Ablation Procedures). Circulation 1995;92:673.

13. Mason JW for the Electrophysiologic Study versus Electrocardiographic Monitoring (ESVEM) Investigators. A comparison of electrophysiologic testing with Holter monitoring to predict antiarrhythmic-drug efficacy for ventricular tachyarrhythmias. N Engl J Med 1993; 329:445.

14. Omoigui NA, Marcus FI, Mason JW, et al. Cost of initial therapy in the electrophysiologic study versus ECG monitoring trial (ESVEM). Circulation 1995;91:1070.

15. Domanski MJ, Zipes DP, Schron E. Treatment of sudden cardiac death. Current understandings from randomized trials and future research directions. Circulation 1997;95:2694.

16. Mason JW for the Electrophysiologic Study versus Electrocardiographic Monitoring (SVEM) Investigators. A comparison of seven antiarrhythmic drugs in patients with ventricular tachyarrhythmias. N Engl J Med 1993;329:452.

17. CASCADE Investigators. The CASCADE Study: Randomized antiarrhythmic drug therapy in survivors of cardiac arrest in Seattle. Am J Cardiol 1993;72:70F.

18. Siebels J, Cappato R, Ruppel R, et al. Preliminary results of the Cardiac Arrest Study Hamburg (CASH). Am J Cardiol 1993;72:109F.

19. Cardiovascular News. NHLBI stops arrhythmia study: implantable cardiac defibrillators reduce deaths. Circulation 1997;95:2456.

20. Bigger JT Jr. Why patients with congestive heart failure die: arrhythmias and sudden cardiac death. Circulation 1987;75(Suppl IV): IV–28.

21. Dec GW, Fuster V. Idiopathic dilated cardiomyopathy. N Engl J Med 1994;331:1564.

22. Doval HC, Nul DR, Grancelli HO, et al. Randomised trial of low-dose amiodarone in severe congestive heart failure. Grupo de Estudio de la Sobrevida en la Insuficiencia Cardiaca en Argentina (GESICA). Lancet 1994;344:493.

23. Singh SN, Fletcher RD, Fisher SG, et al. Amiodarone in patients with congestive heart failure and asymptomatic ventricular arrhythmia. N Engl J Med 1995;333:77.

24. Shen WK, Hammill SC. Survivors of acute myocardial infarction: who is at risk for sudden cardiac death. Mayo Clin Proc 1991;66:950.

25. Gilman JK Jalal S, Naccarelli GV. Predicting and preventing sudden death from cardiac causes. Circulation 1994;90:1083.

26. Kendall MJ, Lynch KP, Hjalmarson A, et al. β-blockers and sudden cardiac death. Ann Intern Med 1995;123:358.

27. Soumerai SB, McLaughlin TJ, Spiegelman D, et al. Adverse outcomes of underuse of β-blockers in elderly survivors of acute myocardial infarction. JAMA 1997;277:115.

28. Hine LK, Laird NM, Chalmers TC. Meta-analysis of empirical long-term antiarrhythmic therapy after myocardial infarction. JAMA 1989; 262:3037.

29. Teo KK, Yusuf S, Furberg CD. Effects of prophylactic antiarrhythmic drug therapy in acute myocardial infarction. An overview of results from randomized controlled trials. JAMA 1993;270:1589.

30. Echt DS, Liebson PR, Mitchell B, et al. Mortality and morbidity in patients receiving encainide, flecainide, or placebo. The Cardiac Arrhythmia Suppression Trial. N Engl J Med 1991;324:781.

31. The Cardiac Arrhythmia Suppression Trial II Investigators: effect of the antiarrhythmic agent moricizine on survival after myocardial infarction. N Engl J Med 1992;327:227.

32. Podrid PJ. Amiodarone: reevaluation of an old drug. Ann Intern Med 1995;122:689.

33. Zamerbski DG, Nolan PE Jr, Slack MK, et al. Empiric long-term amiodarone prophylaxis following myocardial infarction. A meta-analysis. Arch Intern Med 1993;153:2661.

34. Burkart F, Pfisterer M, Kiowski W, et al. Effect of antiarrhythmic therapy on mortality in survivors of myocardial infarction with asymptomatic complex ventricular arrhythmias: Basel Antiarrhythmic Study of Infarct Survival (BASIS). J Am Coll Cardiol 1990;16:1711.

35. Pfisterer M, Kiowski W, Burckhardt D, et al. Beneficial effect of amiodarone on cardiac mortality in patients with asymptomatic complex ventricular arrhythmias after acute myocardial infarction and preserved but not impaired left ventricular function. Am J Cardiol 1992; 69:1399.

36. Cairns JA, Connolly SJ, Gent M, et al: Post-myocardial infarction mortality in patients with ventricular premature depolarizations. Canadian Amiodarone Myocardial Infarction Arrhythmia Trial Pilot Study. Circulation 1991;84:550.

37. Holmes DR Jr, Davis KB, Mock MB, et al. The effect of medical and surgical treatment on subsequent sudden cardiac death in patients

with coronary artery disease. A report from the coronary artery surgery study. Circulation 1986;73:1254.

38. Moss AJ, Hall J, Cannom DS, et al. Improved survival with an implanted defibrillator in patients with coronary disease at high risk for ventricular arrhythmia. N Engl J Med 1996;335:1933.

39. Connolly SJ, Jent M, Roberts RS, et al. Canadian Implantation Defibrillator Study (CIDS): study design and organization. Am J Cardiol 1993;72:103F.

40. Antiarrhythmics versus Implantable Defibrillators (AVID)—rationale, design, and methods. Am J Cardiol 1995;75:470.

Chapter 16

Cardiac Pacemakers

Electrical devices for the heart have changed rapidly during recent years, with both increasing complexity and miniaturization. A basic knowledge of their purposes and modes of operation allow for simple clinical evaluation at time of implantation or follow-up evaluation. This chapter will deal with temporary and permanent pacemakers.

TEMPORARY PACEMAKERS

With the availability of effective external pacemakers and a better understanding of the natural history of conduction system disease, the use of transvenous temporary pacemakers has declined. Indications for their use still include transient inadequate rhythm or clinical situations with a high risk of transient inadequate rhythm. Whenever possible, a patient with an inadequate rhythm with no reversible cause should be considered for direct permanent pacing to avoid the risks and costs of temporary pacing.

Transient bradyarrhythmia is most often seen in **drug toxicity.** Digitalis excess can be treated with antibody therapy but may still require temporary pacing until the degree of underlying conduction disease (and possible need for permanent pacing) is evident. β blockers and calcium channel blockers such as verapamil and diltiazem can induce symptomatic sinus bradycardia or atrioventricular (AV) block, requiring temporary pacing. Less commonly seen are pacemaker-requiring bradycardias caused by amiodarone and class IA drugs.

Prophylactic temporary pacing is indicated in **acute myocardial infarction,** in which development of AV and bundle branch block increases the risk of complete AV block. Situations in which the risk of developing symptomatic complete AV block may be

Table 16.1
Indications for Prophylactic Pacing in Acute Myocardial Infarction

Indicated	Not indicated	Controversial
Mobitz II AV block	1° AV block	New LBBB
Complete AV block	Wenckebach 2° AV block	New RBBB in IMI
New RBBB in AMI	Old LBBB	
RBBB + LAFB	Old RBBB	
RBBB + LPFB		
LBBB + 1° AV block		
Symptomatic bradycardia		

LBBB = left bundle branch block; RBBB = right bundle branch block; LAFB = left anterior fascicular block; LPFB = left posterior fascicular block; AMI = anterior myocardial infarction; IMI = inferior myocardial infarction.

significant (>20%) are summarized in Table 16.1. Most of these patients have large anterior infarctions, and outcome is related more to left ventricular function than the need for pacing. Inferior infarctions may develop AV block above the His bundle. With a stable, narrow QRS junctional rhythm, these patients do not require pacing. Other situations, such as asymptomatic bi-trifascicular block and asymptomatic Wenckebach Type 1 AV block, are not considered indications for prophylactic pacing.

Temporary pacing is indicated in a few other **special circumstances.** Bradycardia-dependent arrhythmia such as torsade de pointes in sinus bradycardia and long QT interval may be managed with temporary transvenous pacing. An internal cardiac recording may help define the source and type of tachyarrhythmia, and overdrive pacing may frequently break up a reentry arrhythmia like atrial flutter, avoiding the need for drug or shock therapy. Recording an His spike before the QRS may separate a supraventricular from ventricular tachycardia and direct appropriate drug and electrical therapy.

APPROACHES TO TEMPORARY PACING

Transvenous temporary pacing remains the standard approach for prolonged patient support; external pacing is suitable only for standby or brief capture of the heart. The transthoracic route is no longer used.

Very emergent transvenous pacing can be accomplished from the right **internal jugular** vein with blind or electrocardiogram (ECG)-guided placement into the right ventricle. When the patient's condition allows, more controlled conditions with full sterility and fluoroscopic guidance is preferred. In the **subclavian** vein approach, the wire can be secured well to the chest wall and subsequent patient mobility is less restricted. The **femoral** vein approach is still used, but leg movement can displace the wire.

Many pacing catheters are available, usually bipolar with both anode and cathode near the wire tip. Semifloating catheters have a fixed curve, whereas floating catheters have an inflatable balloon on the tip to float into the right ventricle. Complications vary with the site, including bleeding, venous arrhythmias, thrombosis, pneumothorax, arterial puncture, and infection. Cardiac perforation with tamponade is a rare problem.

After it has been positioned, the catheter is tied to the skin and a sterile dressing is placed. Usually, a connecting cable is used, with the distal wire connected to the negative pole. All connections must be checked daily with a "tug test," because some connections screw tightly clockwise and seem opposite to normal hardware. Rate and output adjustment are straightforward, with daily check of capture threshold. The output is set at two to three times threshold. The sensitivity dialysis is most sensitive to the far right and least sensitive to the far left. To the extreme left is no sensing, or synchronous pacing.

Elaborate external pacing systems are available. High-output, rapid-burst pacing devices may be used for tachyarrhythmia termination as described above. In some infarctions with complete AV block and low cardiac output, temporary AV pacing may be indicated. AV external generators are used after cardiac surgery with temporary external pacing wires.

TROUBLE-SHOOTING TEMPORARY PACEMAKERS

The patient with a temporary pacemaker is usually very ill and should always be on continuous ECG monitoring. After placement, a chest radiograph should be obtained to check for catheter position, to check for complications, and for future baseline comparison. Daily site dressing change and patient restriction appropriate to the site of insertion is required. Pacing and sensing

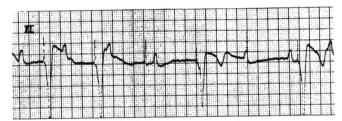

Figure 16.1. Intermittent Failure to Pace. Large P waves are seen in this patient with complete heart block. Ventricular pacing spike fails to capture with the third and fifth spikes.

thresholds should be checked every 24 hours; the rate often should be turned to the lowest possible setting for 24 hours before determining that the pacemaker is no longer needed and can be discontinued.

The most frightening complication of temporary pacing is sudden loss of capture (Fig. 16.1) This is often caused by lead movement or dislodgment and can sometimes be overcome by increasing the generator output. A radiograph should be obtained, and lead repositioning may be necessary.

Sudden loss of pacemaker artifact is usually caused by connection problems. There might be oversensing, and the sensitivity should be turned to the far left for asynchronous pacing.

PERMANENT PACEMAKERS

A letter code, initially established in 1974 and since revised as technology has advanced, standardizes nomenclature for pacing modes. Although there are five positions in the code, the fifth position is rarely used. Table 16.2 includes an explanation of the first four positions and potential abbreviations in each category. Using this table, one should be able to understand the features of any pacing mode. For example, an AAIR is one capable of atrial pacing and atrial sensing, is inhibited by intrinsic atrial activity, and has rate adaptive capability; a VDD pacemaker is one capable of pacing the ventricle and sensing both atrial and ventricular intrinsic activity and responds by inhibition of ventricular pacing in the presence of intrinsic ventricular activity and triggering a paced ventricular beat response to a sensed atrial beat.

Table 16.2
Pacemaker Codes

Position category	I Chamber(s) Paced	II Chamber(s) Sensed	III Modes of Responses	IV Programmable Functions
Letters used	A = Atrium V = Ventricle D = Dual	A = Atrium V = Ventricle D = Dual O = None	I = Inhibited T = Triggered O = Asynchronous	P = Programmable (rate and/or output) M = Multiple programmable R = Rate adaptive

INDICATIONS FOR PERMANENT PACING

The most recent "Guidelines for Implantation of Cardiac Pacemakers" was published in 1991 and is summarized in Table 16.3.

MODE SELECTION OF PERMANENT PACEMAKERS

In the 1970s, it became evident that after ventricular pacemaker placement, some patients became more symptomatic, developing

Table 16.3
Indications for Permanent Pacing

I. Definite indications:
  A. Symptomatic rhythms
    • Second- or third-degree heart blocks
    • Sinus bradycardia
    • Tachycardia-bradycardia syndrome
    • Bundle branch block with prolonged H-V interval and no other cause of symptoms
    • Recurrent syncope with demonstration of carotid sinus hypersensitivity
  B. Asymptomatic rhythms
    • Mobitz II block with demonstration of block below the His
    • Third-degree block within His-Purkinje system
    • Alternating bundle branch block with change in H-V intervals
    • Bifascidular block with H-V >100 msec
II. Pacing is not indicated:
    • Asymptomatic sinus mode dysfunction
    • Asymptomatic block in the A-V node (1° or 2° Mobitz I)
    • Asymptomatic bifascicular block in the absence of evidence of unstable His-Purkinje Conduction

Table 16.4
Common Permanent Pacemakers

Code	Indication	Advantages	Disadvantages
VVI	Intermittent backup pacing Inactive patient	Simplicity, Limited cost	Fixed rate, loss atrial transport, potential pacemaker syndrome
VVIR	Atrial fibrillation	Rate responsiveness	Requires appropriate programming
DDD	Complete heart block	Atrial tracking restores normal physiology	If sick sinus develops no rate responsiveness, requires two leads, more programming
DDDR	Sinus node dysfunction AV block and need for guaranteed rate responsiveness	Universal pacemaker all options available by programming	Complexity, expense, programming, and follow-up

fatigue, dyspnea, and limited exercise output, even to the point of heart failure. This has come to be known as the pacemaker syndrome and occurs in 7–20% of patients with VVI pacemakers. In VVI pacing, the atrial-ventricular synchrony is lost. Losing atrial transport and filling of the ventricles in late diastole may drop cardiac output 20–40%, especially in the noncompliant stiff ventricle. If retrograde ventriculoatrial conduction occurs with retrograde P waves after the ventricular paced event; the atria contract on closed AV valves and send blood backward during early diastole. This may further decrease cardiac output and cause symptomatic cannon waves.

Pacemaker syndrome has been resolved with dual-chamber pacing. The atrial lead is usually placed in high right atrial appendage. Current pacemakers can be effectively programmed for the optimum atrial and ventricular sensing and pacing and AV interval (Table 16.4).

In the 1980s, the first ventricular rate-adaptive pacemaker became available and, later in the decade, the dual-chamber rate-adaptive pacemaker also became available. For patients with

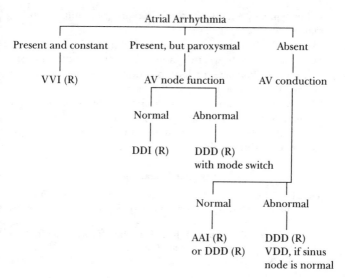

Figure 16.2.

chronotropic incompetence, rate-adaptive pacing is important to provide adequate heart rate response to exercise. The pacing system might be VVIR, DDDR, DDDIR, or AAIR, depending on the presence of associated AV nodal conduction disease and atrial arrhythmia. Up to 40–50% of patients with complete heart block have sinus node dysfunction. Because conduction disease can be progressive, it is important to make certain that patients with complete AV block undergo some evaluation of sinus node function to determine whether rate-adaptive pacing will provide additional benefit.

The algorithm for the selection of optimal pacing system for an individual patient is summarized in Figure 16.2.

PACEMAKER FACTS

- MRI is considered to be contraindicated for patients with pacemakers because MRI can cause inhibition of the pacemaker.
- During radiofrequency ablation in patients with pacemaker, a programmer should be available during the procedure because

radiofrequency energy can result in reprogramming of a pacemaker.

- External defibrillation can result in reprogramming of a permanent pacemaker, transient elevation in pacing/sensing threshold, circuitry damage, or localized myocardial necrosis if the energy is transmitted through the leads.
- Class IC antiarrhythmic drugs are the only ones that result in significant elevation in pacing and/or sensing threshold.
- Hyperkalemia is the most common metabolic disturbance to raise pacing thresholds.

Suggested Reading

Dreifus LS, Fisch C, Griffin JC, et al. Guidelines for implantation of cardiac pacemakers and antiarrhythmic devices. J Am Coll Cardiol 1991; 18:1.

Furman S, Hayes DL, Homes DR Jr. The practice of cardiac pacing. 3rd ed. New York: Futura Publishing Co, 1993.

Kusumoto FM, Goldschlager N. Cardiac pacing. N Engl J Med 1996; 334:89.

Chapter 17

Cardiac Surgery

SURGERY FOR ISCHEMIC HEART DISEASE

Coronary artery bypass grafting remains the most common cardiac surgical procedure performed in the United States; more
than 300,000 operations were completed in 1996. Although there
has been a trend toward operating on patients who are more sick
and elderly, results continue to improve with overall mortality
rates less than 3%. Advanced age continues to be the risk factor
most consistently related to increased mortality.

Improvements in myocardial protection have greatly contrib-
uted to the improved results seen with coronary artery bypass
grafting. Many surgeons routinely use combinations of antegrade
and retrograde (via the coronary sinus) delivery of cardioplegic
solutions to improve delivery to the myocardium. Controversy
still exists regarding warm blood versus cold blood cardioplegia
and intermittent versus continuous perfusion (1).

There is a trend toward increasing the use of arterial grafts,
which have better long-term patency rates when compared with
saphenous vein bypass grafts. It has been recognized for many
years that the left internal mammary is the optimum coronary
artery bypass conduit, with a patency rate higher than 90% at 10-
year follow-up. Furthermore, the use of the left internal mammary artery to the left anterior descending artery (LAD) correlates with improved long-term survival over the use of vein grafts
to the LAD. The increasing use of bilateral internal mammary
artery revascularization has yet to be shown to change survival
statistics, but data on event-free performance should be forthcom-
ing (2). Although frequently subject to arterial spasm, the radial
artery can be used as a graft that is readily available, is easily
obtained, and probably has better long-term patency than saphenous vein grafts (3). The right gastroepiploic artery has also been

successfully grafted to arteries on the diaphragmatic surface of the heart (4).

Minimally invasive techniques for coronary artery bypass grafting are generating an enormous amount of interest in both the medical and lay literature. These techniques allow surgeons to perform single and sometimes multiple coronary bypass operations through small anterior thoracotomy incisions instead of the traditional median sternotomy. With the minimally invasive direct coronary artery bypass (MIDCAB) procedure, the left internal mammary artery is anastomosed to the LAD with the heart beating, thus avoiding the risks of cardiopulmonary bypass and cardiac arrest (5,6). Whereas advantages include shortened hospital stays with the potential for less morbidity and earlier return to normal activity, there is concern that long-term patency rates of these technically more difficult anastomoses will be inferior to those performed with the heart arrested. Furthermore, the MIDCAB procedure tends to be limited to patients with single- or two-vessel disease.

"Port-access" coronary bypass surgery (Heartport Inc.) uses the same approach as the MIDCAB but uses an intra-aortic balloon occlusion catheter inflated in the aortic root to arrest the heart and deliver cardioplegia. Cardiopulmonary bypass is initiated via the femoral artery and vein. Advantages of the approach include the potential for more reliable anastomoses, because the heart is arrested, as well as the ability to perform multivessel grafting. Disadvantages include the risks of cardiopulmonary bypass via the femoral vessels, along with a small but real risk of aortic dissection. It is currently too early to predict what impact minimally invasive coronary surgery will have on the treatment of ischemic heart disease.

Transmyocardial laser revascularization, often with the use of minimally invasive techniques, has been performed successfully on patients with advanced coronary disease who do not have adequate target vessels for coronary artery bypass grafting. The creation of transmyocardial laser channels in ischemic myocardium has been shown to result in symptomatic and functional improvement in selected patients. Studies to determine both the mechanism of action and the applicability of these laser channels are currently under way.

SURGERY FOR CHRONIC CONGESTIVE HEART FAILURE

Surgery for patients with end-stage congestive heart failure is currently limited to heart transplantation, frequently after a period of left ventricular assistance with a mechanical device. More recently, left ventriculoplasty (The Batista Operation) has been proposed as an option for select patients with severe cardiomyopathy (7).

The number of heart transplants performed in the United States each year is limited to approximately 2000 because of the shortage of donor organs. Improved resuscitative techniques have the potential to expand the donor heart pool. As results with cardiac transplantation continue to improve with advances in immunosuppressive therapy and follow-up care, the selection criteria for donors and recipients are being relaxed. Patients older than 60 years of age have been shown to have similar early mortality and length of hospitalization as younger patients. Five-year survival ranges from 71% for older patients to 82% for younger patients (8). Hypercholesterolemia affects 60–80% of recipients and may contribute to coronary vasculopathy. Transplant atherosclerosis is responsible for many late deaths. HMG-CoA reductase inhibitors reduce the level of cholesterol (see Chapter 7) and seem to have the added advantage of decreasing the incidence of cardiac rejection (9).

New devices have been used to provide hemodynamic support to the increasing number of patients awaiting cardiac transplantation. The Heart Mate implantable pneumatic left ventricular assist system (LVAS) has significantly reduced pretransplantation mortality by improving renal and hepatic function and physical capacity (10).

The Batista procedure has created international interest as a surgical approach for patients with end-stage heart failure. This operation involves extensive resection of thinned myocardium to create a more effective chamber geometry with reduced volume. Currently, the best candidates are those with dilated cardiomyopathy with advanced heart failure.

SURGERY FOR VALVULAR HEART DISEASE

Progress continues to be made in the field of cardiac valve surgery. The advantage of durability of mechanical valves has to be weighed against the risks of anticoagulation therapy and problems with thromboembolism. No current mechanical prosthesis is ideal, and all prostheses require chronic anticoagulation. Current mechanical valves offer low profile and superior hemodynamics over the older caged-ball prostheses (Starr-Edwards, Smeloff-Cutter valves). The Medtronic-Hall valve is a pivoting-disk mechanical prosthesis that is extremely low profile. The St. Jude and Carbomedics valves are hinged, bileaflet valves that are extremely popular among cardiac surgeons because of their excellent hemodynamics and ease of implantation (11).

Cryopreserved aortic homografts offer durability for younger patients without the need for anticoagulation. They require special techniques for procurement, storage, and implantation. They are particularly applicable for patients with native or prosthetic valve endocarditis (12).

The Ross procedure is particularly effective for young patients with aortic valve disease. This technique involves replacing the patient's diseased aortic valve and root with his or her own pulmonic valve, reimplanting the coronary arteries into the pulmonary autograft. The pulmonary valve is then replaced with a pulmonary homograft. The Ross procedure offers superior longevity over bioprostheses for younger patients, as well as the advantage of not requiring anticoagulation (13).

Bioprostheses continue to be the valve replacements of choice for older patients, especially those older than 70 years of age. Three popular bioprostheses are available in the United States: the Hancock and Carpentier-Edwards valves, which are both porcine bioprostheses, and the Baxter pericardial valve, which is constructed from bovine pericardium. Bioprostheses are not composed of living tissue but are a combination of chemically treated biologic tissues and artificial material. In general, these valves have a low incidence of thromboembolism, especially in the aortic position. Many patients can go without anticoagulation, but anticoagulation is still advisable for patients with atrial fibrillation, atrial clots, or previous thromboembolism. The primary concern of bioprosthetic valves is valve durability. They are susceptible to primary valve failure caused by calcification and structural deterioration, which tend to be accelerated in patients younger than 40 years of age. Improvements in valve design and calcification-retardant techniques will prove to increase valve durability (14).

Mitral valve repair offers significant advantages over valve replacement in many patients with mitral valve disease. Preservation of the entire mitral apparatus results in improved ventricular function, with improved durability over bioprostheses. Ideal patients for mitral valve repair are those with noncalcified valves and mitral regurgitation. Valve repair can include partial resection of leaflets; lengthening, shortening, transposition, or replacement of chorda tendineae; and placement of valvuloplasty rings to decrease the size of the mitral annulus.

References

1. Rudis E, Gates RN, Laks H, et al. Coronary sinus ostial occlusion during retrograde delivery of cardioplegic solution significantly improves cardioplegic distribution and efficacy. J Thorac Cardiovasc Surg 1995;109:941.

2. Dewar LRS, Jamieson WRE, Jenusz MR, et al. Unilateral versus bilateral internal mammary revascularization: survival and event-free performance. Circulation 1995;92(Suppl II):II–8.

3. Fremes SE, Christakis GT, Del Rizzo DF, et al. The technique of radial artery bypass grafting and early clinical results. J Cardiovasc Surg 1995;10:537.

4. Pyon J, Brown P, Pearson M, et al. Right gastroepiploic to coronary artery bypass. The first decade of use. Circulation 1995;92(Suppl II):II–45.

5. Benetti FJ, Ballester C. Use of thoracoscopy and minimal thoracotomy in mammary-coronary bypass to left anterior descending artery without extracorporeal circulation. J Cardiovasc Surg 1995;36:195.

6. Borst C, Jansen EWL, Tulleken CAF, et al. Coronary artery bypass grafting without cardiopulmonary bypass and without interruption of native coronary flow using a novel anastomosis site restraining device ("Octopus"). J Am Coll Cardiol 1996;27:1356.

7. Batista RJ, Santos JL, Takeshita N, et al. Partial left ventriculectomy to improve left ventricular function in end-stage heart disease. J Cardiovasc Surg 1996;11:96.

8. Bergin P, Rabinov M, Esmore D. Cardiac transplantation in patients over 60 years. Transplant Proc 1995;27:2150.

9. Kobashigawa JA, Katznelson S, Laks H, et al. Effect of pravastatin on outcomes after cardiac transplantation. N Engl J Med 1995;333:621.

10. Frazier OH, Rose EA, McCarthy P, et al. Improved mortality and rehabilitation of transplant candidates treated with long-term implantable left ventricular assist system. Ann Surg 1995;222:327.

11. Carlson D, Stephensen LW. Mechanical cardiac valves: current status. Cardiol Clin 1995;3:439.

12. Kirklin JK, Kirklin JW, Pacifico AD. Homograft replacement of the aortic valve. Cardiol Clin 1995;3:329.

13. Reddy VM, Rajasingke HA, McElhinney DB, et al. Extending the limits of the Ross procedure. Ann Thorac Surg 1995;60(Suppl VI): VI–600.

14. Pupello DF, Bessone LN, Hibo SP, et al. Bioprosthetic valve longevity in the elderly: an 18 year longitudinal study. Ann Thorac Surg 1995; 60:270.

Chapter 18

Cardiac Drug Therapy

This chapter provides a summary and ready reference source for information regarding common drugs mentioned or discussed in some detail in the preceding chapters. The focus of this chapter is on the medications used to treat the more common problems encountered in cardiovascular medicine: ischemic heart disease, congestive heart failure, and arrhythmias.

ANTIARRHYTHMIC DRUGS

Several classifications have been proposed for drugs used for the treatment of cardiac arrhythmias. These classifications are based on the premise that drugs with similar electrophysiologic properties also have similar therapeutic effects as well as toxicities. In practice, the choice of drugs is based largely on the results of controlled trials and clinical experience (Table 18.1). Such studies have demonstrated that although drugs may have similar properties when tested in the experimental laboratory, they may have different effects in the clinical population (Table 18.2). The most common classification of antiarrhythmic drugs is the modified Vaughan-Williams Classification as noted below (1,2).

Modified Vaughan-Williams Classification of Antiarrhythmic Drugs

Class IA

Class IA agents depress or slow the rapid upstroke of the action potential (phase 1), decrease conduction velocity (sodium channel blockade effect), and prolong repolarization (phase 3) (potassium channel blockade).

Examples: quinidine, procainamide, disopyramide.

Table 18.1
Drugs of Choice for Common Arrhythmias

Arrhythmia	Drug of choice	Alternatives
Atrial fibrillation or flutter	Diltiazem, verapamil, or β blocker for urgent ventricular rate control	Ibutilide for conversion Digoxin, β blockers, calcium channel blockers, amiodarone for long-term prevention
Other supraventricular tachycardias	Adenosine, verapamil, or diltiazem for conversion	Esmolol, other β blocker, or digoxin for conversion
PVCs	None indicated for the asymptomatic patient	β blocker for symptomatic patients
Sustained ventricular tachycardia	Lidocaine for acute Rx	Procainamide, bretylium, amiodarone for acute Rx
Ventricular fibrillation	DC cardioversion	Drug therapy is for prevention of recurrence and is the same as for PVCs in acute Rx
Torsades de pointes	Magnesium sulfate	Isoproterenol, pacing

Class IB

Class IB agents slow the action potential upstroke in abnormal tissue and facilitate repolarization. These drugs have little effect on normal myocardial tissue.

Examples: lidocaine, mexiletine, tocainide, moricizine.

Class IC

Class IC agents markedly slow phase 1 of action potential and decrease conduction velocity but exert little effect on phase 3 (repolarization).

Examples: propafenone, encainide (no longer marketed), flecainide, moricizine (moricizine has both class IB and IC properties).

Class II

Class II agents block adrenergic receptors.

Examples: propranolol. metoprolol, atenolol, and others.

Table 18.2
Antiarrhythmic Drugs

Drug	Usual dose	Comments
Adenosine	IV: 6-mg rapid bolus; if no effect, 2 doses of 12 mg at 2-min intervals	Side effects brief Ventricular escape rhythm common
Amiodarone	IV: 150 mg over 10 min infusion: 360 mg over 6 hr maintenance: 540 mg over 18 hr PO: low dose 200 mg q.d.	Higher PO doses needed for ventricular arrhythmias
Bretylium	IV: 5 mg/kg with additional doses of 10 mg/kg (total 30 mg/kg) Infusion: 1–2 mg/min	Preferred over verapamil in patients with left ventricular dysfunction
Diltiazem	IV: 0.25 mg/kg over 2 min, repeat at 0.35 mg/kg in 15–30 min if needed Infusion: 5–15 mg/hr	
Esmolol	see text	
Flecainide	PO: 50–200 mg b.i.d.	PO loading dose required
Ibutilide	IV: 1 mg over 10 min, repeat once in 10 min if needed	Polymorphic VT in 8%
Lidocaine	see text	CNS side effects
Magnesium	IV: 1–2 g over 5–10 min	May give up to 5 mg
Metoprolol	IV: 5 mg every 5 min to total dose 15 mg	Preferred in acute MI
Mexiletine	PO: 150–300 mg every 6–12 hr, maximum dose 1200 mg/day	
Moricizine	PO: 200–300 mg every 8 hr	PO loading dose required
Procainamide	IV: up to 17 mg/kg at 20 mg/min Infusion: 2–4 mg/min PO: 50–100 mg/kg/day	Hypotension may occur with IV loading
Propafenone	PO: 150–300 mg every 8 hr	
Propranolol	IV: 1–5 mg total (1 mg/min) PO: varies with formulation	
Quinidine	PO sulfate: 200–400 mg every 4–6 hr PO gluconate: 324–648 mg every 8–12 hr	
Sotalol	PO: 80–160 mg b.i.d.	Higher doses needed for effect on repolarization
Tocainide	PO: 200–600 mg every 8 hr, maximum dose 2400 mg/day	PO loading doses required
Verapamil	IV: 5–10 mg over 1–3 min, repeat in 15–30 min if needed PO: varies with formulation	Hypotension due to vasodilatation; consider pretreatment with calcium chloride

Class III

Class III agents primarily slow repolarization (phase 3).
   Examples: sotalol, amiodarone, bretylium.

Class IV

Class IV agents block calcium channels.
   Examples: verapamil, diltiazem, nifedipine, and others.

General Comments

Class IA Agents

Quinidine is the most commonly used drug in this group. The dose required to achieve a **therapeutic serum concentration (1.5–5 μg/mL)** varies from patient to patient. When given to a patient in atrial fibrillation, the ventricular response rate may increase as the atrial rate slows; a drug with atrioventricular (AV) node blocking properties (digoxin, a calcium channel blocker, or a blocker) should be given first. Quinidine increases serum digoxin concentrations and digoxin levels should be monitored for a period after this drug combination is initiated. In many instances, the maintenance dose of digoxin will have to be decreased by 50%. Long-term treatment with quinidine has been shown to be associated with a higher risk of cardiovascular mortality, which has been ascribed to its proarrhythmic effect. Torsades de pointes has been implicated and can occur even at low serum concentrations or after single doses of the drug. **Procainamide** is more commonly used in the acute management of arrhythmias. Because hypotension can occur with rapid intravenous loading doses, the loading dose (up to 17 mg/kg) should be given at a rate of 20 mg/min or less. The **therapeutic serum concentration is 4–10 μg/mL.** Long-term use is associated with a lupus-like syndrome in approximately 30% of patients, and many patients will develop antinuclear antibodies within 3–6 months of starting of the drug. N-acetyl procainamide (NAPA) is an active metabolite and may be increased in patients with renal failure. **Disopyramide** has prominent anticholinergic effects and has been associated with a worsening of established heart failure. However, it is sometimes better tolerated than quinidine. All class IA agents have been associated with torsades de pointes (3–6).

Class IB Agents

Prophylactic **lidocaine** is no longer recommended in the management of acute myocardial infarction (MI). A meta-analysis of available literature has, in fact, suggested that it may be detrimental in this setting (7). Lidocaine is given intravenously for the management of symptomatic or life-threatening ventricular arrhythmias (8). The loading dose is usually 1 mg/kg given over 2 minutes, then 0.5 mg/kg over 2 minutes every 8–10 minutes for three doses, if needed, for arrhythmia suppression. An infusion (14 mg/min) is required to maintain **therapeutic serum levels (1.5–5 μg/mL).** The loading dose should be decreased for patients with heart failure, liver dysfunction, and in those older than 70 years of age. Toxicity is manifest primarily as central nervous system (CNS) alterations, particularly seizures. **Mexiletine** and **tocainide** are oral congeners of lidocaine (9). Tocainide is associated with severe hematological effects (agranulocytosis) and is rarely indicated, except for symptomatic patients who have failed to respond to other drugs.

Class IC Agents

These agents are effective in suppressing ventricular arrhythmias in patients who are unresponsive to other drugs. However, these agents have a high proarrhythmia potential and can worsen existing arrhythmias or cause new ones, especially in the setting of chronic ischemic heart disease. When tested in a clinical population of post-MI patients with asymptomatic ventricular arrhythmias, **flecainide, encainide,** and **moricizine** were associated with an increase in mortality when compared to placebo (10,11). **Propafenone** has blocking effects in addition to its class IC electrophysiologic effects (12). Both propafenone and flecainide have been shown to be effective in preventing recurrent episodes of paroxysmal atrial fibrillation and AV nodal reentrant tachyarrhythmias (12,13).

Class II Agents

β blockers are effective in slowing the ventricular response rate in atrial fibrillation, converting reentrant supraventricular tachyarrhythmias, and suppressing ventricular arrhythmias. **Sotalol** is a nonselective blocker that also prolongs the QT interval (14), a property of class III drugs. **Propranolol, acebutolol, sotalol,** and **esmolol** are approved for the treatment of arrhythmias. **Esmolol** is a short-acting intravenous agent with an elimination half-life of approximately 9 minutes and is particularly useful for patients who are at risk for the common complications of blockade because adverse effects are typically brief in duration (<30 min) (15). Chronic treatment with propranolol, metoprolol, or timolol after MI decreases 1-year mortality.

Class III Agents

Amiodarone has been shown to be more effective than class IA agents for the treatment of ventricular arrhythmias (16). However, adverse effects, the most serious of which are proarrhythmia, pulmonary fibrosis, and thyroid dysfunction, can occur with doses commonly used to suppress ventricular ectopy. Low doses have been shown to be effective in suppressing paroxysmal supraventricular arrhythmias and converting new-onset atrial fibrillation (17). This drug has also recently been shown to be effective when given intravenously to suppress sustained ventricular tachycardia and prevent recurrent ventricular fibrillation (18). Low doses of the drug to prevent arrhythmias in patients with congestive heart failure (CHF) have been shown to improve cardiac contractility and possibly survival (19). Its use in post-MI patients to suppress ventricular arrhythmias is currently being evaluated. Amiodarone can increase the serum concentrations of digoxin, diltiazem, quinidine, procainamide, flecainide, and blockers. Intravenous **bretylium** is most commonly used in the acute management of ventricular arrhythmias that are unresponsive to other agents. It is unclear whether it is superior to lidocaine in the cardiac arrest setting for management of recurrent ventricular fibrillation (8). Postural hypotension is a common complication. **Sotalol** is approved only for use in the management of ventricular arrhythmias but has been shown to be effective in the prevention and termination of atrial fibrillation.

Class IV Agents

Verapamil and diltiazem can be given intravenously and are effective in terminating reentrant supraventricular tachyarrhythmias as well as controlling the ventricular response rate in atrial fibrillation (8). Intravenous use can be complicated by hypotension and bradycardia, particularly in patients receiving blockers or other calcium channel blockers. These drugs should be avoided in patients with wide QRS complex tachyarrhythmias when it is unclear whether the rhythm is of ventricular origin or caused by aberrant conduction of a supraventricular rhythm. Chronic oral therapy with these drugs may be useful in preventing reentrant supraventricular tachycardias. Chronic therapy may raise serum digoxin levels.

ANGIOTENSIN-CONVERTING ENZYME (ACE) INHIBITORS

These agents are used primarily in the management of chronic congestive heart failure, systemic hypertension, and the treatment of post-MI patients (20). There are currently eight ACE inhibitors marketed in the United States. The major differences between the drugs are in the zinc ligand portion of the drug, whether the parent drug (prodrug) is converted to an active metabolite, and cost (21). Captopril has a sulfhydryl ligand and fosinopril a phosphodyl ligand; the remainder have a carboxyl ligand. All except captopril and lisinopril are prodrugs. Prodrugs have a longer onset of peak action and a longer duration of action. The sulfhydryl group is believed to be responsible for a higher incidence of side effects. Common doses, comparative costs, and target doses shown to be effective in improving mortality in patients with CHF (22) or for patients after an acute MI are listed in Table 18.3 (23).

These drugs share **common adverse effects,** including *(a)* dry cough; *(b)* rash or rarely angioedema; *(c)* hypotension and worsening of renal function with volume or salt depletion or concomitant use of diuretics; *(d)* hyperkalemia in patients with renal dysfunction, especially diabetics, and in those receiving potassium supplements or potassium-sparing diuretics; *(e)* loss of taste; and *(f)* acute renal failure in patients with bilateral renal artery stenosis.

BETA-ADRENERGIC BLOCKING AGENTS

These drugs differ primarily in their selectivity for β-1 receptors and intrinsic sympathomimetic activity (receptor stimulation by virtue of molecular structure). Agents that are "cardioselective" have a greater effect on cardiac (β-1) adrenoreceptors than on β-2 adrenergic receptors of the bronchi and blood vessels. Selec-

Table 18.3
Angiotensin-Enzyme (ACE) Inhibitors

Drug	Daily dosage	Cost	Target dose
Benazepril—Lotensin	initial: 10 mg usual: 20–40 mg q.d. or b.i.d.	$19	

Captopril—Capoten	initial: 25 mg b.i.d. or
	   t.i.d.
	usual: 25–150 mg
	   b.i.d. or t.i.d.
		$42	50 mg t.i.d.
			
			6.25–50 mg b.i.d.*

Enalapril—Vasotec	initial: 5 mg usual: 10–40 mg q.d. or divided	$30	10 mg b.i.d.
Fosinopril—Monopril	initial: 10 mg usual: 20–40 mg q.d. or b.i.d.	$22	
Lisinopril—Zestril	initial: 10 mg usual: 20–40 mg q.d.	$26	2.5–10 mg q.d.*
Moexipril—Univasc	initial: 10 mg usual: 7.5–30 mg q.d. or divided	$15	
Quinapril—Accupril	initial: 10 mg usual: 20–80 mg q.d. or divided	$27	
Ramipril—Altace	initial: 2.5 mg usual: 2.5–20 mg q.d. or divided	$20	5 mg b.i.d. 2.5–5 mg b.i.d.*

Cost = cost to the pharmacist for 30 days of treatment with the lowest usual dosage according to wholesale price (24); target dose = doses associated with increased survival in CHF clinical trials.
* Target dose for post-MI patients.

tivity is dose-dependent, and these drugs become less selective as the dosage is increased and even in low doses can cause bronchospasm in patients with asthma. Selectivity is an advantage for patients with diabetes because selective β blockers are less likely to mask the symptoms of hypoglycemia, to delay recovery from hypoglycemia, or cause severe hypertension when hypoglycemia leads to increased circulating catecholamines. Agents with intrinsic sympathomimetic activity (ISA) produce less of a decrease in heart rate at rest and may be preferred for patients who develop symptomatic bradycardia with other β blockers. They have not, however, been shown to lower mortality after myocardial infarction. These agents also do not increase serum triglyceride concentrations or decrease high-density lipoprotein (HDL) cholesterol levels as noted with other β blockers.

The bioavailability, protein binding, lipid solubility, and metabolism of these drugs vary widely. Drugs that are primarily metabolized by the liver are subjected to a "first-pass" phenomenon, which has a substantial impact on bioavailability. For drugs with >90% hepatic metabolism (e.g., labetalol, metoprolol, propranolol), the bioavailability of an oral dose of drug ranges from 10 to 50%. Drugs metabolized by the liver have shorter half-lives than drugs excreted primarily by the kidney. This is important in the management of patients with renal or hepatic dysfunction, for whom dosages of β blockers may have to be adjusted, especially because the pharmacodynamic effects of β blockers are longer than their pharmacologic half-lives.

The β-1 selectivity and ISA for commonly used blockers and the usual doses are summarized in Table 18.4 (25,26).

Labetalol also has α-adrenoreceptor blocking properties, which make it particularly useful in the management of selected cardiovascular emergencies (e.g., hypertensive crisis, acute aortic dissection) when given intravenously. The usual intravenous dose is 20 mg, then 40–80 mg every 10 min until the desired effect on blood pressure and heart rate is achieved or a total dose of 300 mg is given.

Table 18.4
β-Adrenergic Blocking Agents

Drug	Relative β-1 selectivity	ISA	Membrane stabilizing activity	Dose
Acebutolol	+	+	+	100–1200 mg in 1 or 2 doses
Atenolol	+	0	0	25–100 mg in 1 or 2 doses
Labetalol	0	+ (?)	0	200–1200 mg in 1 or 2 doses
Metoprolol	+	0	0	50–200 mg in 1 or 2 doses
Nadolol	0	0	0	20–240 mg q.d.
Pindolol	0	+ +	+	10–60 mg in 2 doses
Propranolol	0	0	+ +	40–240 mg in 2 doses LA—80–240 mg q.d.
Sotalol	0	0	0	80–160 mg b.i.d.
Timolol	0	0	0	10–40 mg in 2 doses

The **most frequent or severe side effects** associated with these drugs are *(a)* fatigue, *(b)* decreased exercise tolerance, *(c)* precipitation of CHF in patients with marginal left ventricular function, *(d)* bronchospasm in patients with asthma, *(e)* bradycardia and heart block, (f) impotence, *(g)* acute mental disorders including acute delirium, *(h)* changes in triglyceride and HDL cholesterol levels, and *(i)* exacerbation of angina and acute infarction with sudden withdrawal or cessation of therapy.

Atenolol, metoprolol, and timolol have been shown to decrease short- and long-term mortality in acute MI. Intravenous and oral dosing are discussed in Chapter 9.

CALCIUM CHANNEL-BLOCKING AGENTS

Calcium channel-blocking drugs cause selective inhibition of transmembrane flux of calcium in excitable tissue. Their ability to block calcium-mediated electromechanical coupling in contractile tissue reduces the contractile activity of heart (decreasing myocardial oxygen demand) and also produces arterial dilatation in both the coronary (increased myocardial oxygen supply) and peripheral vascular bed (decreased afterload). Their inhibition of transmembrane cellular flow of calcium during the slow inward current of cardiac action potentials decreases sinus node automaticity and slows both sinoatrial and atrioventricular conduction, thereby increasing refractoriness. This wide range of effects has led to the use of these drugs in the management of chronic angina pectoris, cardiac arrhythmias (particularly AV nodal reentrant tachyarrhythmias), and hypertension.

These agents are most commonly classified based on structure. However, there seems to be little or no simple structure–activity relationship for the different classes of drugs (27,28).

Structural Classification

Benzothiazepine derivative—diltiazem
Dihydropyridine derivative—nifedipine, nicardipine, isradipine, nisoldipine, nimodipine, felodipine
Phenylalkylamine derivative—verapamil
Other—bepridil

Five other classifications have been proposed. The most useful would be one based on tissue specificity, because it would correlate most closely with clinical indications for use (29). Table

Table 18.5
Pharmacologic Effects of Calcium Antagonists

Drug	Systemic vasodilatation	Neg inotropic effects	Neg dromotropic effects	Vasodilatory side effects
Diltiazem	+	+	+	+
Nifedipine	+ + +	+	0	+ + +
Verapamil	+	+ + +	+ +	+
Felodipine	+ +	+	+	+ +
Nicardipine	+ +	0	0	+ +
Nisoldipine	+ +	0	0	+ +
Isradipine	+ +	0	0	+ +

18.5 represents a simplified version of pharmacologic or physiologic classification.

Selected drugs, usual daily adult dose, and costs are shown in the Table 18.6.

Frequent or severe adverse effects of these agents include *(a)* dizziness, *(b)* headache, *(c)* bradycardia and AV block, *(d)* precipitation of heart failure in patients with marginal left ventricular function, *(e)* peripheral edema, and *(f)* flushing. Verapamil and diltiazem can raise serum digoxin concentration and precipitate digoxin toxicity.

Calcium channel blockers should be avoided for patients who have had a Q-wave infarction because these drugs have been shown to worsen 1-year mortality when compared to placebo.

ORAL NITRATES

Oral nitrates have an established history in the management of stable and unstable angina pectoris (31). Despite this extensive history, there is no evidence that nitrates improve mortality caused by ischemic heart disease. However, they have been shown to improve exercise tolerance and the quality of life for patients with coronary artery disease.

Recent advances in nitrate therapy have included a better understanding of the phenomenon of nitrate tolerance and the introduction of extended-release preparations. The usual maintenance dose of isosorbide dinitrate is 30 mg 3 times a day for the immediate-release preparation and 40 mg 2 times a day for the

Table 18.6
Calcium Blockers

Diltiazem		
Cardizem SR	120–360 mg in 2 doses	$49
Cardizem CD	120–360 mg in 1 dose	$31
Dilacor XR	120–480 mg in 1 dose	$28
Tiazac	120–480 mg in 1 dose	$24
Verapamil	120–480 mg in 2 or 3 doses	
Generic		$26
Calan		$31
Isoptin		$28
Calan SR	120–480 mg in 1 or 2 doses	$28
Isoptin SR		$27
Verelan	120–480 in 1 dose	$41
Amlodipine—Norvac	2.5–10 mg in 1 dose	$37
Felodipine—Plendil	2.5–10 mg in 1 dose	$26
Isradipine—DynaCirc	5–10 mg in 1 or 2 doses	$25
Nicardipine—Cardene	60–120 mg in 3 doses	$40
Cardene SR	60–120 mg in 2 doses	$40
Nifedipine—extended release	30–90 mg in 1 dose	
Adalat CC		$26
Procardia XL		$38
Nisoldipine—Sular	20–60 mg in 1 dose	$25

Cost = cost to pharmacist for 30 days of treatment with lowest recommended dosage, based on wholesale price (30).

Table 18.7
Nitrate Pharmacokinetics and Common Dosing Schedules

Drug	Usual dose (mg)	Action onset (min)	Duration of action
Sublingual			
NTG	0.3–0.8	2–5	20–30 min
ISDN	2.5–10.0	5–20	45–120 min
Oral			
NTG-SR	6.5–19.5 b.i.d./t.i.d.	20–45	2–6 hr
ISDN	10–60 b.i.d./t.i.d.	15–45	2–6 hr
ISMN	20 bid	30–60	3–6 hr
ISDN-SR	40–60 b.i.d.	60–90	10–14 hr
ISMN-SR	60–120 q.d.	60–90	10–14 hr
NTG			
Ointment (2%)	0.5–2.0 inches t.i.d.	15–60	3–8 hr
Patch	10–20 mg	30–60	8–12 hr

NTG = nitroglycerin; ISDN = isosorbide dinitrate; ISMN = isosorbide mononitrate; SR = sustained release.

extended-release preparation. Isosorbide mononitrate is the major active metabolite of isosorbide dinitrate and is available in an immediate-release preparation (20 mg 2 times a day) or an extended-release preparation (120 mg every day) (32,33) (Table 1.7).

All nitrates cause rapid development of tolerance, but a dosing interval of 3 times a day versus every day and a drug-free overnight interval can largely reverse the tolerance that develops during the day. Transdermal nitroglycerin preparations, although initially greeted with enthusiasm, are being replaced by extended-release oral preparations. However, they can be effective if they are removed for 10–12 hours daily. Patients who have frequent angina or angina at night during the nitrate-free period should be treated with a second drug such as a β blocker or a calcium channel blocker (34).

References

1. Vaughan Williams EM. A classification of antiarrhythmic actions reassessed after a decade of new drugs. J Clin Pharmacol 1984;24:129.
2. Harrison DC. Antiarrhythmic drug classification: new science and practical applications. Am J Cardiol 1985;56:185.
3. Morganroth J, Goin JE. Quinidine-related mortality in the short-to-medium-term treatment of ventricular arrhythmias. A meta-analysis. Circulation 1991;84:1977.
4. Coplen SE, Antman EM, Berlin JA, et al. Efficacy and safety of quinidine therapy for maintenance of sinus rhythm after cardioversion: a meta-analysis of randomized control trials. Circulation 1990;82:1106.
5. Levine JH, Morganroth J, Kadish AH. Mechanisms and risk factors for proarrhythmia with type IA compared with IC antiarrhythmic drug therapy. Circulation 1989;80:1063.
6. Tan HL, Hou CJY, Lauer MR, et al. Electrophysiologic mechanisms of the long QT interval syndromes and torsade de pointes. Ann Intern Med 1995;122:701.
7. Antman EM, Lau J, Kupelnick B, et al. A comparison of results of meta-analyses of randomized control trials and recommendations of clinical experts. Treatments of myocardial infarction. JAMA 1992; 268:240.
8. Guidelines of Cardiopulmonary Resuscitation and Emergency Cardiac Care. Adult advanced cardiac life support. JAMA 1992;268:2199.
9. Kreeger RW, Hammill SC. New antiarrhythmic drugs: tocainide, mexiletine, flecainide, encainide, and amiodarone. Mayo Clin Proc 1987; 62:1033.
10. Echt DS, Liebson PR, Mitchell B, et al. Mortality and morbidity in

patients receiving encainide, flecainide, or placebo. The Cardiac Arrhythmia Suppression Trial. N Engl J Med 1991;324:781.

11. The Cardiac Arrhythmia Suppression Trial II Investigators. Effect of the antiarrhythmic agent moricizine on survival after myocardial infarction. N Engl J Med 1992;327:227.

12. Funck-Brentano C, Kroemer HK, Lee JT, et al. Propafenone. N Engl J Med 1990;322:518.

13. The Flecainide Supraventricular Tachycardia Study Group. Flecainide acetate for paroxysmal supraventricular tachyarrhythmias. Am J Cardiol 1994;74:578.

14. Hohnloser SH, Woosley RL. Sotalol. N Engl J Med 1994;331:31.

15. Gray RJ. Managing critically ill patients with esmolol, an ultra short-acting beta-adrenergic blocker. Chest 1988;93:398.

16. Podrid PJ. Amiodarone: reevaluation of an old drug. Ann Intern Med 1995;122:689.

17. Kerin NZ, Faitel K, Naini M. The efficacy of intravenous amiodarone for the conversion of chronic atrial fibrillation. Arch Intern Med 1996;156:49.

18. Naccarelli GV, Jalal S. Intravenous amiodarone. Another option in the acute management of sustained ventricular tachyarrhythmias. Circulation 1995;92:3154.

19. Singh SN, Fletcher RD, Fisher SG, et al. Amiodarone in patients with congestive heart failure and symptomatic ventricular arrhythmias. N Engl J Med 1995;333:77.

20. Gavras H. Angiotensin converting enzyme inhibition and its impact on cardiovascular disease. Circulation 1990;81:381.

21. Materson BJ, Preston RA. Angiotensin-converting enzyme inhibitors in hypertension. A dozen years of experience. Arch Intern Med 1994; 154:513.

22. Cohn JN. The management of chronic heart failure. N Engl J Med 1996;335:490.

23. Latini R, Maggioni AP, Flather M, et al. ACE inhibitor use in patients with myocardial infarction. Summary of evidence from clinical trials. Circulation 1995;92:3132.

24. Moexipril: another ACE inhibitor for hypertension. The Medical Letter 1995;37:75.

25. Frishman WH. Clinical differences between beta-adrenergic blocking agents: implications for therapeutic substitution. Am Heart J 1987; 113:1190.

26. Drugs for hypertension. The Medical Letter 1995;37:45.

27. Man In'T Veld AJ. Calcium antagonists in hypertension. Am J Med 1989;86(Suppl 4A):6.

28. Wood AJJ. Calcium antagonists. Pharmacologic differences and similarities. Circulation 1989;80(Suppl IV):IV–184.

29. Parmley WW. New calcium antagonists: relevance of vasoselectivity. Am Heart J 1990;120:1408.

30. Nisoldipine—a new calcium channel blocker for hypertension. The Medical Letter 1996;38:13.

31. Abrams J. The role of nitrates in coronary heart disease. Arch Intern Med 1995;155:357.

32. Extended-release isosorbide mononitrate for angina. The Medical Letter 1994;36:13.

33. Abrams J. The role of nitrates in coronary heart disease. Arch Intern Med 1995;155:357.

34. Abrams J. Use of nitrates in ischemic heart disease. Curr Probl Cardiol 1992;17:483.

Index

Page numbers in *italics* denote figures; those followed by a t denote tables.